NOVEL THERAPEUTIC CONCEPTS IN TARGETING GLIOMA

Edited by **Faris Farassati**

Novel Therapeutic Concepts in Targeting Glioma
Edited by Faris Farassati

Published by InTech

Janeza Trdine 9, 51000 Rijeka, Croatia

Publishing Process Manager Petra Nenadic

Technical Editor Teodora Smiljanic

Cover Designer InTech Design Team

Additional hard copies can be obtained from orders@intechopen.com

Novel Therapeutic Concepts in Targeting Glioma, Edited by Faris Farassati
p. cm.
ISBN 978-953-51-0491-9

For EU product safety concerns:
IN TECH d.o.o., Prolaz Marije Krucifikse Kozulić 3, 51000 Rijeka, Croatia,
info@intechopen.com or visit our website at intechopen.com.

Meet the editor

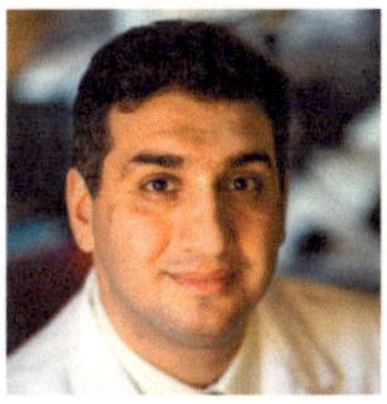

Dr. Farassati was trained as a Molecular Oncologist and Cancer Gene Therapist at the University of Calgary, Harvard Medical School and Mayo Clinic. His Research is mainly focused on understanding the features of pro-oncogenic cell signaling events in cancer cells and utilizing this knowledge to design gene and drug therapy strategies to target them. He currently directs the Molecular Medicine Laboratory at the University of Kansas Medical Center (Kansas City, KS, USA) where a group of clinicians and scientists study a range of human malignancies including brain tumors in adults and children under his leadership. Concepts pursued by this team to target brain tumors include gene therapy strategies using oncolytic viruses, identification and intervention with novel cell signaling pathways involved in generation of brain malignancies and designing gene therapy strategies to target cancer stem cells.

Contents

Preface

Brain, the source of human's ingenuity, passion, motivation and emotions holds a world of mystery and promises for scientists, biologists, physicians, philosophers and poets! It is, therefore, not surprising that Gliomas, as the most common form of the malignant brain tumors, impose such a strong impact on our society at different levels.

Despite a series of significant improvements in our understanding about the molecular etiology of Gliomas, the road lays long in front of us to reach the ultimate goal of elimination of the burden delivered to human health by these deadly diseases. But, in this mix, there are also good news: First, the rate of malignant brain tumors in men seems to be declining. Secondly, the overall incidence rate of Glioblastomas has been stable suggesting that external risk factors may not influence the origination of these malignancies*.

Novel Therapeutic Concepts for Targeting Glioma offers a comprehensive collection of current information and the upcoming possibilities for designing new therapies for Glioma by an array of experts ranging from Cell Biologists to Oncologists and Neurosurgeons. A variety of topics cover therapeutic strategies based on Cell Signaling, Gene Therapy, Drug Therapy and Surgical methods providing the reader with a unique opportunity to expand and advance his knowledge of the field.

We remain grateful to the efforts of our colleagues at *INTECH* for providing such an accessible and efficient platform for dissemination of science. Our hopes are raised and our spirits are lifted because of endeavors of the people who not only seek but one day will deliver human race's freedom from Cancer.

Faris Farassati, PhD, PharmD,
Department of Medicine-Molecular Medicine Laboratory
The University Of Kansas Medical Center, Kansas City, Kansas,
USA

**Kohler BA, Ward E, McCarthy BJ, Schymura MJ, Ries LAG, Eheman C, Jemal A, Anderson RA, Ajani UA, Edwards BK. Report to the Nation on the Status of Cancer, 1975-2007, Featuring Tumors of the Brain and Other Nervous System. JNCI; May 4, 2011.*

Part 1

Surgical Therapy of Glioma

1

Innovative Surgical Management of Glioma

Dave Seecharan[1], Faris Farassati[1] and Ania Pollack[2]
[1]*Department of Neurosurgery,*
[2]*Department of Medicine, Molecular Medicine Laboratory,*
The University of Kansas Medical Centre, Kansas City, KS,
USA

1. Introduction

Glioma is one of the most common primary brain tumors accounting for 30 to 40% of all intracranial tumors. Gliomas can be divided into two types based upon histopathalogic diagnosis according to the World Health Organization (WHO) classification, low grade (WHO I and II) and high grade (WHO III and IV). High grade malignant glioblastoma accounts for the majority of diagnoses and carries the worst prognosis. Prognosis with glioma depends on the patient's age and Karnofsky performance score (KPS) as well as the histological grade of the tumor. For the United States in 2010 there were 6.8 new cases of glioblastoma for every 100,000 people[1]. The current standard of care for patients with newly diagnosed high-grade glioma is surgical resection followed by fractionated external beam radiation therapy and systemic chemotherapeutic treatment mostly with temozolomide[2].

The single best therapeutic option in the treatment of glioma is extensive surgical resection, and the extent of resection directly correlates with the greatest survival benefit. Despite our best efforts however, the outcomes for malignant glioblastoma are still very poor with less than 5% of patients surviving five years post diagnosis even with the best current treatment3. In light of these poor results there is significant room for innovation and improvement in the area of surgical management particularly with an objective to increase the extent of surgical resection. Throughout this chapter we will discuss the importance of surgical resection in the treatment of glioma as well as emerging innovative surgical methods and technologies for increasing the extent of resection and improving upon the associated survival benefit. We will also explore adjuvant therapies in glioma management and the important role that surgery plays in maximizing the potential benefit of these adjuvant therapies.

2. Current surgical management of glioma

Three options are available for the surgical management of gliomas. The first option is to refrain from surgery for as long as possible, sometimes referred to as the "wait and see" approach. The second option involves biopsy of the lesion or subtotal resection of surgically accessible areas within the tumor in order to obtain histopathology diagnosis. Biopsy and subtotal resection are often followed by adjuvant therapies (radiation or chemotherapy). The best surgical option is gross total resection (GTR), usually defined as removal of all areas of contrast enhancement on T1 weighted MRI obtained postoperatively. GTR provides the best surgical treatment and is associated with the best survival rates; however, it also carries the greatest risks of postoperative neurologic deficits and disability.

Current treatment for glioma, particularly high grade lesions, is not curative and the majority of patients experience reoccurrence following initial resection. Reoccurrence is due to the infiltrative nature of these lesions and the inability of current treatment modalities to fully remove and destroy all tumor cells. The rationale behind surgical management of these aggressive lesions is based on the Gompertzian phenomenon. In 1825, the English mathematician Benjamin Gompertz postulated that the biological growth of normal organs and malignancies follows a characteristic curve and that cell number increases with time, but the relative rate of increase falls exponentially as the mass reaches a "plateau phase" of a very slow actual growth[4]. Therapy can induce regression in tumor volume, however, there is always regrowth between cycles of treatment and this "regrowth" will follow the same Gompertzian growth curve. The only escape from Gompertzian phenomenon is complete tumor cell eradication. Therefore, the ultimate goal of surgical therapy in these tumors should be the complete eradication of all abnormal neoplastic cells. With the currently available surgical techniques we are still unable to fully resect most of these tumors. Therefore we need new techniques to improve surgical resection as well as adjuvant therapies to eradicate remaining tumor cells and thereby maximize the survival benefit of surgery.

Low grade gliomas (WHO I and II) are a broad group of tumors that are clinically, histologically and molecularly diverse. WHO grade I tumors comprise the group of pilocytic astrocytoma and subependymal giant cell astrocytoma the more common being pilocytic. Management of WHO grade I glioma consists of gross total resection as the treatment of choice and carries an excellent prognosis. Following resection, 25-year survival rates of 50-94% have been reported[5]. Grade I lesions are the only glioma subtype where gross total resection is considered curative.

WHO grade II gliomas consist of diffuse fibrillary astrocytoma, oligodendrogliomas, and oligoastrocytomas, all of which have similar invasive and malignant potential. Grade II gliomas that are symptomatic and surgically accessible should undergo maximal cytoreductive surgery as the treatment of choice. Predictors of incomplete tumor resection in low grade lesions include tumor involvement of the cortico-spinal tract, large tumor volume, and oligodendroglioma histopathologic type. 5 year survival of up to 95-97% has been reported following gross total resection in these lesions[6]. In 2008, Smith and colleagues reported a large series of 216 patients with biologically aggressive grade II lesions and examined the extent of resection and the effect on overall survival[7]. Patients with at least 90% resection showed 5 and 8 year survivals of 97% and 91% respectively compared to those with less than 90% resection who showed survival rates of 76% and 60% at 5 and 8 years.

For both grade I and grade II tumors, maximal surgical resection is the single best treatment for obtaining increased survival. In cases where there is progressive tumor growth following resection or progressive neurological symptoms in unresectable tumors, adjuvant chemotherapy or radiation treatment may be used.

High grade glioma's (WHO III and IV) consist of anaplastic astrocytoma (Grade III), and glioblastoma (Grade IV). These tumors are malignant and carry a significantly poorer prognosis than the low grade lesions. The first line therapy for high-grade glioma is cytoreductive surgery with the goal of removing as much abnormal tissue as possible without causing further damage to normal parenchyma. The reduction in tumor volume results in improved survival and quality of life by delaying recurrence and malignant progression.

There are many studies over the past two decades that examine the extent of cytoreductive surgery; gross total resection verses biopsy and subtotal resection in regards to increasing patient survival. Tumor location as well as extent of neurologic deficits plays a large role in the decision making process for surgical management. One retrospective study in 1996 showed significant increased mean survival time of 292 days vs 184 days between a group undergoing cytoreductive surgery and a group undergoing stereotactic biopsy respectively[8]. However quality of life measured by KPS was not significantly different between the two groups.

A prospective study utilizing 60 patients, examined the extent of resection compared to survival. These authors found median survival of 64 weeks for the group who underwent gross total resection compared to 36 weeks for the group undergoing subtotal resection[9]. They concluded that patients undergoing subtotal resection have 6.6 times higher risk of death. Another large prospective of study 645 patients showed that patients undergoing total resection had a median survival of 11.3 months compared to 10.4 months for subtotal resection, both of which were significant increases in survival compared to 6.6 months for patients with biopsy only[10].

Increased survival with resection holds true even for the elderly. A study by Vuorienen, focusing specifically on elderly patients over the age of 65 showed median survival of 5.7 months with open craniotomy and surgical resection compared to 2.8 months with stereotactic biopsy alone for an increased estimated survival time of 2.7 times longer in the resection group[11]. However, this increased survival time is modest in this patient population providing only a 2-3 month survival benefit. The role of aggressive surgical management in the elderly population is still a controversial subject. Chronological age however, is not necessarily the most important factor to consider in deciding to pursue an aggressive surgical course. Rather biological age which takes into account the patients general health and functional level should be used as a guideline.

A recent review article from 2008 examined over thirty published articles from the neurosurgical and neuro-oncologic literature regarding extent of resection and the effects on survival for malignant glioma. Only one study failed to support the idea that extent of surgical resection correlates with an increased survival advantage[12]. These authors recommend that based on the current prospective and retrospective data that for newly diagnosed malignant glioma in adults, maximal cytoreductive surgery should be undertaken provided that postoperative neurological deficits are minimized.

Studies have also been performed in order to quantify exactly what percent of tumor resection is necessary to provide maximal survival benefit. The original landmark study was published in 2001 by Lacroix and colleagues in which they performed a retrospective analysis of 416 patients with glioblastoma treated with surgical resection[13]. Patients who received resection of greater than 98% had a mean survival of 13 months compared to patients receiving resection of less than 98% with mean survival of 8.8 months.

A more recent 2011 retrospective study by Sanai and colleagues also quantified the percent of tumor resection required for maximal survival benefit[14]. 500 patients with gliobastoma were treated with surgical resection followed by standard radiation and chemotherapy. They found a survival benefit with extent of surgical resection of as low as 78%. However, for maximal survival benefit, resection of greater than 95% was observed

Overall, these studies demonstrate that prolonged survival time correlates with the extent of surgical resection. The data also suggests that for high grade lesions, resection of greater than 95% of the tumor volume should be performed in order to provide the maximal survival benefit. In some cases, however, such a high level of resection is unable to be obtained. This is usually due to tumor involvement in areas of eloquent brain tissue (areas involved with speech production, motor function and sensory perception), and is associated with a high risk of postoperative deficits. Maximizing the extent of tumor resection while preserving normal brain function and optimizing quality of life postoperatively represents a major challenge in neurosurgery. Several strategies and innovative techniques have been developed to assist the surgeon in safely resecting tumors located in these eloquent areas, particularly in the areas of neuroimaging, neuronavigation, functional mapping, and photodynamics. Theses new developments provide for greater resection volumes and better survival rates.

3. Neuronavigation

Image guided neuronavigation utilizes the principle of stereotaxis. The brain is considered as a geometric volume which can be divided by three imaginary intersecting spatial planes based on a Cartesian coordinate system. Any point within the brain can be specified by measuring its distance along these three planes. This provides a precise surgical guidance by referencing this coordinate system of the brain with a parallel coordinate system of the three-dimensional image data of the patient that is displayed on a computer-workstation so that the medical images become point-to-point maps of the corresponding actual locations within the brain[15]. Neuronavigation provides intraoperative orientation to the surgeon, helps in planning a precise surgical approach to the targeted lesion and defines the surrounding neurovascular structures. Conventional neuronavigation typically utilizes a preoperative MRI which is registered to the patients skull at the beginning of the procedure and is used throughout the case without any update in imaging or reregistration of the imaging to the corresponding brain tissue. Conventional neuronavigation is readily available at most centers providing neurosurgical care and is not particularly cost prohibitive. (Figure 1)

Intraoperative MRI (iMRI) guided intracranial surgery improves upon the benefits of conventional stereotactic guided neurosurgery by providing a real time updated view of the anatomic relationship between tumor and normal brain structures. During surgical resection utilizing traditional cranial neuronavigation, the brain parenchyma becomes distorted due to changes in tumor volume, edema and volume of cerebrospinal fluid resulting in brain shift, which is not reflected in the preoperatively obtained MRI. This results in less reliability of the stereotactic guidance as the surgery progresses. Intraoperatively obtained MRI allows updating of the images used for neuronavigation as well as updated visualization of the contrast enhancing tissue that remains.

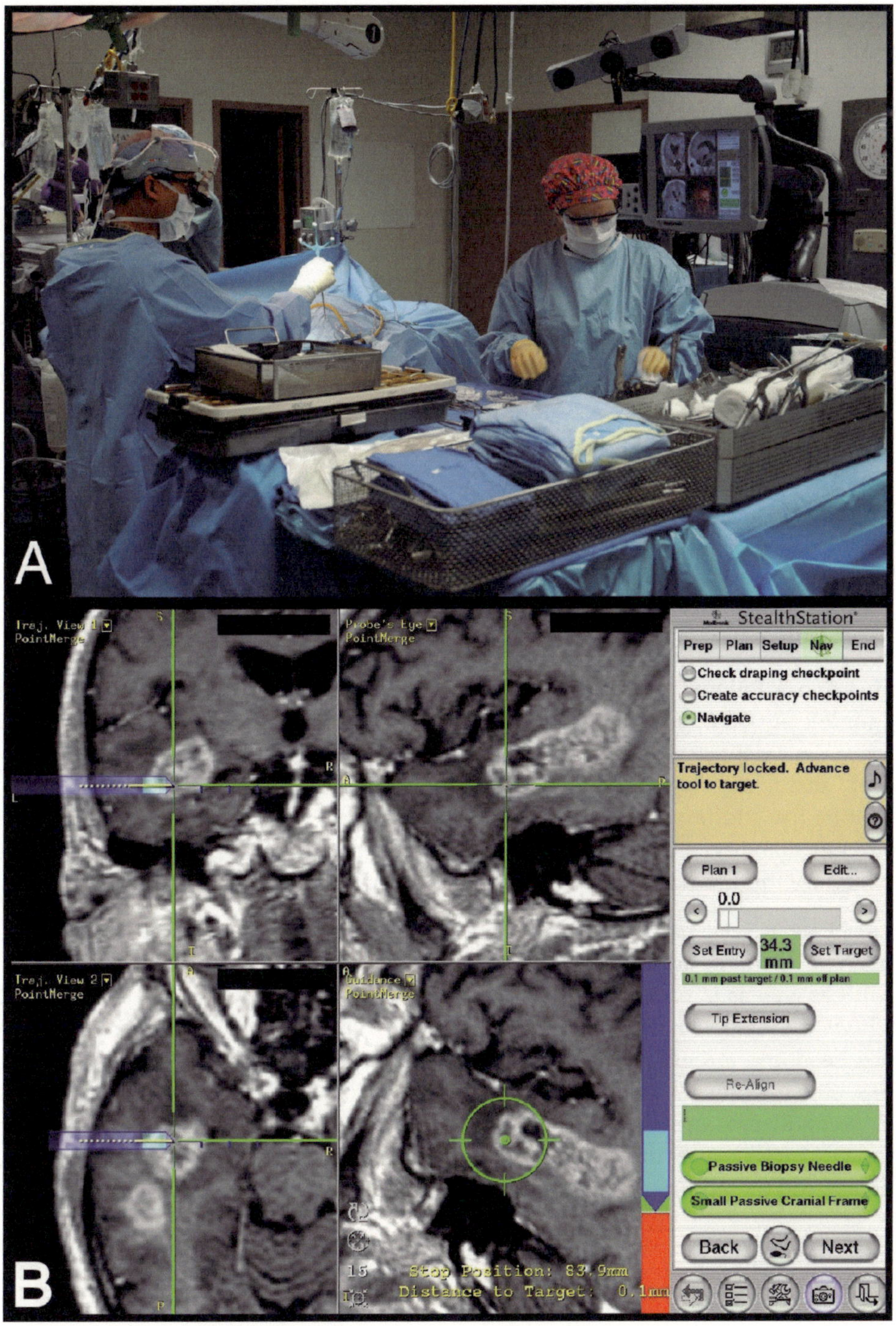

Fig. 1. Neuronavigation. Operating room setup with patient positioned and neuronavigational stereotactic equipment (A). Neuronavigational MRI for stereotactic guided biopsy showing a temporal lobe glioma in three planes.

Over the past decade several studies have looked at iMRI guided resection vs conventional neuronavigation in patients with glioma. In 2000, Wirtz and colleagues examined 68 cases of high grade glioma resected with iMRI[16]. Of the 68 cases, 27% of showed GTR on the first iMRI scan and 66% percent underwent continued resection. Median survival was 13.3 months for GTR vs 9.2 months for subtotal resection.

In 2005, Hisrschberg and colleagues examined the use of iMRI in 32 patients with glioblastoma compared to a matched control group of 32 patients using conventional neuronavigation. They found a mean survival time of 14.5 months in the iMRI group vs 12.1 months in the control group. They also saw a significant increase in length of surgical time with iMRI 5.1 hours vs 3.4 with conventional navigation. They also reported postoperative functional performance results, which were not significantly different between the two groups. Neurologic improvement was seen in 16% of patients, 55% showed no change, and 19% showed some worsening of symptoms.

In 2010, Senft and colleagues reported on 41 patients with glioblastoma, 10 of whom underwent resection with iMRI and 31 who received resection by conventional means[17]. GTR was seen in all 10 iMRI cases and 19 of the conventional group. Median survival was 88 weeks for the iMRI group and 68 weeks for the conventional group. Median survival in regards to the extent of resection was 74 weeks for the 29 patients who obtained GTR vs 46 weeks for the 12 patients who obtained subtotal resection.

A recent 2011 review article of 12 studies from the current literature examined the benefits of iMRI vs conventional stereotactic surgery for glioblastoma. The authors concluded that iMRI guided surgery is more effective that conventional neuronavigational surgery in increasing the extent of resection and prolonging survival in patients with glioblastoma[18]. However there are currently no randomized trials with validated endpoints that demonstrate the additional value of iMRI guided surgery. Intraoperative MRI is currently of limited availability, adds significant expense and prolongs surgical time. Therefore, the decision to use this modality should be made judiciously on a case by case basis.

These systems are not perfect and continued improvements are needed. Advances in real time surgical imaging are important to reduce the neuronavigational inaccuracies due to brain shift as well as to provide a clearer more accurate representation of the tumor margins throughout the case. Currently these systems still rely heavily on a rigid fixation of the patient's head and a registration landmark. Movement of the patient's head, pin slippage, and loss of registration can drastically limit the utility of these surgical tools and more robust technologies are needed. Despite these limitations, the use of improved neuroimaging and newer methods of neuronavigation can significantly improve the extent of resection and thereby increase the survival rates for patients with glioma.

4. Functional mapping

Functional mapping is another tool that is changing the surgical management of glioma therapy. These new techniques allow the protection of eloquent areas of the brain while permitting the extent of surgical resection to be maximized. With this technology, lesions that were previously thought to be inoperable due to location are now often resectable. One such procedure is awake craniotomy. Intraoperative direct electrostimulation under awake anesthesia is the best technique to locate eloquent domains as well as to distinguish functional area from nonfunctional area. In 2008, Duffau and colleagues, reported the largest experience with cortical and subcortical mapping of gliomas affecting the language area[19]. They performed resection using awake craniotomy and direct electrical stimulation in 115 patients. 98% of patients improved or returned to their preoperative baseline following resection guided by direct electrostimulation. Awake craniotomy however presents several challenges in regards to anesthesia, patient comfort and anxiety as well as prolongation of operative time.

Functional magnetic resonance imaging (fMRI) is another improving technology that shows promise for increasing the extent of surgical resection while minimizing neurological deficits by providing functional mapping with the use of newly developed imaging modalities. The use of functional magnetic resonance imaging (fMRI) allows information regarding the location of specific brain functions such as speech, motor function, and sensory perception to be mapped to three-dimensional reconstructed MRI images. Blood oxygen level dependent (BOLD) fMRI is one of the most commonly used forms of fMRI. BOLD fMRI provides functional information based on cerebral hemodynamic responses by measuring changes in the ratio of blood oxyhemoglobin and deoxyhemoglobin during the presentation of a various stimuli to the patient. This data can then be used to map task-driven regional cortical activity in patients to noninvasively locate the brains essential eloquent areas and guide surgical planning. (Figure 2)

In 2010, Talacchi and colleges retrospectively examined the use of preoperative fMRI and neuronavigation compared to traditional intraoperative neurostimulation in 171 patients[20]. They found that preoperative fMRI provided equivalent rate of GTR when compared to the invasive neurostimulation 71% vs 73%c compared to 40% in resections not utilizing either modality. Similar findings have been demonstrated by additional authors[21,22]. Together these studies support fMRI as a viable alternative to awake craniotomy and functional neurostimulation with the benefit of reduced operative time as well as elimination of the challenges associated with awake craniotomy.

Diffusion tensor imaging (DTI) is an additional form of functional magnetic resonance imaging used to delineate white matter anatomy. DTI is based upon the principle that water preferentially diffuses along the long axis of white matter tracts and the degree and direction of water diffusion can be measured. Tractography uses algorithms to process this data and to reconstruct three-dimensional maps representing subcortical fiber tracts[23]. Tractography can be used in surgical planning to show the relationship between white matter tracts and tumor. It can reveal whether tracts are displaced, disrupted, or infiltrated by tumor. (Figure 3)

In 2007, Wu and colleges reported a large prospective randomized controlled trial of 238 patients with gliomas[24]. A randomized study group of 118 patients underwent resection with DTI tractography and neuronavigation while a control group of 120 patients underwent resection with neuronavigation alone. They found a significant increase in the ability to achieve GTR with the use of DTI tractography with 74.4 % of patients in the study group achieving GTR compared to 33.3% of patients in the control group. This translated into an increased mean survival time 21.2 months in the study group compared to 14.0 months mean survival in the control group. They also found better outcomes with DTI tractography with motor strength deterioration occurring in 15.3% of patients in the study group compared to 32.8% in the control group. Improved outcome was also demonstrated in 6 month Karnofsky Performace Scale scores with a mean score of 77 for study group patients and 53 for the control group. When combined, fMRI, neuronavigation, and DTI allows precise surgical resection of the maximal tumor volume while sparing intact fiber tracts as well as eloquent areas of the brain. This results increased patient survival and improved functional outcomes.

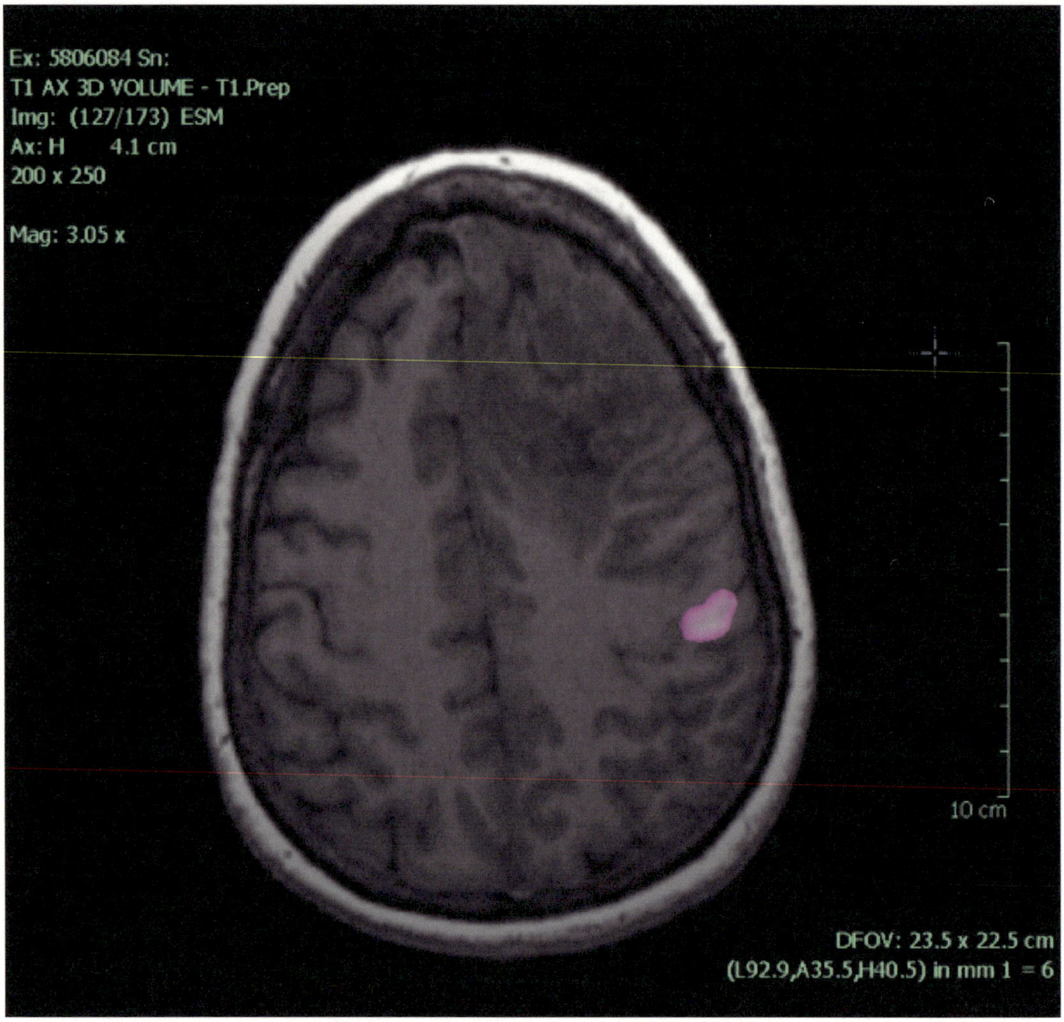

Fig. 2. Functional MRI. MRI generated from BOLD data in a patient with large frontal lobe glioma showing areas of activation during a sentence completion task.

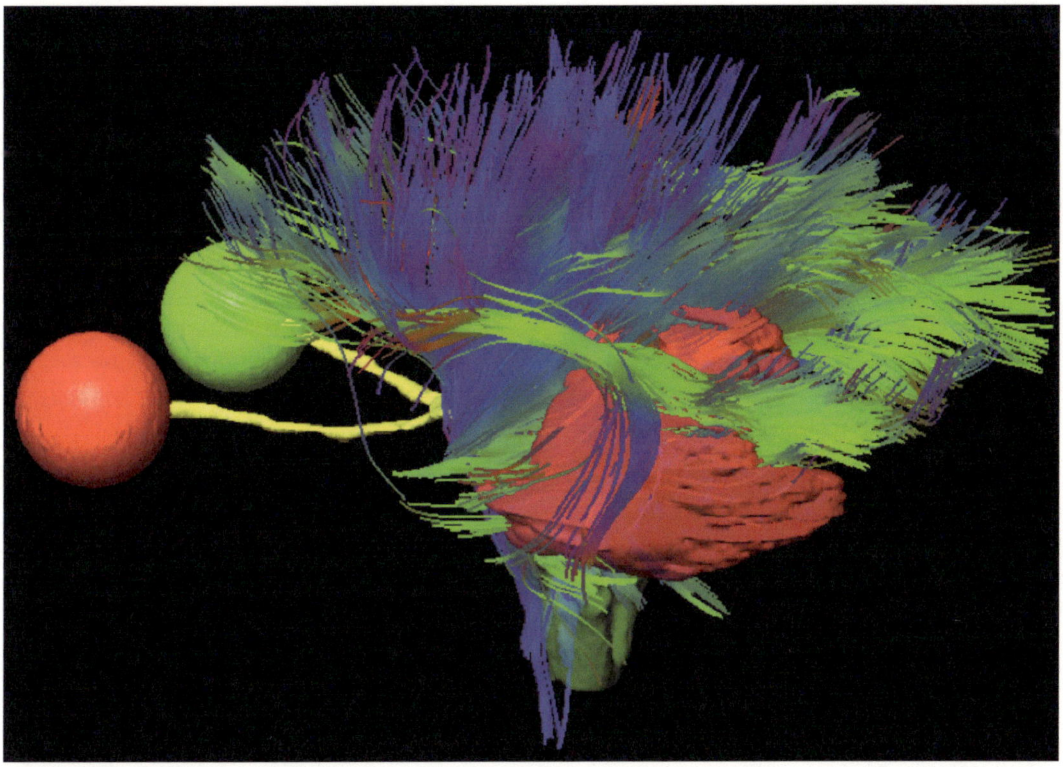

Fig. 3. Tractography. 3-Dimensional reconstruction showing fiber tracts generated from DTI MRI sequence in a patient with large glioblastoma multiforme.

5. Florescence guided resection

Another problem arises in surgery when dealing with the infiltrating malignant cells present at the tumor margins. These cells often lie outside the area of enhancement on neuroimaging and intraoperatively appear grossly and microscopically indistinguishable from normal brain tissue. These areas of infiltrating cells contribute to reoccurrence and negatively effect long-term tumor control if not resected.

Fluorescence image guided surgical resection (FIGS) is another innovative surgical technique which uses fluorescence intraoperatively to enhance the visualization of abnormal tumor cells intraoperatively and allow for maximal extent of resection. 5-Aminolevulinic acid (ALA) is injected systemically prior to surgery. High grade gliomas and other metabolically active tumors take up ALA at a rapid rate. After gross resection of the visible tumor, a specially filtered blue light can illuminate the areas of high uptake within the cavity allowing selective resection of the residual areas[25].

In 2000, Stummer and colleagues reported an initial study of the efficacy of FIGS which demonstrated FIGS to be quite specific (only 0.4 % of fluorescent biopsy sites did not contain tumor cells) and quite sensitive (81.6% of fluorescent biopsy sites contained tumor cells)[26]. In 2006 this same author reported a multicenter phase III trial comparing FIGS to placebo and found 64% complete surgical excision with fluorescence guided resection compared to 38%

complete excision in the placebo group[27]. In 2007 Stepp and colleagues reported similar findings with GTR in 65% of patients undergoing FIGS compared to 36% in placebo group[28]. They also demonstrated improved 6 month progression free survival in 41% of patients in the study group vs 21% in the control group.

Despite the positive initial results with FIGS, there are several limitations of this modality. The blue light used to illuminate 5-ALA has a depth of penetration of only a few millimeters and is easily obscured by blood products. Also 5-ALA has minimal uptake in tumors that have minimal contrast enhancement or that do not enhance at all, such as low grade glioma[29,30]. Advances in florescence guidance, particularly in its use for resection of these low grade, non-enhancing lesions are needed. As this technology continues to progress it will allow for greater extent of resection and increased survival in patients with glioma.

6. Photodynamic treatment

Photodynamic treatment (PDT) is another novel surgical method for the treatment of malignant glioblastoma. It utilizes the selective uptake of a photosensitizer by the individual tumor cells followed by irradiation of the tumor with light of a specific wavelength during surgery, which activates the photosensitizer to destroy the tumor cells selectively via oxidative reactions. Many different photosensitisers have been studied with the most promising being haematoporphyrin derivative (HPD). One of the greatest benefits with PDT is that it is a localized treatment, which lacks the systemic side effects associated with chemotherapy and radiation. The major side effect associated with PTD is cerebral edema in the irradiated area which can usually be managed with steroids.

In 2005, Stylli and colleagues reported one of the largest series of PDT for high grade glioma in 136 patients[31]. They utilized HPD administered IV preoperatively followed by irradiation with laser light during surgery. Median survival time following treatment for the 78 patients with glioblastoma was 14.3 months and median survival for the patients with anaplastic astrocytoma was 76.5 months. The same authors have also reported a review of the literature examining 10 studies, which show similar results although with fewer numbers of patients[32]. They conclude that PDT shows potential as a novel adjuvant therapy for glioma treatment along with chemotherapy and radiation therapy. However, further controlled clinical trials are needed to standardize HPD dosage as well as type and dose of light irradiation.

7. Radiation therapy

Following surgical resection, radiation therapy (RT) is considered the next step in the treatment of glioma. The principal goal of RT is to destroy residual tumor cells that were not removed with surgery, therefore preventing or postponing tumor reoccurrence. RT is most affective on smaller lesions and is therefore an adjuvant therapy in addition to surgical resection. Resection of maximal tumor bulk results in smaller residual volumes which are more responsive to RT and thereby increase the efficacy of RT. Historically, conventional radiation therapy using external beam radiation has been the main modality of radiotherapy used for glioma. Due to the risk of radiation induced injury to normal brain tissue, conventional radiation therapy is fractionated and the total dose is delivered over several treatments. Standard therapy usually consists of a total radiation dose in the range of 50–60 Gy administered over 20-30 fractions each with a dose of 1.8–2.0 Gy [33].

Novel methods of administering radiation therapy are also being developed. Following optimal surgical resection, image guided stereotactic radiosurgery (SRS) is now being evaluated for treatment these lesions. This new modality utilizes a single high doses of radiation specifically targeted to a well-defined lesions using detailed neuroimaging. This allows delivery of focused radiation to the tumor with a much lower dose to adjacent non-targeted tissue which results in reduced side effects compared with traditional methods.

For low grade gliomas, adjuvant RT following resection has failed to show a survival benefit. In cases of disease progression or inoperable lesions with neurologic symptoms, delayed RT appears to provide the same survival advantage as postoperative RT[34]. For newly diagnosed high grade gliomas studies have demonstrated that SRS does not provide a significant survival advantage over conventional radiotherapy[35,36]. The use of SRS has also been explored as a treatment for recurrent high grade lesions. A recent article by Romanelli and colleagues reviewed 17 retrospective studies examining the role of SRS in the treatment of recurrent high grade glioma. This review demonstrated that SRS is associated with prolonged survival in patients with recurrent GBM with median survival times ranging from 7.5 to 30 months[37]. SRS has been shown to have no significant advantage as a first line radiation therapy for glioma and the results for recurrent glioma are inconclusive, therefore further study on the role of SRS in glioma treatment is needed.

In addition to externally administered sources of radiation therapy, interstitial brachytherapy is another form of radiation therapy used to treat glioma, which refers to surgical placement of the radioactive source a short distance from or within the tumor being treated. Brachytherapy was developed due to the observation that 80% of malignant gliomas reoccur within 2cm of the initial tumor site following resection. By placing the radioactive source directly in the tumor or tumor bed, continuous high dose radiation increases damage to nearby proliferating tumor cells located at the margin with a rapid fall off in the dose delivered to normal cells which are located farther from the source.

There are multiple surgical methods for delivering the radiation source to the tumor. During surgery, temporary implants can be placed which provide a source of radiation for a specified duration and are then removed at a later time, however this usually requires multiple procedures. To avoid multiple procedures, small radioactive seed have been developed which are surgically implanted and are left permanently to gradually decay over a period of weeks to months to a state of zero radiation emission. Another novel approach uses a surgically implanted catheter system with an expandable balloon reservoir implanted at the site of resection and a catheter connecting to a subcutaneous access port. A radioactive solution can then be injected percutaneously into the implanted reservoir and retrieved at a later time. The most commonly radiation sources used for glioma brachytherapy are iodine-125 and iridium-192.

Brachytherapy is usually reserved for cases of high grade gliomas which have shown reoccurrence since several studies have shown no significant survival benefit for brachytherapy in newly diagnosed glioma[38,39]. One large randomized study by Selker and colleagues with 270 patients examined the use of interstitial brachytherapy in newly diagnosed high grade glioma[40]. Patients were randomized to two groups, one receiving resection, external beam radiation, and chemotherapy with the other group receiving resection, external beam radiation, chemotherapy, and ^{125}I permanent interstitial brachytherapy. They found no statistical difference in the median survival time between the two groups for newly diagnosed high grade glioma.

The results for brachytherapy in the case of recurrent high grade glioma appear to show improved survival[41-43]. One large study with 95 patients by Gabayan and colleagues examined the use of the GliaSite Radiation Therapy System in the treatment of recurrent high grade glioma. This system utilizes ^{125}I administered via a surgically implanted balloon catheter system. All patient were initially treated with resection followed by external beam radiation. Following reoccurrence, patients underwent maximal surgical debulking followed by implantation of an expandable balloon catheter system. Radioactive solution was then administered between 2-6 weeks following the debulking procedure. Patient undergoing this treatment showed median survival of 36.3 weeks from the time of the debulking surgery with a 1 year survival of 31.1%. Although no control group was used in this study, survival times were compared to matched patients from another published study matched for age, KPS, and surgical management. These control patients showed a median survival of 23 weeks following resection for reoccurrence. The results from the brachytherapy group compare favorably with the control group. Further studies including randomized trials are still needed but brachytherapy appears to show promise as adjuvant therapy in recurrent glioma.

8. Chemotherapy

In addition to surgical resection and radiation therapy the other mainstay of treatment for malignant glioma is chemotherapeutics. Chemotherapy is another adjuvant therapy to be utilized along with surgical resection. As with radiation therapy, chemotherapy is more effective in treating smaller tumor volumes and therefore maximizing the extent of surgical resection is important in order to provide a more favorable response to chemotherapy[44]. Two main classes of drugs are currently used, alkylating agents (carmusitine, temozolomide) and antiangiogenic agents (bevacizumab).

9. Blood brain barrier

The blood brain barrier (BBB) presents difficulty in the chemotherapuetic treatment of gliomas as many agents that are effective for the treatment of systemic disease are unable to cross the BBB. There have been several developments designed to open the BBB and provide direct treatment of the central nervous system. Initial therapies to open the BBB made use of small lipophilic molecule drugs administered systemically for increased permeation across the BBB. This approach was limited by drug binding to plasma protein as well as extravasation of the drug back across the BBB into the systemic circulation. Other early treatments used osmotic modification of the BBB with agents such as mannitol given intra-arterially to disrupt the BBB followed by the chemotherapeutic agent of choice. The effectiveness of these early methods were limited due to the transient elevation of drug concentration within the brain tissues and short drug half-life which did not allow for accumulation of the drug at a therapeutic concentration. Over the past decade, several innovative surgical methods of opening the BBB have been developed to provide longer acting and direct treatment to the tumor cells.

10. Implantable polymers

One advancement has come in the area of surgically implantable polymers, which are infused with chemotherapeutic agents. These polymers are then placed into the surgical cavity following resection to provide direct application of the chemotherapeutic agent to the tumor bed over a prolonged period of time as the polymer degrades and releases the agent.

The most widely studied therapy of this nature utilizes a polyanhydride wafer embedded with carmustine (gliadel wafers). Gliadel is currently the only interstitial chemotherapy treatment approved for use with malignant glioma. Wafers can be implanted at the time of initial surgery or reserved for episodes of reoccurrence. Several trials have demonstrated increased survival following the use of implantable wafers. For initial tumor treatment, increased survival has been shown of 13.9 months compared to 11.6 months in non-treatment group. Wafer usage for treatment of tumor reoccurrence provided increased survival of 31 weeks compared to 23 weeks in non-treated patients[45–47].

Overall, these studies show a 35% risk reduction of death with the use of gliadel, with a median survival of 14 months, which is a 2.5 month improvement over placebo. 1 year survival is approximately 10% better with use of gliadel[48]. Care must be taken with the use of this therapy as side effects of necrosis, cerebral edema, and seizure are common but can be controlled with steroid and antiepliptic therapy.

Use of gliadel can also exclude from further clinical trials and newer treatments. It can cause confounding effects on another trial because all of these are so new. Improvement of surgical resection can eliminate these problems.

11. Nanoparticles

Another novel approach still in the early phases of development is the use of surgically implantable nanoparticles to deliver chemotherapeutic agents. Small spherical particles 7 to 10 nanometers in size comprised of polymers or liposomes are non-covalently attached to slow sustained release formulations of chemotherapeutic drugs for delivery. These nanoparticles are small enough to cross the blood brain tumor barrier (BBTB) and transmit drug directly into individual tumor cells[49].

Nanoparticles can be administered intravascularly or directly into the brain via a surgically implanted catheter. Delivery of nanoparticles via surgically implanted catheter has the benefit of greater volume of distribution directly to the brain tissue compared with diffusion alone[50]. Development of these nanoparticle systems for treatment of malignant brain tumors is currently in the animal model phase and no human studies are currently available. Rat models of glioblastoma have shown increased survival using doxorubicin bonded to cyanoacrylate nanoparticles for delivery to tumor cells. The drug transport across the BBB by nanoparticles appears to be due to a receptor-mediated interaction with the brain capillary endothelial cells, which is facilitated by certain plasma apolipoproteins adsorbed by nanoparticles in the blood. Nanoparticle uptake appears selective to tumor cells in these models as the animals did not manifest signs of neurotoicity[51].

In addition to drug delivery, nanoparticles are being investigated for use in neuroimaging. Current imaging techniques have a maximum resolution of 1 mm. Nanoparticles could improve the resolution by a factor of ten or more, allowing detection of smaller tumors and more precise surgical resection. Several nanoparticle-based contrast materials have been used to enhance MRI imaging. One iron oxide nanoparticle currently under study has shown an innocuous toxicity profile as well as sustained retention in mouse tumors[52]. These fluorescent nanoparticles improved the contrast between the tumor tissue and the normal tissue in both MRI and optical imaging, which can be used during surgery to see the tumor boundary more precisely.

Another promising role of nanoparticle in the treatment of glioma involves hyperthermia treatment. The heating of cancerous tissues between 41 and 45°C, has been shown to improve the efficacy of cancer therapy when used in conjunction with chemotherapy and radiation[52]. Magnetic nanocomposites based on iron oxide can be used as implantable biomaterials for thermal cancer therapy applications at the time of surgery. These implanted particles can then be remotely heated by exposure to an external alternating magnetic field.

In 2011, Maier-Hauff and colleagues reported a trial of magnetic nanoparticle thermotherapy in conjunction with radiation treatments in 59 patients with recurrent glioblastoma[53]. Magnetic fluid was instilled within the tumor site using a neuronavigational procedure comparable to a brain needle biopsy and an external magnetic field was then applied for multiple treatments. Patients undergoing this procedure showed a mean survival time of 13.4 months after the first re-occurrence. Thermotherapy using magnetic nanoparticles in conjunction with a reduced radiation dose is safe and effective and leads to longer overall survival compared with conventional therapies in the treatment of recurrent GBM.

12. Immunotherapies

Using the body's own immune system to fight glioma, immunotherapy, is a new field which has seen significant advancements over the past decade. There are two categories of immunotherapy for glioma that are currently undergoing clinical research. Passive immunotherapy involves the activation of cytotoxic effector cells ex vivo and thee transfer of these activated cells back into the patient's body. Active immunotherapy, on the other hand, uses an exogenous trigger which causes activation of endogenous effector cells within the patients own body to target tumor cells. Active immunotherapy is generally employed in the tumor vaccine model. Surgery plays a large role in these therapies, as sizeable volumes of tumor tissue must be surgically obtained in order to construct the immunotherapeutic agents. Also several of these therapies utilize direct delivery of these agents into the brain during surgery.

Current clinical trials utilizing passive immunotherapy focus on the activation of effector cytotoxic T lymphocytes, natural killer cells, or lymphokine activated killer cells sensitized to glioma-associated antigens. Once such trial for glioblastoma treatment uses donor cytotoxic T lymphoyctes which are sensitized ex vivo to recognize patient human leukocyte antigen (HLA) groups expressed on the surface of glioma cells but not on normal neurons or glia. After surgical resection, the sensitized CTL cells are placed in the resection cavity as well as surgical placement of an intraparanchemal catheter and reservoir system to allow future delivery of CTL cells. An initial pilot study with this model showed significant survival benefit in 3 of 6 patients with 2 patients surviving >15 years since beginning immunotherapy[54].

Treatments using active immunotherapy via cell-based and peptide vaccines are also under study. Cells from glioma tumors are thought to be poor antigen-presenting cells because they often secrete immunosuppressive cytokines as well as growth factors such as transforming growth factor and vascular endothelial growth factor which can have a negative effect on T cell and natural killer cell activity. Tumor vaccines are designed to augment tumor-specific cellular immunity and enhance low-level immunity by stimulating the production of higher-avidity T cells specific to a tumor[55].

Chang and colleagues published results from one vaccine based phase II clinical trial in 2011. 16 patients with glioblastoma (8 newly diagnosed, 8 recurrent) underwent craniotomy for maximal cytoreduction followed by standard external beam radiation therapy in the newly diagnosed patients. Tumor cells obtained from the surgical resection were cultured in the laboratory and combined with autologous dendritic cells to produce vaccine. The vaccine was administered to patients via subcutaneous injection over lymph nodes for a total of 10 treatments over a 6 month period. Median survival and 5 year survival was 381 days and 12.5% for the newly diagnosed group, 966 days and 25% for the recurrent group compared to 380 days mean survival and 0% five years survival for a 16 patient age and sex matched historical control group.

Although most published results are from preliminary studies with small numbers of patients, immunotherapy for the treatment of glioma is a promising area currently undergoing multiple phase II and phase III trials for FDA approval[54]. Once the basic efficacy of these initial studies have been verified as a plausible modality for the treatment of glioma, randomized and controlled clinical trials can be undertaken to further explore the full potential of this therapy.

13. Gene therapy

Gene therapy is another novel modality used in the treatment of glioma, which focuses on the delivery of apoptotic genes at the time of surgical intervention and implantation in the surgical cavity. One of the most effective methods of in vivo gene delivery is the use of viral vectors as gene carriers. Retroviruses, adenovirus, and herpes simplex virus-1 (HSV-1) are all currently undergoing trials as vectors for viral brain tumor therapy Replication competent retroviruses have been shown to have infection rates of 97% with specificity for tumor cells without significant effects on non-tumor cells[56]. Adenovirus and HSV-1 are used in both replication competent and replication defective forms and have shown high transgenic capacity and persistent gene expression[57].

In 2003, Germano and colleagues reported a series of 11 patients with high grade glioma treated with gene therapy using adenovirus as a viral vector[57]. Adenovirus was used to transfer the herpes simplex-thymidine kinase gene into malignant glioma cells. This gene then phosphorylates ganciclovir, a non-cytotoxic nucleotide analog, into a compound that halts the transcription of DNA in dividing cells. Since normal brain cells are not rapidly dividing they are not affected. At the time of surgery, following gross total resection, the viral solution was injected directly into the tumor bed. This was followed by administration of ganciclovir systemically over 7 days. Of the 11 patients 10 had a survival of > 52 weeks following treatment. This survival time was associated with maintaining quality of life. 8 patients maintained a KPS of greater than 70 after 3 months and 5 patients 6 months after treatment.

Oncolytic viruses are also currently being used for clinical trials. These virus replicate selectively within tumor cells and can lead to increased intratumoral viral titers and cell death[58]. In 2004, Harrow and colleges used a modified herpes simplex virus with an affinity for glioblastoma cells which replicates only in rapidly diving cells causing cell lysis while sparing normal terminally differentiated cells. Twelve patients, 6 with newly diagnosed glioblastoma and 6 with recurrent glioblastoma, underwent craniotomy and surgical resection. Following resection during the same surgical procedure they were injected with the modified herpes virus at 8-10 sights adjacent to the tumor bed. Four patients, 2 newly diagnosed and 2 with recurrent disease showed survival of greater than 15 months following treatment.

Viral vectors, although promising, do have several limitations. Viral vectors suffer from low levels of gene incorporation due to limited diffusion into the brain parenchyma as well as low transfection rates of some cell types. Formation of antigenicity to vectors and introduced gene products causes additional difficulties. Also the use of retroviruses that incorporate genes into the host chromosome can result in insertional mutagenesis and propensity to form new tumors. The use of genetically modified cells to deliver gene therapy to the CNS may avoid some of these limitations. The use of stem cells is one area of research being used to avoid these limitations seen with traditional gene therapy.

Neural stem cells (NSC) are self-renewing multipotent cells found in the fetal brain within the ventricular zone, midbrain and spinal cord. These cells have the ability to repopulate a degenerated CNS region and can migrate toward pathologically altered tissues, including stroke, trauma and tumors. Genetic changes in NSCs may result in tumorigenesis by activation of oncogenes and/or inactivation of tumor suppressor genes.

Within brain tumors, a population of cells known brain tumor stem cells (BTSC) have been found. They are resistant to current treatments and capable of maintaining and propagating these tumors[59]. BTSCs are thought to arise from aberrant NSCs or from mature cells that have undergone mutation and dedifferentiation. BTSCs are similar to normal stem cells with regards to self-renewal, capacity, multi-potentiality, tumorigenicity as well as migratory capability. Transformation of these neural stem cells and their progenitor cells may therefore lead to the formation of BTSCs and eventually malignancy[60]. Gene therapies focusing on preventing the malignant transformation of

NSCs into BTSCs as well as the use of normal stem cells as a method of targeted delivery of therapeutic agents to glioma cells are currently under investigation.

Genetic modification of NSCs to secrete anti-tumor agents allows targeted delivery as well as provides a high level of active compounds at the local site of neoplasm. These types of therapies are still in the early stages and have not been evaluated in human glioma patients, however there are studies which have shown good results using animal models. One model using neural stem cells modified to produce high quantities of interleukin-4 in vivo was examined in Spraque-Dawley rats[61]. They implanted the modified NSCs into the brain tissue of rats affected with malignant gliobastoma and found a long term survival of 50% compared to control animals.

Another rat study used immortalized neural progenitor stem cells to express a eukaryotic catalytic enzyme that converts the nontoxic compound 5-flourocytosine into the highly toxic drug 5-flourouracil[62]. These stem cells were then implanted in rats with induced glioblastoma and the animals were subsequently treated with the nontoxic compound. After 10 days, the animals treated with the modified NSCs showed significant 50% decrease in tumoral mass compared to a control group. After histopathological examination of the treated tissue, they also found high levels of the toxic 5-flourouracil drug in adjacent tissue demonstrating in vivo conversion of the nontoxic compound to the toxic drug with therapeutic benefit.

Neural stem cells are also being used as vehicles for the tracking and suppression of glioblastoma. These methods exploit the tendency of NSCs to preferentially migrate towards brain tumors. This allows NSCs to be labeled and used as diagnostic imaging tools to identify extent of tumor invasion. One such animal model used NSCs modified to express the firefly luciferase gene[63]. These cells were then implanted into the contralateral brain parenchyma as well as injected into the ventricles of mice with intracranial gliomas. Over a period of 3 weeks, serial bioluminescence imaging was performed, which showed migration of the implanted cell across the corpus callosum with a maximal density at the site of the tumors. A subsequent study using the same model but with the addition of an apoptosis-promoting gene to the NSCs was performed to evaluate the therapeutic possibilities of this model. NSCs were modified not only to express the luciferase gene but also the tumor necrosis factor related apoptosis inducing ligand S-TRAIL. The transformed NSCs were then stereotactically implanted into the left frontal lobe of mice and glioma cells were stereotactically injected into the right frontal lobe of the same animals. Serial imaging was again performed which initially showed increased tumor volumes at the site of glioma injection as well as migration of the NSCs towards the tumor areas. After 16 days however there was a considerable decrease in tumor growth and a significant reduction in tumor cells on quantitative analysis compared to control animals. They also found expression of the S-TRAIL gene product at the tumor site on histopathological examination. These studies demonstrate the promising role that stem cells can play in the treatment of glioma.

14. Conclusion

Surgical resection remains the single most important primary treatment in the management of patients with glioma and extent of surgical resection directly correlates with increased patient survival. In this chapter we reviewed several innovative technologies and surgical methods for increasing the extent of resection as well as several adjuvant therapies and the important role that surgery plays in maximizing the potential benefit of these therapies in the treatment of glioma. As our ability to increase the extent of resection improves and new innovative technologies are perfected, we will continue to see improvements in long term survival in patients affected with glioma.

15. References

[1] Jemal A, Siegel R, Xu J, Ward E. Cancer statistics, 2010. *CA Cancer J Clin*. 2010;60(5):277-300.

[2] Schneider T, Mawrin C, Scherlach C, Skalej M, Firsching R. Gliomas in adults. *Deutsches \Ärzteblatt International*. 2010;107(45):799.

[3] CBTRUS. CBTRUS Statistical Report:Primary Brain and Central Nervous System Tumors Diagnosed in the United States in 2004-2007. 2011. Available at: http://www.cbtrus.org/.

[4] Norton L. Conceptual and practical implications of breast tissue geometry: toward a more effective, less toxic therapy. *Oncologist*. 2005;10(6):370-381.

[5] Piepmeier J, Baehring JM. Surgical resection for patients with benign primary brain tumors and low grade gliomas. *J. Neurooncol*. 2004;69(1-3):55-65.

[6] McGirt MJ, Chaichana KL, Attenello FJ, et al. Extent of surgical resection is independently associated with survival in patients with hemispheric infiltrating low-grade gliomas. *Neurosurgery*. 2008;63(4):700-707; author reply 707-708.

[7] Smith JS, Chang EF, Lamborn KR, et al. Role of extent of resection in the long-term outcome of low-grade hemispheric gliomas. *J. Clin. Oncol.* 2008;26(8):1338-1345.

[8] Kiwit JC, Floeth FW, Bock WJ. Survival in malignant glioma: analysis of prognostic factors with special regard to cytoreductive surgery. *Zentralbl. Neurochir.* 1996;57(2):76-88.

[9] Albert FK, Forsting M, Sartor K, Adams HP, Kunze S. Early postoperative magnetic resonance imaging after resection of malignant glioma: objective evaluation of residual tumor and its influence on regrowth and prognosis. *Neurosurgery*. 1994;34(1):45-60; discussion 60-61.

[10] Simpson JR, Horton J, Scott C, et al. Influence of location and extent of surgical resection on survival of patients with glioblastoma multiforme: results of three consecutive Radiation Therapy Oncology Group (RTOG) clinical trials. *Int. J. Radiat. Oncol. Biol. Phys.* 1993;26(2):239-244.

[11] Vuorinen V, Hinkka S, Färkkilä M, Jääskeläinen J. Debulking or biopsy of malignant glioma in elderly people - a randomised study. *Acta Neurochir (Wien)*. 2003;145(1):5-10.

[12] Ryken TC, Frankel B, Julien T, Olson JJ. Surgical management of newly diagnosed glioblastoma in adults: role of cytoreductive surgery. *J Neurooncol*. 2008;89(3):271-286.

[13] Lacroix M, Abi-Said D, Fourney DR, et al. A multivariate analysis of 416 patients with glioblastoma multiforme: prognosis, extent of resection, and survival. *J. Neurosurg.* 2001;95(2):190-198.

[14] Sanai N, Polley M-Y, McDermott MW, Parsa AT, Berger MS. An extent of resection threshold for newly diagnosed glioblastomas. *J. Neurosurg.* 2011;115(1):3-8.

[15] Ganslandt O, Behari S, Gralla J, Fahlbusch R, Nimsky C. Neuronavigation: concept, techniques and applications. *Neurol India*. 2002;50(3):244-255.

[16] Wirtz CR, Knauth M, Staubert A, et al. Clinical evaluation and follow-up results for intraoperative magnetic resonance imaging in neurosurgery. *Neurosurgery*. 2000;46(5):1112-1120; discussion 1120-1122.

[17] Senft C, Franz K, Blasel S, et al. Influence of iMRI-guidance on the extent of resection and survival of patients with glioblastoma multiforme. *Technol. Cancer Res. Treat.* 2010;9(4):339-346.

[18] Kubben PL, Ter Meulen KJ, Schijns OE, et al. Intraoperative MRI-guided resection of glioblastoma multiforme: a systematic review. *Lancet Oncol*. 2011. Available at:
http://www.ncbi.nlm.nih.gov/pubmed/21868286. Accessed September 6, 2011.

[19] Duffau H, Peggy Gatignol ST, Mandonnet E, Capelle L, Taillandier L. Intraoperative subcortical stimulation mapping of language pathways in a consecutive series of 115 patients with Grade II glioma in the left dominant hemisphere. *J. Neurosurg*. 2008;109(3):461-471.

[20] Talacchi A, Turazzi S, Locatelli F, et al. Surgical treatment of high-grade gliomas in motor areas. The impact of different supportive technologies: a 171-patient series. *J. Neurooncol*. 2010;100(3):417-426.

[21] Leclercq D, Duffau H, Delmaire C, et al. Comparison of diffusion tensor imaging tractography of language tracts and intraoperative subcortical stimulations. *J. Neurosurg*. 2010;112(3):503-511.

[22] Roux F-E, Boulanouar K, Lotterie J-A, et al. Language functional magnetic resonance imaging in preoperative assessment of language areas: correlation with direct cortical stimulation. *Neurosurgery*. 2003;52(6):1335-1345; discussion 1345-1347.

[23] Awasthi R, Verma SK, Haris M, et al. Comparative evaluation of dynamic contrast-enhanced perfusion with diffusion tensor imaging metrics in assessment of corticospinal tract infiltration in malignant glioma. *J Comput Assist Tomogr*. 2010;34(1):82-88.

[24] Wu J-S, Zhou L-F, Tang W-J, et al. Clinical evaluation and follow-up outcome of diffusion tensor imaging-based functional neuronavigation: a prospective, controlled study in patients with gliomas involving pyramidal tracts. *Neurosurgery*. 2007;61(5):935-948; discussion 948-949.

[25] Eljamel S. Photodynamic applications in brain tumors: A comprehensive review of the literature. *Photodiagnosis and Photodynamic Therapy*. 2010;7(2):76–85.

[26] Stummer W, Novotny A, Stepp H, et al. Fluorescence-guided resection of glioblastoma multiforme by using 5-aminolevulinic acid-induced porphyrins: a prospective study in 52 consecutive patients. *J. Neurosurg*. 2000;93(6):1003-1013.

[27] Stummer W, Pichlmeier U, Meinel T, et al. Fluorescence-guided surgery with 5-aminolevulinic acid for resection of malignant glioma: a randomised controlled multicentre phase III trial. *Lancet Oncol*. 2006;7(5):392-401.

[28] Stepp H, Beck T, Pongratz T, et al. ALA and malignant glioma: fluorescence-guided resection and photodynamic treatment. *J. Environ. Pathol. Toxicol. Oncol*. 2007;26(2):157-164.

[29] Widhalm G, Wolfsberger S, Minchev G, et al. 5-Aminolevulinic acid is a promising marker for detection of anaplastic foci in diffusely infiltrating gliomas with nonsignificant contrast enhancement. *Cancer*. 2010;116(6):1545-1552.

[30] Floeth FW, Sabel M, Ewelt C, et al. Comparison of (18)F-FET PET and 5-ALA fluorescence in cerebral gliomas. *Eur. J. Nucl. Med. Mol. Imaging*. 2011;38(4):731-741.

[31] Stylli SS, Kaye AH, MacGregor L, Howes M, Rajendra P. Photodynamic therapy of high grade glioma - long term survival. *J Clin Neurosci*. 2005;12(4):389-398.

[32] Stylli SS, Kaye AH. Photodynamic therapy of cerebral glioma - a review. Part II - clinical studies. *J Clin Neurosci*. 2006;13(7):709-717.

[33] Laperriere N, Zuraw L, Cairncross G. Radiotherapy for newly diagnosed malignant glioma in adults: a systematic review. *Radiother Oncol*. 2002;64(3):259-273.

[34] Mirimanoff RO, Stupp R. Radiotherapy in low-grade gliomas: Cons. *Semin. Oncol.* 2003;30(6 Suppl 19):34-38.

[35] Souhami L, Seiferheld W, Brachman D, et al. Randomized comparison of stereotactic radiosurgery followed by conventional radiotherapy with carmustine to conventional radiotherapy with carmustine for patients with glioblastoma multiforme: report of Radiation Therapy Oncology Group 93-05 protocol. *Int. J. Radiat. Oncol. Biol. Phys.* 2004;60(3):853-860.

[36] Tsao MN, Mehta MP, Whelan TJ, et al. The American Society for Therapeutic Radiology and Oncology (ASTRO) evidence-based review of the role of radiosurgery for malignant glioma. *Int. J. Radiat. Oncol. Biol. Phys.* 2005;63(1):47-55.

[37] Romanelli P, Conti A, Pontoriero A, et al. Role of stereotactic radiosurgery and fractionated stereotactic radiotherapy for the treatment of recurrent glioblastoma multiforme. *Neurosurg Focus*. 2009;27(6):E8.

[38] Laperriere NJ, Leung PM, McKenzie S, et al. Randomized study of brachytherapy in the initial management of patients with malignant astrocytoma. *Int. J. Radiat. Oncol. Biol. Phys.* 1998;41(5):1005-1011.

[39] Videtic GM, Gaspar LE, Zamorano L, et al. Use of the RTOG recursive partitioning analysis to validate the benefit of iodine-125 implants in the primary treatment of malignant gliomas. *Int. J. Radiat. Oncol. Biol. Phys.* 1999;45(3):687-692.

[40] Selker RG, Shapiro WR, Burger P, et al. The Brain Tumor Cooperative Group NIH Trial 87-01: a randomized comparison of surgery, external radiotherapy, and carmustine versus surgery, interstitial radiotherapy boost, external radiation therapy, and carmustine. *Neurosurgery*. 2002;51(2):343-355; discussion 355-357.

[41] Gaspar LE, Zamorano LJ, Shamsa F, et al. Permanent 125iodine implants for recurrent malignant gliomas. *Int. J. Radiat. Oncol. Biol. Phys.* 1999;43(5):977-982.

[42] Larson DA, Suplica JM, Chang SM, et al. Permanent iodine 125 brachytherapy in patients with progressive or recurrent glioblastoma multiforme. *Neuro-oncology*. 2004;6(2):119.

[43] Patel S, Breneman JC, Warnick RE, et al. Permanent iodine-125 interstitial implants for the treatment of recurrent glioblastoma multiforme. *Neurosurgery*. 2000;46(5):1123-1128; discussion 1128-1130.

[44] Keles GE, Lamborn KR, Chang SM, Prados MD, Berger MS. Volume of residual disease as a predictor of outcome in adult patients with recurrent supratentorial glioblastomas multiforme who are undergoing chemotherapy. *J. Neurosurg.* 2004;100(1):41-46.

[45] Lawson HC, Sampath P, Bohan E, et al. Interstitial chemotherapy for malignant gliomas: the Johns Hopkins experience. *J Neurooncol*. 2006;83(1):61-70.

[46] Valtonen S, Timonen U, Toivanen P, et al. Interstitial chemotherapy with carmustine-loaded polymers for high-grade gliomas: a randomized double-blind study. *Neurosurgery*. 1997;41(1):44-48; discussion 48-49.

[47] Westphal M, Ram Z, Riddle V, et al. Gliadel® wafer in initial surgery for malignant glioma: long-term follow-up of a multicenter controlled trial. *Acta Neurochir (Wien)*. 2006;148(3):269-275.

[48] Silagy CA, Middleton P, Hopewell S. Publishing Protocols of Systematic Reviews. *JAMA: the journal of the American Medical Association*. 2002;287(21):2831.

[49] Sarin H. Recent progress towards development of effective systemic chemotherapy for the treatment of malignant brain tumors. *J Transl Med*. 2009;7(1):77.

[50] Roger M, Clavreul A, Venier-Julienne MC, et al. The potential of combinations of drug-loaded nanoparticle systems and adult stem cells for glioma therapy. *Biomaterials*. 2010.

[51] Jain KK. Use of nanoparticles for drug delivery in glioblastoma multiforme. *Expert Rev Neurother*. 2007;7(4):363-372.

[52] Jain KK. Role of nanobiotechnology in the personalized management of glioblastoma multiforme. *Nanomedicine (Lond)*. 2011;6(3):411-414.

[53] Maier-Hauff K, Ulrich F, Nestler D, et al. Efficacy and safety of intratumoral thermotherapy using magnetic iron-oxide nanoparticles combined with external beam radiotherapy on patients with recurrent glioblastoma multiforme. *J. Neurooncol*. 2011;103(2):317-324.

[54] Hickey MJ, Malone CC, Erickson KL, et al. Cellular and vaccine therapeutic approaches for gliomas. *J Transl Med*. 8:100-100.

[55] Yamanaka R. Dendritic-cell- and peptide-based vaccination strategies for glioma. *Neurosurg Rev*. 2009;32(3):265-273.

[56] Rainov NG, Kramm CM. Recombinant retrovirus vectors for treatment of malignant brain tumors. *Int. Rev. Neurobiol*. 2003;55:185-203.

[57] Germano IM, Fable J, Gultekin SH, Silvers A. Adenovirus/herpes simplex-thymidine kinase/ganciclovir complex: preliminary results of a phase I trial in patients with recurrent malignant gliomas. *J. Neurooncol*. 2003;65(3):279-289.

[58] Harrow S, Papanastassiou V, Harland J, et al. HSV1716 injection into the brain adjacent to tumour following surgical resection of high-grade glioma: safety data and long-term survival. *Gene Ther*. 2004;11(22):1648-1658.

[59] Singh SK, Clarke ID, Terasaki M, et al. Identification of a cancer stem cell in human brain tumors. *Cancer Res*. 2003;63(18):5821-5828.

[60] Achanta P, Roman NI., Qui\ nones-Hinojosa A. Gliomagenesis and the use of neural stem cells in brain tumor treatment. *Anti-cancer agents in medicinal chemistry*. 2010;10(2):121.

[61] Benedetti S, Pirola B, Pollo B, et al. Gene therapy of experimental brain tumors using neural progenitor cells. *Nat. Med*. 2000;6(4):447-450.

[62] Barresi V, Belluardo N, Sipione S, et al. Transplantation of prodrug-converting neural progenitor cells for brain tumor therapy. *Cancer Gene Ther*. 2003;10(5):396-402.

[63] Tang Y, Shah K, Messerli SM, et al. In vivo tracking of neural progenitor cell migration to glioblastomas. *Hum. Gene Ther.* 2003;14(13):1247-1254.

Part 2

EGFR and Glioma Therapy

2

Advances in the Development of EGFR Targeted Therapies for the Treatment of Glioblastoma

Terrance Johns
Monash University,
Australia

1. Introduction

The epidermal growth factor receptor (EGFR) is receptor tyrosine kinase (RTK) dysregulated in glioblastoma (GBM) through overexpression, mutation or inappropriate expression of ligand. Activation of the EGFR by these mechanisms contributes to the development and progression of GBM by engaging downstream targets, such as the PI3K pathway. The de2-7 EGFR (or EGFRvIII), a naturally occurring mutation of the EGFR frequently expressed in GBM, preferentially activates this pathway. Clinical trials with EGFR-specific tyrosine kinase inhibitors (TKIs) have been disappointing with very little antitumor activity observed. The outcome of controlled clinical trials with EGFR-specific antibodies is yet to be reported. Encouraging preclinical and preliminary clinical data suggests that the combination of EGFR therapeutics and compounds that target molecules downstream of EGFR might have increased efficacy. Finally, the identification of biomarkers that predict those patients most likely to respond to EGFR inhibition is desperately needed.

2. Expression of EGFR and its ligands in GBM

The EGFR is frequently expressed in GBM (Jungbluth et al., 2003), the most common and deadly form of malignant brain cancer (DeAngelis, 2001). Extensive co-expression of EGFR ligands such as EGF and TGF-α has also been reported (Ekstrand et al., 1991), suggesting the existence of a robust autocrine loop in many cases of GBM. Furthermore, overexpression of the EGFR has been reported in up to 60% of GBM cases depending on the technique used (Libermann et al., 1985; Schlegel et al., 1994; Jungbluth et al., 2003), with overexpression leading to ligand-independent activation of the receptor (Thomas et al., 2003). The activation and subsequent phosphorylation of EGFR stimulates several downstream pathways including Ras/MAPK, PI3K/Akt, PLC-gamma and STAT3 (Halatsch et al., 2006; Nakamura, 2007). All four pathways contribute to the tumorigenicity of GBM, but the PI3K/Akt pathway appears to have a central role in the development and maintenance of this cancer (Chakravarti et al., 2004). Indeed, inactivation/deletion/mutation of PTEN, an endogenous inhibitor of the PI3K pathway, is also a common event in GBM (Rasheed et al., 1997). Of note, there is an emerging role for EGFR-mediated activation of STAT3 in the development of GBM (Weissenberger et al., 2004; Mizoguchi et al., 2006; Sherry et al., 2009).

3. Amplification of the EGFR gene in GBM

Amplification of the *EGFR* gene was the first reported genetic alteration in GBM (Libermann et al., 1985). Subsequent studies have confirmed that approximately 40% of GBMs display amplification of the *EGFR* gene (Wong et al., 1987). Gene amplification invariably leads to overexpression of the EGFR at the cell surface (Wong et al., 1987), although given that overexpression of the receptor occurs in 60% of GBMs, gene amplification is not the only route to increased expression. The majority of GBMs develop rapidly, without evidence of pre-existing malignant lesion, and are known as primary (or *de novo*) GBMs, while secondary GBMs arise from low-grade diffuse astrocytomas or anaplastic astrocytomas (Furnari et al., 2007; Ohgaki & Kleihues, 2007). *EGFR* gene amplification is more commonly associated with primary GBMs than secondary GBMs, where it occurs at a frequency of less than 10% (Watanabe et al., 1996; Ohgaki & Kleihues, 2007). Overexpressed EGFR not only activates in a ligand-independent manner, but shows enhanced signaling through the STATs, including STAT3 (Thomas et al., 2003; Pedersen et al., 2005), which in turn can induce expression of IL-6. Since IL-6 autocrine loops and amplification of the *IL6* gene have been reported at high frequency in GBM (Weissenberger et al., 2004; Tchirkov et al., 2007), this could be an important, but largely overlooked, consequence of EGFR overexpression.

Recent studies have shown that GBM can be classified into at least 4 distinct molecular sub-types; classical, pro-neural, neural and mesenchymal (Brennan et al., 2009; Verhaak et al., 2010). Pro-neural GBMs largely constitutes the secondary GBMs and therefore does not display EGFR amplification and/or overexpression. In contrast nearly all GBM in the classical sub-type overexpress EGFR (Verhaak et al., 2010). Furthermore, the GBM specific mutation, de2-7 EGFR, is found almost exclusively in the classical sub-type. Neural and mesenchymal GBMs have variable levels of EGFR with some showing increased expression and others decreased expression.

4. Mutations of EGFR described in GBM

Amplification of the *EGFR* gene in GBM is associated with gene rearrangements. The first rearrangement to be described in detail was an extracellular domain (ECD) deletion producing a mutant known as the de2-7 EGFR (or EGFRvIII) (Sugawa et al., 1990; Yamazaki et al., 1990; Ekstrand et al., 1992; Wong et al., 1992). Several other deletion mutants have since been described and categorized (Table 1) (Ekstrand et al., 1992; Frederick et al., 2000). Numerous subsequent studies have shown that the most common mutation is the de2-7 EGFR, occurring in about 50% of cases where the *EGFR* gene is amplified (Wikstrand et al., 1998; Frederick et al., 2000; Pedersen et al., 2001). This cancer-specific EGFR mutant has a specific deletion between exons 2 and 7 of *EGFR* (Sugawa et al., 1990). The truncation of exons 2–7 leads to the elimination of 267 amino acids from the ECD and the insertion of a novel glycine at the fusion junction. This renders the mutant EGFR unable to bind any known ligand (Sugawa et al., 1990; Wikstrand et al., 1998; Pedersen et al., 2001). Despite this, the de2-7 EGFR is capable of low-level constitutive signaling, which is augmented by the mutant receptor's impaired internalization and downregulation (Nishikawa et al., 1994; Schmidt et al., 2003).

GBM cell lines transfected with the de2-7 EGFR display enhanced tumorigenicity when grown as xenografts in nude mice, but only a marginal effect on growth is observed *in vitro*

(Nishikawa et al., 1994). Furthermore, expression of the de2-7 EGFR is consistently lost when GBM cell lines are established *in vitro* using serum, yet is retained if GBM samples are implanted and subsequently passaged directly in nude mice (Sarkaria et al., 2007). Taken together, this indicates that the de2-7 EGFR contributes primarily to aspects of *in vivo* growth. While the increased tumorigenicity mediated by the de2-7 EGFR is primarily due to the receptor's constitutive tyrosine kinase activity (Huang et al., 1997), attempts to identify intracellular molecules and signaling pathways associated with its growth advantage remain ongoing. Transfection of the de2-7 EGFR into U87MG human GBM cells results in an increase in PI3K activity that is important to the growth advantage mediated by the mutant receptor, an observation confirmed by several papers (Moscatello et al., 1998; Li et al., 2004; Luwor et al., 2004). U87MG cells transfected with the de2-7 EGFR also co-express wild-type (wt) EGFR, a scenario that probably mimics the situation in GBM patients. The significance of a possible interaction between the de2-7 EGFR and wtEGFR is not fully known, but it has been shown that the de2-7 EGFR can directly activate PI3K in the absence of the wtEGFR in non-GBM cell lines (Moscatello et al., 1998). We reported that the de2-7 EGFR and the wt EGFR can heterodimerize leading to increased PI3K signaling (Luwor et al., 2004), suggesting that an interaction between the mutant and wt receptor could enhance de2-7 EGFR signaling. One clear consequence of PI3K activation by de2-7 EGFR is the increased production of VEGF, both under normoxic and hypoxic conditions (Feldkamp et al., 1999), ascribing a pro-angiogenic function to this receptor.

Mutation	**Frequency (%)**	**Biological Effect**
Δ6–273	30	**Ligand-independent, failure to down-regulate**
Δ521–603	<10	**Unknown**
Δ959–1186	<10	**Increased ligand-dependant kinase activity**
Δ959–1030 and Δ959-1043	<10	**Increased basal activity especially Δ959–1030 but responds to ligand**
R84K	<5	**Increased basal activity but responds to ligand**
T239P	<5	**Increased basal activity but responds to ligand**
A265V/D/T	<5	**Increased basal activity but responds to ligand**
G574V	<1	**Increased basal activity but responds to ligand**
Kinase mutation (L861Q)	<1	**Increased basal activity, failure to downregulate**

Table 1. Selected mutations of the EGFR expressed in GBM

Very recently de2-7 EGFR has been shown to stimulate the production of cytokines, including IL-6 and LIF, which signal through the gp130 complex (Inda et al., 2010). Importantly these cytokines were shown to activate the wtEGFR when it is overexpressed in neighboring GBM cells, through a mechanism involving cross-talk between gp130 and

EGFR. Activation of the wtEGFR in this manner leads to enhanced proliferation. Thus, de2-7 EGFR contributes to the growth of surrounding GBM cells through this field effect. This work also shows the functional link between EGFR and IL-6. More generally this indicates that the de2-7 EGFR actively contributes to the heterogeneity of GBM by acting indirectly with neighboring de2-7 EGFR negative cells (Inda et al., 2010). This hypothesis is entirely consistent with the observation that wtEGFR amplification and de2-7 EGFR expression are usually seen together. It may also explain why the pronounced growth advantage mediated by the de2-7 EGFR does not lead in patients to a homogenous population of cells in patients all expressing the receptor.

Lee *et al* sequenced the entire *EGFR* gene in a panel of eight GBM cell lines and 132 GBM samples (Table 1) (Lee et al., 2006). Interestingly, they identified a series of missense mutations in the ECD of the EGFR expressed in 14% of the GBM samples and 12% of the cell lines (Lee et al., 2006). In general, the missense mutations were found to be independent of the de2-7 EGFR but were associated with *EGFR* gene amplification; approximately 60% of samples with missense mutations also had *EGFR* gene amplification. Subsequent studies showed that these single amino acid mutations led to ligand-independent activation of the EGFR, and unlike the wtEGFR, were transforming in NR6 cells; a variant of mouse 3T3 cells lacking the EGFR (Lee et al., 2006). However, unlike the de2-7 EGFR, these mutants could also respond to ligand stimulation. Recently, we extended these studies and showed that some of these mutations also provide a significant advantage to *in vivo* growth (Ymer et al., 2011).

The presence of activating kinase mutations, such as those commonly found in lung cancer (Sharma et al., 2007), is extremely rare in GBM, with only one sample displaying this type of mutation (Lee et al., 2006). Interestingly, a subsequent analysis of 119 lung cancer samples failed to find a single missense mutation in the ECD, although 13% of the samples contained kinase domain mutations, as expected (Lee et al., 2006). Thus, mutations of the EGFR in GBM appear to cluster in the ECD and lead to ligand independence. Therefore, the lessons learned with respect to EGFR therapeutics for the treatment of lung cancer are probably of minimal value in the context of GBM. Finally, these mutations further emphasize just how frequently the EGFR is perturbed in GBM; in fact, taking into account EGFR autocrine loops, activation of the EGFR probably occurs in over 70% of GBMs.

5. EGFR as a therapeutic target in GBM

Given that the EGFR is activated or dysregulated in a large percentage of GBM cases it is a rational target for therapeutic intervention in this disease. There are two major classes of EGFR inhibitors either currently approved or being evaluated for the treatment of various cancers; antibodies that target the ECD and small molecule TKIs that target the intracellular kinase domain (Marshall, 2006). No specific agent from either class has been approved for the treatment of GBM, but as described below, a number of clinical trials have been reported or are ongoing.

5.1 Antibodies directed to the EGFR

Overexpression of the de2-7 EGFR on the cell surface, the unique junctional peptide created by the deletion and the aggressive phenotype associated with this receptor, suggests that targeting the de2-7 EGFR with antibodies that are cancer-specific is an attractive therapeutic strategy. In fact, antibodies specific for the de2-7 EGFR have been generated; the monoclonal antibodies (mAbs) DH8.3 (Hills et al., 1995), L8A4 and Y10 (Wikstrand et al., 1995) all preferentially recognize the unique junctional peptide. DH8.3 and Y10 have been shown to specifically target cells expressing the de2-7 EGFR (i.e. they do not bind the wtEGFR) (Hills et al., 1995; Wikstrand et al., 1995). Although DH8.3 has been shown to target de2-7 EGFR-expressing xenografts *in vivo* (Johns et al., 2002), its efficacy has not been reported. The Y10 antibody has been shown to have *in vivo* antitumor activity against murine B16 melanoma cells transfected with a murine homolog of the human de2-7 EGFR (Sampson et al., 2000), an unusual system for its evaluation since expression of the de2-7 EGFR has not been reported in melanoma. Furthermore, the antitumor activity seen was completely dependent on the Fc function of the Y10 antibody and not a direct inhibitory effect on de2-7 EGFR signaling (Sampson et al., 2000). There have been no reports to date of clinical trials using de2-7 EGFR-specific antibodies. These antibodies are internalized and could be used for delivery of radiotherapy or cytotoxics given their specificity (Foulon et al., 2000), but this approach has not been examined clinically.

Numerous therapeutic antibodies to the wtEGFR have been described and several have been used in the context of GBM (Quang & Brady, 2004; Belda-Iniesta et al., 2006). These antibodies all function in a similar manner by interacting with the L2 domain of the EGFR and inhibiting the binding of ligand. Structural studies with Cetuximab suggest that these antibodies also prevent EGFR dimerization, a crucial step in its activation (Li et al., 2005). Antibodies directed to the wtEGFR do show antitumor activity in GBM xenograft models even when the tumors are grown intracranially (Eller et al., 2002; Perera et al., 2005). Furthermore, these antibodies can bind the de2-7 EGFR and can inhibit GBM cells co-expressing the de2-7 and wtEGFR (Perera et al., 2005). However, the large intratumoral pressure found in GBM, the 'remnants' of a blood brain barrier (BBB) and the inefficient nature of GBM vascularization have all raised concerns about the effective targeting of antibodies to GBM following systemic administration. Despite these concerns, three antibodies targeting wtEGFR are have been tested in GBM using systemic administration, including mAb 425. ^{131}I-mAb 425 has been used in several clinical trials and clearly demonstrates targeting to GBM following systemic administration (Quang & Brady, 2004). Unfortunately, this antibody is of murine origin and can only be administered on a few occasions before immune responses render it ineffective.

Cetuximab is a chimeric antibody directed to the EGFR that has been approved in several human cancers including that of the colon (Moosmann & Heinemann, 2007). There are anecdotal reports of this antibody being used for the treatment of GBM, but no rigorously controlled studies have been implemented to date (Belda-Iniesta et al., 2006). Preclinical *in vitro* and *in vivo* studies suggest that cetuximab and related antibodies have significant antitumor activity in GBM, encouraging the establishment of a Phase I/II clinical trial (Combs et al., 2006). In this trial, cetuximab will be co-administered with a combination of temozolomide and radiotherapy, which is the standard of care following initial resection of a GBM (Trial Number: NCT00311857). Outcomes from this trial should be reported shortly. Recently cetuximab was trialed with a combination with bevacizumab (i.e. avastin) and irinotecan but did not increase the efficacy of this combination in GBM patients (Hasselbalch et al., 2010). There are several other EGFR-directed antibodies either approved or in development including Panitumumab (Rivera et al., 2008); however, there have been no reports of their systematic evaluation in GBM.

A novel EGFR antibody (mAb 806) was generated against cells expressing the de2-7 EGFR but, unexpectedly, was also found to bind to a small proportion of the wtEGFR in GBM samples that overexpress the receptor (Jungbluth et al., 2003). mAb 806 does not bind the unique junctional peptide found in the de2-7 EGFR; rather, it binds to a short cysteine loop on the ECD that is only transiently exposed as the wtEGFR moves from its inactive to active conformation (Johns et al., 2004). The loop is constitutively exposed in the de2-7 EGFR, consistent with our original desire to generate a de2-7 EGFR-specific antibody. Thus, mAb 806 reactivity is found only in cells with favorable conditions for receptor activation, such as the presence of mutations (e.g. de2-7 EGFR), overexpression of the wt receptor or increased presence of EGFR ligands. In the case of EGFR overexpression, there is increased activation as a result of ligand-independent EGFR activation and changes in glycosylation (Johns et al., 2005). These conditions are common in malignant cells but are rare in normal tissues, thereby allowing mAb 806 to preferentially target malignancy such as GBM but not normal organs such as the liver. Our recent Phase I clinical trial confirmed that a chimeric version of mAb 806 did not bind normal tissue and could target GBM following systemic administration (Scott et al., 2007). Since mAb 806, unlike Cetuximab, does not target organs such as the liver it is easier to deliver a therapeutically relevant dose to the site of the GBM. Furthermore, the lack of normal tissue uptake will allow the labeling of mAb 806 with cytotoxic compounds or radioisotopes to enhance its already substantial antitumor efficacy (Johns et al., 2007). This antibody has been licensed and has re-entered clinical trial.

5.2 Tyrosine kinase inhibitors that target the EGFR

TKIs are small molecules that specifically target the kinase domain of tyrosine kinases, preventing binding of ATP and subsequent activation (Marshall, 2006). Two EGFR-specific TKIs have been approved for the treatment of certain cancers (Mendelsohn & Baselga, 2006), while several others are in clinical trials. Similar to EGFR-specific antibodies, these compounds have shown antitumor activity in *in vitro* and *in vivo* preclinical models (Mendelsohn & Baselga, 2006). They are active against both the wtEGFR and the de2-7 EGFR (Stea et al., 2003; Halatsch et al., 2006; Sarkaria et al., 2007), although they might be less effective against the latter, especially if the de2-7 EGFR is expressed in the absence of the wtEGFR (Learn et al., 2004). Given that there are fewer concerns with regard to delivery of TKIs to the site of GBM when compared with antibodies, the development of these reagents for the treatment of GBM is more advanced. In fact, excellent targeting of these agents to the site of GBM has been well demonstrated (Hofer et al., 2006; Hegi et al., 2011).

The two clinically approved EGFR TKIs, erlotinib and gefitinib, have been used as monotherapy or in combination with temozolomide and/or radiotherapy in clinical trials of GBM patients (Table 2 lists selected Phase II trials). No significant clinical activity has been observed for either erlotinib or gefitinib in either primary or recurrent GBM when used as monotherapies (Table 2). Surgery, followed by temozolomide/radiotherapy is standard of care in primary GBM. The addition or erlotinib to this standard of care has been assessed in 3 different Phase II trials (Table 2). Two of these trials failed to show any benefit when erlotinib was added to standard of care and was associated with significant toxicity (Brown et al., 2008; Peereboom et al., 2010). In a third trial however, the authors reported encouraging PFS and median survival when compared to their previous studies using other agents (Prados et al., 2009). All three studies were conducted in newly diagnosed patients.

Why these trials have produced conflicting outcomes is not clear, but a comprehensive Phase III study is probably required to finally determine if erlotinib improves standard therapy. Overall though the data suggests that erlotinib's benefits are relatively small at best.

Trial	Patients (*n*)	Objective Response#	PFS	Median OS (months)
Gefitinib (single agent, recurrent)				
Rich *et al* (Rich et al., 2004)	**53**	**0**	**13% (6 months)**	**10**
Franceschi *et al* (Franceschi et al., 2007)	**16**	**0**	**12% (6 months)**	**6**
Gefitinib (single agent, primary)				
Uhm *et al* (Uhm et al., 2011)	**98**	**N/A**	**17% (12 months)**	**12**
Erlotinib (single agent, recurrent)				
Raizer *et al (Raizer et al., 2010)*	**38**	**0**	**3% (6 months)**	**6**
Erlotinib (plus standard care, primary)				
Peereboom *et al* (Peereboom et al., 2010)	**27**	**5 patients remain on study**	**3 months (median)**	**9†**
Prados *et al* (Prados et al., 2009)	**65**	**N/A**	**8 months (median)**	**19**
Brown *et al* (Brown et al., 2008)	**97**	**N/A**	**7 months (median)**	**15†**

Abbreviations: CR, complete response; PR, partial response; N/A not available; PFS, progression-free survival; OS, overall survival. *Abstract form only. #Excludes stable disease. †Significant toxicity

Table 2. Selected Phase II clinical trials of EGFR TKI's in GBM

A group of GBM patients treated with erlotinib or gefitinib who had responded or failed to respond to therapy was analyzed retrospectively to determine factors that might explain the different responses (Mellinghoff et al., 2005). The majority of responders expressed the de2-7 EGFR. Furthermore, loss of PTEN, an endogenous inhibitor of PI3K that leads to reduced phosphorylated AKT (Akt), was highly predictive of treatment failure. Not surprisingly, the co-expression of de2-7 EGFR and PTEN was predictive of response to EGFR-specific TKI therapy. A panel of human GBMs directly established as xenografts in nude mice retains expression of de2-7 EGFR in some cases (Sarkaria et al., 2006). This model system also confirmed that the presence of de2-7 EGFR and PTEN in a xenograft was predictive of response (Sarkaria et al., 2007). The mechanistic reasons for this observation remain unknown, but it provides a potential method for screening for patients likely to respond to TKI therapy. Finally, none of the current trials have shown a correlation between response to EGFR TKIs and *EGFR* gene amplification (Brown et al., 2008), although one immunohistochemical study reported a correlation between response to erlotinib and high expression of EGFR in combination with low levels of pAkt (Haas-Kogan et al., 2005). Once again this supports the notion that activated EGFR in the presence of low pAkt may be indicative of increased levels of response to EGFR inhibition.

Recently bevacizumab (i.e. avastin) was approved for the treatment of recurrent GBM. A Phase II trial of erlotinib and bevacizumab showed that this combination was adequately tolerated, but provided no additional benefit to that seen in other bevacizumab containing regimens (Sathornsumetee et al., 2010). mTOR is downstream of the PI3K/Akt pathway and therefore represents a therapeutic target in GBM. The combination of sirolimus (a mTor inhibitor), and erlotinib has been reported in recurrent GBM patients (Reardon et al., 2010). While the combination was well tolerated, it displayed negligible anti-tumor activity.

6. Future developments

Both Cetuximab and Panitumumab have been approved for the treatment of colon cancer and erlotinib and gefitinib are approved for non-small cell lung cancer (NSCLC), validating the EGFR as a genuine therapeutic target (Van den Eynde et al., 2011). Given the dysregulation of the EGFR in GBM through the range of mechanisms described above, the failure of these agents to show significant anti-tumor activity in this cancer is somewhat surprising. The possibility that the BBB is responsible for this lack of activity has been conclusively discounted for EGFR TKI's and appears not to be a factor for anti-EGFR antibodies, although formal demonstration of this is still required for antibodies. Future research should focus the identification of patients more likely to respond to EGFR inhibition and identifying other targeted therapies that might work synergistically with EGFR inhibitors. Further classification of GBM into unique molecular sub-types beyond the four already described (Verhaak et al., 2010) will hopefully help identify EGFR levels of tumor subtypes more likely to respond to EGFR inhibition.

6.1 Lessons from other cancers

In NSCLC the sub-set of patients most likely to respond to EGFR TKI's are those containing activating mutations in the kinase domain of *EGFR (da Cunha Santos et al., 2011)*. Significant clinical and laboratory evidence suggests that these mutations lead to "oncogenic addiction"; the phenomenon whereby a tumor becomes largely dependent on a single activated kinase. Interestingly, *EGFR* amplification is not strongly associated with response to TKI's in NSCLC (De Luca & Normanno, 2010). In contrast, EGFR activation in GBM is most often driven by gene amplification and/or mutations found in the ECD domain of the receptor (Lee et al., 2006), although a recent report described several c-terminal deleted EGFR molecules that are constitutively active (Pines et al., 2010). The clinical data in GBM implies that mutations of this nature do not lead to EGFR addiction. The reason for this remains speculative but suggests that the primary role of EGFR in GBM may not be tumor proliferation or survival but some other important biological function that supports, but is not essential to, GBM growth. A recent paper showing that inactive EGFR has a critical role in upregulating glucose transport highlights other unanticipated roles for this receptor (Weihua et al., 2008). Importantly inhibition of EGFR does not block this activity, rather EGFR needed to be removed from the cell surface. This result suggests at least one mechanism by which the presence of inactive EGFR may contribute to GBM development in a non-critical manner. Indeed, we have very recently shown that de2-7 EGFR has a role in regulating GBM response to low glucose (Cvrljevic et al, *in press*).

EGFR antibodies do not have any efficacy in colon cancer in patients containing mutations in Ras or Raf (Laurent-Puig et al., 2009). While mutations in these molecules are comparatively rare in GBM (McLendon et al., 2008), and thus cannot be used to stratify patients, the pathways associated with Ras/Raf can be activated by other RTKs on the cell surface. The activation of Ras/Raf by these RTKs might cause *de novo* resistance to EGFR therapeutics. Raf can be targeted directly by TKIs already in the clinic, however Ras cannot be inhibited by this approach. However, the signalling of both kinases can be targeted by blocking downstream targets such as ERK and MEK (Pratilas & Solit, 2010). If the toxicity issues can be managed, targeting these kinases in combination with EGFR inhibitors is a logical next step in GBM. This is not a problem in NSCLC as EGFR and ras mutations are mutually exclusive in this cancer type.

Recent data suggests that mutations in PI3K may also cause resistance to EGFR antibodies in colon cancer (Weickhardt et al., 2010). This is highly relevant to GBM as the PI3K pathway appears to be dysregulated in most GBMs through direct mutation of PI3K, the deletion or mutation of the negative PI3K regulator PTEN or activation through other RTKs (McLendon et al., 2008). Indeed, as discussed above, the absence of PTEN was associated with clinical resistance to EGFR TKIs in GBM patients expressing the de2-7 EGFR while responsiveness was associated with co-expression of PTEN and de2-7 EGFR. The recent translation of PI3K inhibitors into the clinic provides a strategy for overcoming PI3K-mediated resistance to EGFR inhibitors. All the evidence suggests that this combinational approach might finally unleash the potential of EGFR inhibitors for the treatment of GBM (Fan & Weiss, 2010); once again management of toxicity remains as a concern.

6.2 Combination of EGFR inhibitors with other targeted therapies

Since most RTKs can activate Ras/Raf and/or PI3K, the dual inhibition of EGFR and additional activated RTKs is an obvious therapeutic approach. Stommel *et al* clearly showed that multiple RTKs can be activated in GBM and that these RTKs activate overlapping downstream pathways causing resistance to TKIs that only targeting a single RTK (Stommel et al., 2007). The RTK c-Met is also commonly activated in GBM through a number of mechanisms and also has an important role in angiogenesis (Abounader & Laterra, 2005). We recently showed that co-expression of de2-7 EGFR and c-Met in GBM xenografts causes therapeutic resistant to single agents directed to either of these RTK. However, the combination of EGFR and c-Met inhibitors produced synergistic anti-tumor activity (Pillay et al., 2009), confirming that dual inhibition of RTKs is a valid approach in GBM. A number of other RTKs have been shown to be activated in GBM including the FGFR family, Axl, ErbB2/3/4, EphA2/7, VEGFR2 and PDGFRα/β (Ren et al., 2007; Pillay et al., 2009). Given the range of potential RTKs activated in a given patient, the most effective therapeutic strategy may have to be determined by screening patient tissues for RTK mutation and/or activation (i.e. phosphorylation) before commencing treatment.

We recently showed that EGFR and Src-family kinases (SFK) are frequently coactivated in GBM (Lu et al., 2009). Furthermore, the de2-7 EGFR physically associated with SFKs and this interaction increased tumor growth and invasion. This association was also confirmed in clinical samples. Treatment of GBM xenografts with the EGFR antibody mAb 806 and dasatinib, a SFK inhibitor, resulted in synergistic anti-tumor activity compared to either agent alone (Lu et al., 2009). These results suggest that the combination of EGFR inhibition and SFK blockade may be efficacious in GBM. As such, a trial of evaluating the combination of erlotinib and dasatinib has commenced in recurrent GBM (Trial No. NCT00609999).

7. Conclusion

The seemingly central role of EGFR in GBM biology would suggest that it should be an excellent therapeutic target in GBM; clinical trials clearly show that this is not the case when EGFR is targeted alone or in combination with standard GBM therapy. The further development of EGFR inhibitors in GBM must be underpinned by additional studies into the biology of EGFR in this cancer and the identification of signalling events associated with resistance to EGFR therapeutics. On-going rational trials using EGFR inhibitors in combination with other TKIs are justified, possibly underpinned by some basic stratification of patients based on mutations present in tumors. Finally, a prospective study formally proving that therapeutic antibodies do actually enter the GBMs and bind target cells would be informative. In conclusion, inhibition of the EGFR pathway in GBM is ineffective as a therapeutic strategy even when used in combination with current therapies. However, their effectiveness in combination with other targeted therapeutics should form the next stage of their development as a therapeutic target.

8. References

Abounader, R. and J. Laterra (2005). Scatter factor/hepatocyte growth factor in brain tumor growth and angiogenesis. *Neuro Oncol*, Vol. 7, No. 4, (Oct) pp. 436-451.

Belda-Iniesta, C., et al. (2006). Long term responses with cetuximab therapy in glioblastoma multiforme. *Cancer Biol Ther*, Vol. 5, No. 8, (Aug) pp. 912-914.

Brennan, C., et al. (2009). Glioblastoma subclasses can be defined by activity among signal transduction pathways and associated genomic alterations. *PLoS One*, Vol. 4, No. 11, pp. e7752.

Brown, P. D., et al. (2008). Phase I/II trial of erlotinib and temozolomide with radiation therapy in the treatment of newly diagnosed glioblastoma multiforme: North Central Cancer Treatment Group Study N0177. *J Clin Oncol*, Vol. 26, No. 34, (Dec 1) pp. 5603-5609.

Chakravarti, A., et al. (2004). The prognostic significance of phosphatidylinositol 3-kinase pathway activation in human gliomas. *J Clin Oncol*, Vol. 22, No. 10, (May 15) pp. 1926-1933.

Combs, S. E., et al. (2006). Treatment of primary glioblastoma multiforme with cetuximab, radiotherapy and temozolomide (GERT)--phase I/II trial: study protocol. *BMC Cancer*, Vol. 6, No., pp. 133.

da Cunha Santos, G., et al. (2011). EGFR mutations and lung cancer. *Annu Rev Pathol*, Vol. 6, No., (Feb 28) pp. 49-69.

De Luca, A. and N. Normanno (2010). Predictive biomarkers to tyrosine kinase inhibitors for the epidermal growth factor receptor in non-small-cell lung cancer. *Curr Drug Targets*, Vol. 11, No. 7, (Jul) pp. 851-864.

DeAngelis, L. M. (2001). Brain tumors. *N Engl J Med*, Vol. 344, No. 2, (Jan 11) pp. 114-123.

Ekstrand, A. J., et al. (1991). Genes for epidermal growth factor receptor, transforming growth factor alpha, and epidermal growth factor and their expression in human gliomas in vivo. *Cancer Res*, Vol. 51, No. 8, (Apr 15) pp. 2164-2172.

Ekstrand, A. J., et al. (1992). Amplified and rearranged epidermal growth factor receptor genes in human glioblastomas reveal deletions of sequences encoding portions of the N- and/or C-terminal tails. *Proc Natl Acad Sci U S A*, Vol. 89, No. 10, (May 15) pp. 4309-4313.

Eller, J. L., et al. (2002). Activity of anti-epidermal growth factor receptor monoclonal antibody C225 against glioblastoma multiforme. *Neurosurgery*, Vol. 51, No. 4, (Oct) pp. 1005-1013; discussion 1013-1004.

Fan, Q. W. and W. A. Weiss (2010). Targeting the RTK-PI3K-mTOR axis in malignant glioma: overcoming resistance. *Curr Top Microbiol Immunol*, Vol. 347, No., pp. 279-296.

Feldkamp, M. M., et al. (1999). Normoxic and hypoxic regulation of vascular endothelial growth factor (VEGF) by astrocytoma cells is mediated by Ras. *Int J Cancer*, Vol. 81, No. 1, (Mar 31) pp. 118-124.

Foulon, C. F., et al. (2000). Radioiodination via D-amino acid peptide enhances cellular retention and tumor xenograft targeting of an internalizing anti-epidermal growth factor receptor variant III monoclonal antibody. *Cancer Res*, Vol. 60, No. 16, (Aug 15) pp. 4453-4460.

Franceschi, E., et al. (2007). Gefitinib in patients with progressive high-grade gliomas: a multicentre phase II study by Gruppo Italiano Cooperativo di Neuro-Oncologia (GICNO). *Br J Cancer*, Vol. 96, No. 7, (Apr 10) pp. 1047-1051.

Frederick, L., et al. (2000). Diversity and frequency of epidermal growth factor receptor mutations in human glioblastomas. *Cancer Res*, Vol. 60, No. 5, (Mar 1) pp. 1383-1387.

Furnari, F. B., et al. (2007). Malignant astrocytic glioma: genetics, biology, and paths to treatment. *Genes Dev*, Vol. 21, No. 21, (Nov 1) pp. 2683-2710.

Haas-Kogan, D. A., et al. (2005). Epidermal growth factor receptor, protein kinase B/Akt, and glioma response to erlotinib. *J Natl Cancer Inst*, Vol. 97, No. 12, (Jun 15) pp. 880-887.

Halatsch, M. E., et al. (2006). Epidermal growth factor receptor inhibition for the treatment of glioblastoma multiforme and other malignant brain tumours. *Cancer Treat Rev*, Vol. 32, No. 2, (Apr) pp. 74-89.

Hasselbalch, B., et al. (2010). Cetuximab, bevacizumab, and irinotecan for patients with primary glioblastoma and progression after radiation therapy and temozolomide: a phase II trial. *Neuro Oncol*, Vol. 12, No. 5, (May) pp. 508-516.

Hegi, M. E., et al. (2011). Pathway Analysis of Glioblastoma Tissue after Preoperative Treatment with the EGFR Tyrosine Kinase Inhibitor Gefitinib - A Phase II Trial. *Mol Cancer Ther*, Vol., No., (Apr 6).

Hills, D., et al. (1995). Specific targeting of a mutant, activated FGF receptor found in glioblastoma using a monoclonal antibody. *Int J Cancer*, Vol. 63, No. 4, (Nov 15) pp. 537-543.

Hofer, S., et al. (2006). Gefitinib accumulation in glioblastoma tissue. *Cancer Biol Ther*, Vol. 5, No. 5, (May) pp. 483-484.

Huang, H. S., et al. (1997). The enhanced tumorigenic activity of a mutant epidermal growth factor receptor common in human cancers is mediated by threshold levels of constitutive tyrosine phosphorylation and unattenuated signaling. *J Biol Chem*, Vol. 272, No. 5, (Jan 31) pp. 2927-2935.

Inda, M. M., et al. (2010). Tumor heterogeneity is an active process maintained by a mutant EGFR-induced cytokine circuit in glioblastoma. *Genes Dev*, Vol. 24, No. 16, (Aug 15) pp. 1731-1745.

Johns, T. G., et al. (2004). Identification of the epitope for the epidermal growth factor receptor-specific monoclonal antibody 806 reveals that it preferentially recognizes an untethered form of the receptor. *J Biol Chem*, Vol. 279, No. 29, (Jul 16) pp. 30375-30384.

Johns, T. G., et al. (2005). The antitumor monoclonal antibody 806 recognizes a high-mannose form of the EGF receptor that reaches the cell surface when cells over-express the receptor. *Faseb J*, Vol. 19, No. 7, (May) pp. 780-782.

Johns, T. G., et al. (2007). The efficacy of epidermal growth factor receptor-specific antibodies against glioma xenografts is influenced by receptor levels, activation status, and heterodimerization. *Clin Cancer Res*, Vol. 13, No. 6, (Mar 15) pp. 1911-1925.

Johns, T. G., et al. (2002). Novel monoclonal antibody specific for the de2-7 epidermal growth factor receptor (EGFR) that also recognizes the EGFR expressed in cells containing amplification of the EGFR gene. *Int J Cancer*, Vol. 98, No. 3, (Mar 20) pp. 398-408.

Jungbluth, A. A., et al. (2003). A monoclonal antibody recognizing human cancers with amplification/overexpression of the human epidermal growth factor receptor. *Proc Natl Acad Sci U S A*, Vol. 100, No. 2, (Jan 21) pp. 639-644.

Laurent-Puig, P., et al. (2009). Analysis of PTEN, BRAF, and EGFR status in determining benefit from cetuximab therapy in wild-type KRAS metastatic colon cancer. *J Clin Oncol*, Vol. 27, No. 35, (Dec 10) pp. 5924-5930.

Learn, C. A., et al. (2004). Resistance to tyrosine kinase inhibition by mutant epidermal growth factor receptor variant III contributes to the neoplastic phenotype of glioblastoma multiforme. *Clin Cancer Res*, Vol. 10, No. 9, (May 1) pp. 3216-3224.

Lee, J. C., et al. (2006). Epidermal Growth Factor Receptor Activation in Glioblastoma through Novel Missense Mutations in the Extracellular Domain. *PLoS Med*, Vol. 3, No. 12, (Dec 19) pp. e485.

Li, B., et al. (2004). Mutant epidermal growth factor receptor displays increased signaling through the phosphatidylinositol-3 kinase/AKT pathway and promotes radioresistance in cells of astrocytic origin. *Oncogene*, Vol. 23, No. 26, (Jun 3) pp. 4594-4602.

Li, S., et al. (2005). Structural basis for inhibition of the epidermal growth factor receptor by cetuximab. *Cancer Cell*, Vol. 7, No. 4, (Apr) pp. 301-311.

Libermann, T. A., et al. (1985). Amplification, enhanced expression and possible rearrangement of EGF receptor gene in primary human brain tumours of glial origin. *Nature*, Vol. 313, No. 5998, (Jan 10-18) pp. 144-147.

Lu, K. V., et al. (2009). Fyn and SRC are effectors of oncogenic epidermal growth factor receptor signaling in glioblastoma patients. *Cancer Res*, Vol. 69, No. 17, (Sep 1) pp. 6889-6898.

Luwor, R. B., et al. (2004). The tumor-specific de2-7 epidermal growth factor receptor (EGFR) promotes cells survival and heterodimerizes with the wild-type EGFR. *Oncogene*, Vol. 23, No. 36, (Aug 12) pp. 6095-6104.

Marshall, J. (2006). Clinical implications of the mechanism of epidermal growth factor receptor inhibitors. *Cancer*, Vol. 107, No. 6, (Sep 15) pp. 1207-1218.

McLendon, R., et al. (2008). Comprehensive genomic characterization defines human glioblastoma genes and core pathways. *Nature*, Vol., No., (Sep 4).

Mellinghoff, I. K., et al. (2005). Molecular determinants of the response of glioblastomas to EGFR kinase inhibitors. *N Engl J Med*, Vol. 353, No. 19, (Nov 10) pp. 2012-2024.

Mendelsohn, J. and J. Baselga (2006). Epidermal growth factor receptor targeting in cancer. *Semin Oncol*, Vol. 33, No. 4, (Aug) pp. 369-385.

Mizoguchi, M., et al. (2006). Activation of STAT3, MAPK, and AKT in malignant astrocytic gliomas: correlation with EGFR status, tumor grade, and survival. *J Neuropathol Exp Neurol*, Vol. 65, No. 12, (Dec) pp. 1181-1188.

Moosmann, N. and V. Heinemann (2007). Cetuximab in the treatment of metastatic colorectal cancer. *Expert Opin Biol Ther*, Vol. 7, No. 2, (Feb) pp. 243-256.

Moscatello, D. K., et al. (1998). Constitutive activation of phosphatidylinositol 3-kinase by a naturally occurring mutant epidermal growth factor receptor. *J Biol Chem*, Vol. 273, No. 1, (Jan 2) pp. 200-206.

Nakamura, J. L. (2007). The epidermal growth factor receptor in malignant gliomas: pathogenesis and therapeutic implications. *Expert Opin Ther Targets*, Vol. 11, No. 4, (Apr) pp. 463-472.

Nishikawa, R., et al. (1994). A mutant epidermal growth factor receptor common in human glioma confers enhanced tumorigenicity. *Proc Natl Acad Sci U S A*, Vol. 91, No. 16, (Aug 2) pp. 7727-7731.

Ohgaki, H. and P. Kleihues (2007). Genetic pathways to primary and secondary glioblastoma. *Am J Pathol*, Vol. 170, No. 5, (May) pp. 1445-1453.

Pedersen, M. W., et al. (2001). The type III epidermal growth factor receptor mutation. Biological significance and potential target for anti-cancer therapy. *Ann Oncol*, Vol. 12, No. 6, (Jun) pp. 745-760.

Pedersen, M. W., et al. (2005). Analysis of the epidermal growth factor receptor specific transcriptome: effect of receptor expression level and an activating mutation. *J Cell Biochem*, Vol. 96, No. 2, (Oct 1) pp. 412-427.

Peereboom, D. M., et al. (2010). Phase II trial of erlotinib with temozolomide and radiation in patients with newly diagnosed glioblastoma multiforme. *J Neurooncol*, Vol. 98, No. 1, (May) pp. 93-99.

Perera, R. M., et al. (2005). Treatment of human tumor xenografts with monoclonal antibody 806 in combination with a prototypical epidermal growth factor receptor-specific antibody generates enhanced antitumor activity. *Clin Cancer Res*, Vol. 11, No. 17, (Sep 1) pp. 6390-6399.

Pillay, V., et al. (2009). The plasticity of oncogene addiction: implications for targeted therapies directed to receptor tyrosine kinases. *Neoplasia*, Vol. 11, No. 5, (May) pp. 448-458, 442 p following 458.

Pines, G., et al. (2010). EGFRvIV: a previously uncharacterized oncogenic mutant reveals a kinase autoinhibitory mechanism. *Oncogene*, Vol. 29, No. 43, (Oct 28) pp. 5850-5860.

Prados, M. D., et al. (2009). Phase II study of erlotinib plus temozolomide during and after radiation therapy in patients with newly diagnosed glioblastoma multiforme or gliosarcoma. *J Clin Oncol*, Vol. 27, No. 4, (Feb 1) pp. 579-584.

Pratilas, C. A. and D. B. Solit (2010). Targeting the mitogen-activated protein kinase pathway: physiological feedback and drug response. *Clin Cancer Res*, Vol. 16, No. 13, (Jul 1) pp. 3329-3334.

Quang, T. S. and L. W. Brady (2004). Radioimmunotherapy as a novel treatment regimen: 125I-labeled monoclonal antibody 425 in the treatment of high-grade brain gliomas. *Int J Radiat Oncol Biol Phys*, Vol. 58, No. 3, (Mar 1) pp. 972-975.

Raizer, J. J., et al. (2010). A phase II trial of erlotinib in patients with recurrent malignant gliomas and nonprogressive glioblastoma multiforme postradiation therapy. *Neuro Oncol*, Vol. 12, No. 1, (Jan) pp. 95-103.

Rasheed, B. K., et al. (1997). PTEN gene mutations are seen in high-grade but not in low-grade gliomas. *Cancer Res*, Vol. 57, No. 19, (Oct 1) pp. 4187-4190.

Reardon, D. A., et al. (2010). Phase 2 trial of erlotinib plus sirolimus in adults with recurrent glioblastoma. *J Neurooncol*, Vol. 96, No. 2, (Jan) pp. 219-230.

Ren, H., et al. (2007). Receptor tyrosine kinases as therapeutic targets in malignant glioma. *Rev Recent Clin Trials*, Vol. 2, No. 2, (May) pp. 87-101.

Rich, J. N., et al. (2004). Phase II trial of gefitinib in recurrent glioblastoma. *J Clin Oncol*, Vol. 22, No. 1, (Jan 1) pp. 133-142.

Rivera, F., et al. (2008). Current situation of Panitumumab, Matuzumab, Nimotuzumab and Zalutumumab. *Acta Oncol*, Vol. 47, No. 1, pp. 9-19.

Sampson, J. H., et al. (2000). Unarmed, tumor-specific monoclonal antibody effectively treats brain tumors. *Proc Natl Acad Sci U S A*, Vol. 97, No. 13, (Jun 20) pp. 7503-7508.

Sarkaria, J. N., et al. (2006). Use of an orthotopic xenograft model for assessing the effect of epidermal growth factor receptor amplification on glioblastoma radiation response. *Clin Cancer Res*, Vol. 12, No. 7 Pt 1, (Apr 1) pp. 2264-2271.

Sarkaria, J. N., et al. (2007). Identification of molecular characteristics correlated with glioblastoma sensitivity to EGFR kinase inhibition through use of an intracranial xenograft test panel. *Mol Cancer Ther*, Vol. 6, No. 3, (Mar) pp. 1167-1174.

Sathornsumetee, S., et al. (2010). Phase II trial of bevacizumab and erlotinib in patients with recurrent malignant glioma. *Neuro Oncol*, Vol. 12, No. 12, (Dec) pp. 1300-1310.

Schlegel, J., et al. (1994). Amplification and differential expression of members of the erbB-gene family in human glioblastoma. *J Neurooncol*, Vol. 22, No. 3, pp. 201-207.

Schmidt, M. H., et al. (2003). Epidermal growth factor receptor signaling intensity determines intracellular protein interactions, ubiquitination, and internalization. *Proc Natl Acad Sci U S A*, Vol. 100, No. 11, (May 27) pp. 6505-6510.

Scott, A. M., et al. (2007). A phase I clinical trial with monoclonal antibody ch806 targeting transitional state and mutant epidermal growth factor receptors. *Proc Natl Acad Sci U S A*, Vol. 104, No. 10, (Mar 6) pp. 4071-4076.

Sharma, S. V., et al. (2007). Epidermal growth factor receptor mutations in lung cancer. *Nat Rev Cancer*, Vol. 7, No. 3, (Mar) pp. 169-181.

Sherry, M. M., et al. (2009). STAT3 is required for proliferation and maintenance of multipotency in glioblastoma stem cells. *Stem Cells*, Vol. 27, No. 10, (Oct) pp. 2383-2392.

Stea, B., et al. (2003). Time and dose-dependent radiosensitization of the glioblastoma multiforme U251 cells by the EGF receptor tyrosine kinase inhibitor ZD1839 ('Iressa'). *Cancer Lett*, Vol. 202, No. 1, (Dec 8) pp. 43-51.

Stommel, J. M., et al. (2007). Coactivation of receptor tyrosine kinases affects the response of tumor cells to targeted therapies. *Science*, Vol. 318, No. 5848, (Oct 12) pp. 287-290.

Sugawa, N., et al. (1990). Identical splicing of aberrant epidermal growth factor receptor transcripts from amplified rearranged genes in human glioblastomas. *Proc Natl Acad Sci U S A*, Vol. 87, No. 21, (Nov) pp. 8602-8606.

Tchirkov, A., et al. (2007). Interleukin-6 gene amplification and shortened survival in glioblastoma patients. *Br J Cancer*, Vol. 96, No. 3, (Feb 12) pp. 474-476.

Thomas, C. Y., et al. (2003). Spontaneous activation and signaling by overexpressed epidermal growth factor receptors in glioblastoma cells. *Int J Cancer*, Vol. 104, No. 1, (Mar 10) pp. 19-27.

Uhm, J. H., et al. (2011). Phase II Evaluation of Gefitinib in Patients With Newly Diagnosed Grade 4 Astrocytoma: Mayo/North Central Cancer Treatment Group Study N0074. *Int J Radiat Oncol Biol Phys*, Vol. 80, No. 2, (Jun 1) pp. 347-353.

Van den Eynde, M., et al. (2011). Epidermal growth factor receptor targeted therapies for solid tumours. *Acta Clin Belg*, Vol. 66, No. 1, (Jan-Feb) pp. 10-17.

Verhaak, R. G., et al. (2010). Integrated genomic analysis identifies clinically relevant subtypes of glioblastoma characterized by abnormalities in PDGFRA, IDH1, EGFR, and NF1. *Cancer Cell*, Vol. 17, No. 1, (Jan 19) pp. 98-110.

Watanabe, K., et al. (1996). Overexpression of the EGF receptor and p53 mutations are mutually exclusive in the evolution of primary and secondary glioblastomas. *Brain Pathol*, Vol. 6, No. 3, (Jul) pp. 217-223; discussion 223-214.

Weickhardt, A. J., et al. (2010). Strategies for overcoming inherent and acquired resistance to EGFR inhibitors by targeting downstream effectors in the RAS/PI3K pathway. *Curr Cancer Drug Targets*, Vol. 10, No. 8, (Dec) pp. 824-833.

Weihua, Z., et al. (2008). Survival of cancer cells is maintained by EGFR independent of its kinase activity. *Cancer Cell*, Vol. 13, No. 5, (May) pp. 385-393.

Weissenberger, J., et al. (2004). IL-6 is required for glioma development in a mouse model. *Oncogene*, Vol. 23, No. 19, (Apr 22) pp. 3308-3316.

Wikstrand, C. J., et al. (1995). Monoclonal antibodies against EGFRvIII are tumor specific and react with breast and lung carcinomas and malignant gliomas. *Cancer Res*, Vol. 55, No. 14, (Jul 15) pp. 3140-3148.

Wikstrand, C. J., et al. (1998). The class III variant of the epidermal growth factor receptor (EGFRvIII): characterization and utilization as an immunotherapeutic target. *J Neurovirol*, Vol. 4, No. 2, (Apr) pp. 148-158.

Wong, A. J., et al. (1987). Increased expression of the epidermal growth factor receptor gene in malignant gliomas is invariably associated with gene amplification. *Proc Natl Acad Sci U S A*, Vol. 84, No. 19, (Oct) pp. 6899-6903.

Wong, A. J., et al. (1992). Structural alterations of the epidermal growth factor receptor gene in human gliomas. *Proc Natl Acad Sci U S A*, Vol. 89, No. 7, (Apr 1) pp. 2965-2969.

Yamazaki, H., et al. (1990). A deletion mutation within the ligand binding domain is responsible for activation of epidermal growth factor receptor gene in human brain tumors. *Jpn J Cancer Res*, Vol. 81, No. 8, (Aug) pp. 773-779.

Ymer, S. I., et al. (2011). Glioma Specific Extracellular Missense Mutations in the First Cysteine Rich Region of Epidermal Growth Factor Receptor (EGFR) Initiate Ligand Independent Activation. *Cancers*, Vol. 3, No. 2, pp. 2032-2049.

3

Future Perspectives of Enhancing the Therapeutic Efficacy of Epidermal Growth Factor Receptor Inhibition in Malignant Gliomas

Georg Karpel-Massler and Marc-Eric Halatsch
University of Ulm School of Medicine, Ulm, Germany

1. Introduction

In adults, glioblastoma multiforme (GBM) represents the most common malignant brain tumor (Karpel-Massler et al., 2009). Unfortunately, even with the best available standard of care, patients with this disease still face a poor clinical outcome (Stupp et al., 2005). Based on the discovery of molecular targets that are involved in tumorigenesis and maintenance of the malignant cellular phenotype, new therapeutic strategies were developed. In about half of all glioblastomas, the epidermal growth factor receptor (HER1/EGFR) was shown to be amplified and overexpressed, rendering it an outstanding target in this disease (Libermann et al., 1985; Ekstrand et al., 1991). Thus, great interest was generated in the creation of HER1/EGFR-targeted agents. The clinically most advanced compounds that were developed to target HER1/EGFR for the treatment of GBM are small-molecule tyrosine kinase (TK) inhibitors such as erlotinib (Tarceva®, Genentech Inc., San Francisco, CA, U.S.A.). TK inhibitors reversibly bind to the intracellular catalytic TK domain of HER1/EGFR followed by the inhibition of autophosphorylation of the receptor as well as further downstream signaling involving phosphatidylinositol 3-kinase/murine thymoma viral oncogene homolog (PI3-K/AKT) and mitogen-activated protein kinase (MAPK) pathways (Arteaga, 2001; Busse et al., 2000; Scagliotti et al., 2004). Erlotinib does not only inhibit HER1/EGFR but also EGFRvIII, the most frequent mutant form of HER1/EGFR which is characterized by ligand-independent activation (Chu et al., 1997). In experimental studies, erlotinib was shown to inhibit the expression of genes encoding pro-invasive proteins and to significantly diminish EGFRvIII expression in transfected glioblastoma cells (Lal et al., 2002). Moreover, the extent of erlotinib-mediated inhibition of anchorage-independent growth of glioblastoma-derived cell lines was shown to correlate inversely with the cellular capability to induce *HER1/EGFR* mRNA (Halatsch et al., 2004). However, clinical studies examining the therapeutic efficacy of erlotinib in the setting of GBM have so far failed to prove a therapeutic benefit (Raizer et al., 2010; van den Bent et al., 2009). In a randomized, controlled phase II trial, only 11.4% of the patients with recurrent glioblastoma treated with erlotinib were free of progression after 6 months compared to 24.1% of the patients treated with temozolomide or carmustine (van den Bent et al., 2009). In addition, overall survival of the two treatment groups was found to be similar (7.7 months for the erlotinib group versus 7.3 months for the temozolomide/carmustine group).

In addition, several studies examined the therapeutic efficacy of erlotinib when combined with standard radiochemotherapy (Brown et al., 2008; Peereboom et al., 2010; Prados et al., 2009). Overall, the results of these studies appear unfavorable and discourage the use of erlotinib in combination with temozolomide and radiotherapy.

Combined inhibition of HER1/EGFR and downstream key regulators such as mammalian target of rapamycin (mTOR) and PI3-K represents another approach that has been evaluated. In an experimental study, combined treatment with erlotinib and rapamycin, an mTOR inhibitor, resulted in significantly increased anti-proliferative effects on phosphatase and tensin homolog deleted on chromosome 10 (PTEN)-deficient U87 and SF295 glioblastoma cells when compared to cells receiving erlotinib alone (Wang et al., 2006). Moreover, additional inhibition of PI3-K using a dual mTOR/PI3-K inhibitor (PI-103) was shown to result in even more pronounced antineoplastic effects when combined with erlotinib in comparison to erlotinib combined with either mTOR or PI3-K inhibition (Fan et al., 2007). In the clinical setting, in a pilot study, a 6-month progression-free survival of 25% was reported for 22 recurrent glioblastoma patients who were treated with erlotinib or gefitinib in combination with sirolimus (rapamycine, Rapamune®, Wyeth Pharmaceuticals Inc., Ayerst, PA, U.S.A.) (Doherty et al., 2006). In a phase II clinical trial, no complete or partial responses were observed in 32 patients with recurrent glioblastoma treated with erlotinib and sirolimus in combination (Reardon et al., 2010). Median progression-free survival and median overall survival were shown to be 6.9 weeks and 33.8 weeks, respectively.

The therapeutic efficacy of a combined treatment with erlotinib and bevacizumab, a humanized anti-vascular endothelial growth factor (VEGF) monoclonal antibody, on patients with recurrent high-grade glioma was recently evaluated by a phase II clinical trial (Sathornsumetee et al., 2010). For glioblastoma patients, median 6-month progression-free survival and overall survival were reported as 28% and 42 weeks, respectively. In addition, for 48% of the glioblastoma patients radiographic response was reported. However, progression-free survival and radiographic response were similar to historical data of patients treated with bevacizumab alone.

In conclusion, current data suggest that the targeted therapeutic approach against HER1/EGFR may require a synergistic drug combination strategy involving other targeted agents in addition to HER1/EGFR-targeted TK inhibitors. This chapter focuses on innovative therapeutic strategies combining HER1/EGFR-targeted TK inhibitors with novel agents aiming to enhance the antineoplastic effect exerted by erlotinib. Most of the agents discussed in this chapter have not been evaluated for the treatment of GBM yet but constitute worthy candidates for further evaluation in this setting.

2. Promising candidates for enhancing the antineoplastic activity of erlotinib

2.1 Inhibitors of Kit

Kit (CD117) is a receptor tyrosine kinase which is related to the macrophage colony-stimulating factor receptor (c-fms) and to the platelet-derived growth factor receptor (PDGFR) (Heinrich et al., 2002; Yarden et al., 1987). Its physiologic ligand is stem cell factor, also known as mast cell factor or steel factor (Nocka et al., 1990). Ligand-binding is followed by receptor dimerization, autophosphorylation and activation of downward signaling pathways such as MAPK, JAK/STAT and PI3K/AKT pathways (Duensing et al., 2004; Mol et al., 2003). Kit was found to be expressed by a variety of cell types including the interstitial cells of Cajal, mast cells, haemopoietic progenitor cells or melanocytes (Natali et al., 1992; Nocka et al., 1989; Turner et al., 1992; Ishikawa et al., 1997), and its dysregulation has been associated with the pathogenesis of various different human malignancies (Duensing & Duensing, 2010; Heinrich et al., 2002; Woodman & Davies, 2010).

In glioma, about 75% of the tumors were reported to express Kit (Cetin et al., 2005). Interestingly, amplification and expression of Kit were shown to be significantly higher in high-grade gliomas when compared to low-grade gliomas (Joensuu et al., 2005; Puputti et al., 2006). These findings suggest that Kit may be involved in the tumorigenesis and malignant transformation of gliomas.

Different mutational changes of Kit have been described, such as the D816V mutation conferring an enhanced catalytic activity and an increased affinity for adenosine triphosphate or small in-frame deletions or insertions in the inhibitory juxtamembrane region causing ligand-independent activation of the receptor (Heinrich et al., 2002). Such genetic alterations of Kit have not been reported for gliomas yet. In other human malignancies including gastrointestinal stromal tumors (GIST) or mast cell leukemia, these mutations are quite frequently encountered (Duensing & Duensing, 2010). As a consequence, Kit-targeted agents such as imatinib mesylate (Gleevec®, Novartis, East Hanover, NJ, U.S.A.), a small molecule tyrosine kinase inhibitor, were developed. Imatinib was shown to significantly increase median overall survival of patients with GIST from 19 months to more than 50 months (Blanke et al., 2008a, 2008b; Gold et al., 2007).

Imatinib was shown to inhibit the proliferation of certain glioblastoma cell lines *in vitro* (Hagerstrand et al., 2006). In another experimental study, imatinib significantly inhibited the proliferation of human U87 glioblastoma cells and significantly increased the radiosensitivity of this glioma cell line *in vitro* and *in vivo* (Oertel et al., 2006). However, in clinical phase I and II trials, imatinib was shown to exert only moderate antitumor activity (Razis et al., 2009; Wen et al., 2006). In a phase I/II study, 34 patients with glioblastoma were treated with imatinib monotherapy at a dose of 800 mg/d (Wen et al., 2006). Progression-free survival at 6 months was only 3%, no patient achieved complete response and only 6 patients reached stable disease while 2 patients showed partial response. In a different phase II study, 20 patients with glioblastoma were diagnosed by tumor biopsy and treated with 400 mg imatinib administered twice a day for a period of 7 days prior to re-biopsy or tumor resection. Molecular examination of the tumor specimens showed that treatment with imatinib did not significantly change Ki67 expression, suggesting that treatment with imatinib did not affect tumor proliferation (Razis et al., 2009).

The fact that inhibition of Kit and co-targeted tyrosine kinases such as the platelet-derived growth factor (PDGFR), alone, does not sufficiently suppress tumor growth in glioblastoma might be explained by co-activation of other growth factor receptors such as HER1/EGFR. Cellular signaling derived from activated HER1/EGFR might interfere with the inhibitory effects of imatinib on Kit and preserve the cancerous cellular phenotype. In this regard, additional inhibition of HER1/EGFR by erlotinib might prove beneficial in terms of a more pronounced therapeutic efficacy. To date, no experimental or clinical data exist with respect to a combined therapeutic approach with erlotinib and an inhibitor of Kit in this disease.

However, in the setting of recurrent glioblastoma, encouraging results were reported by a phase II study evaluating the therapeutic efficacy of a combination therapy with imatinib and hydroxyurea, a ribonucleotide reductase inhibitor (Reardon et al., 2005). Median overall survival, progression-free survival at 6 months and median progression-free survival were 48.9 weeks, 27% and 14.4 weeks, respectively. Nine percent of the patients achieved radiographic response and 42% had stable disease within a median follow-up of 58 weeks.

In conclusion, despite rather discouraging results of Kit inhibitors used as single agent therapies in clinical trials, Kit inhibitors may prove as valuable partners for the treatment of glioblastoma when combined with other agents such as erlotinib.

2.2 Histone deacetylase (HDAC) inhibitors

In humans, 18 HDACs with different tissue distributions and functions have been identified. Class I, IIa and IV HDACs are found in the brain (Marsoni et al., 2008). HDACs induce an increased packaging of chromatin and subsequent suppression of transcription (Lane & Chabner, 2009; Svechnikova et al., 2008). Modulation of the chromatin state through enzymatic histone modification may alter the transcriptional activity of genes involved in cell cycle control which is considered to be an important factor in tumorigenesis (Yoo & Jones, 2006). HDACs were shown to be overexpressed in a variety of human cancers including breast cancer, hematologic malignancies, colorectal cancer or pancreatic carcinoma (Lane & Chabner, 2009; Nakagawa et al., 2007). Moreover, inhibition of HDAC was shown to induce apoptosis by different mechanisms (Insinga et al., 2005; Nebbioso et al., 2005; Zhang et al., 2006; Zhao et al., 2005). In addition, inhibition of HDAC was shown to disrupt the function of the heat shock protein 90 which promotes the degradation of oncogenic proteins such as HER1/EGFR, AKT or BCR-ABL (Bolden et al., 2006; Kovacs et al., 2005; Whitesell & Lindquist, 2005). Thus, HDAC inhibition may constitute a promising approach in cancer therapy.

Romidepsin is a bicyclic peptide that was shown to have anti-microbial, immunosuppressive and antineoplastic activities (Ritchie et al., 2009; Ueda et al., 1994). It was shown to selectively inhibit deacetylases such as HDAC or tubulin deacetylase and represents one of the best studied HDAC inhibitors in the clinical setting (Yoo & Jones, 2006). The clinical experience with HDAC inhibitors is most advanced for the treatment of cutaneous T-cell lymphoma (CTCL) and hematologic malignancies (Lane & Chabner, 2009; Prince et al., 2009). In an early phase I trial, 10 patients with chronic lymphocytic leukemia (CLL) and 10 patients with acute myeloid leukemia (AML) were treated with romidepsin at a dose of 13 mg/m^2 on day 1, 8, and 15 of a 4-week cycle (Byrd et al., 2005). Despite absence of formal complete or partial responses, all seven CLL patients who had elevated leukocyte counts at the beginning of the therapy showed an improvement in peripheral leukocyte counts, while in the AML group one patient developed a tumor lysis syndrome. Moreover, in a phase II clinical trial, treatment with romidepsin resulted in a decrease of bone marrow blasts in 5 of 7 patients with AML (Odenike et al., 2008). However, within a month after achieving their best response towards romidepsin, these 5 patients developed disease progression. In the clinical setting of refractory CTCL, two phase II clinical trials examining the therapeutic efficacy of romidepsin were recently published (Piekarz et al., 2009; Whittaker et al., 2010). In 71 patients with treatment-refractory or advanced CTCL treated with a starting dose of 14 mg/m^2 romidepsin administered as a 4-h intravenous infusion on days 1, 8, and 15 of a 28-day cycle, an overall response rate of 34% was found (Piekarz et al., 2009). Partial response, complete response and stable disease were reported as 26%, 7% and 38%, respectively. Similar findings were reported by a different group (Whittaker et al., 2010). Overall, the safety profile of romidepsin has been favorable, and serious adverse events were shown to be rare (Byrd et al., 2005; Odenike et al., 2008; Piekarz et al., 2009; Prince et al., 2009; Whittaker et al., 2010).

There is no clinical data on romidepsin in glioblastoma and only little data on other HDAC inhibitors in this setting. However, in experimental studies, a radiosensitizing effect was observed in glioblastoma cells treated with HDAC inhibitors. The fraction of surviving SF539 and U251 glioblastoma cells that were treated with valproic acid (VA), an anticonvulsive drug known to also inhibit HDACs, and radiation was significantly lower in comparison to cells that were treated with radiation only (Camphausen et al., 2005). Moreover, in a murine heterotopic U251 xenograft model, treatment with VA and irradiation was shown to result in a significantly greater delay of tumor growth when compared to animals treated with either VA or irradiation alone. These findings were confirmed by other groups using different HDAC inhibitors (Entin-Meer et al., 2007; Lucio-Eterovic et al., 2008). In another experimental study, treatment with the HDAC inhibitor trichostatin A or 4-phenyl-butyrate was shown to induce cellular differentiation of different human glioblastoma cell lines (Svechnikova et al., 2008). In addition, both HDAC inhibitors were shown to inhibit cellular proliferation and to promote apoptosis in glioblastoma cell lines.

In the setting of glioblastoma, so far only one experimental study was published examining the effects of romidepsin. In that study, treatment with romidepsin at a concentration of 1 ng/ml was shown to significantly reduce proliferation of T98G, U251MG and U87MG glioblastoma cells (Sawa et al., 2004). In addition, U251MG cells treated with romidepsin were shown to be significantly less invasive when compared to controls. Moreover, in a heterotopic xenograft model, mice treated with romidepsin were shown to have significantly reduced tumor growth of subcutaneously inoculated EGFRvIII-bearing U87MG glioblastoma cells.

Both erlotinib and romidepsin are promising anticancer agents fitting a reasonable safety profile. However, further studies are needed to elucidate if combining the antineoplastic effects of erlotinib and HDAC inhibitors such as romidepsin may result in a significant improvement of the current clinical course of glioblastoma.

2.3 Vascular disrupting agents

Tumor angiogenesis stands for cancers' development of their own blood supply. This process was found to be crucial for the growth and metastasis of solid tumors and can be achieved by different mechanisms such as sprouting angiogenesis, recruitment of bone marrow-derived endothelial progenitor cells or the longitudinal splitting of existing blood vessels called intussusception (reviewed in Heath & Bicknell, 2009).

Different anti-angiogenic agents were developed for the treatment of human malignancies including high-grade glioma. One such agent is bevacizumab (Avastin®, Genentech Inc., San Francisco, CA, U.S.A.), a humanized monoclonal antibody targeted to VEGF. Numerous clinical studies were conducted evaluating the therapeutic efficacy of bevacizumab in glioblastoma. In a phase II study, 20 of 35 patients (57%) with recurrent glioblastoma who were treated with bevacizumab in combination with irinotecan showed at least partial response. The 6-month progression-free survival and 6-month overall survival rates were 46% and 77%, respectively (Vredenburgh et al., 2007). Similar findings were reported for patients with recurrent World Health Organization (WHO) grade III gliomas (Desjardins et al., 2008). More recently, Friedman et al. reported the results of a phase II multicenter clinical trial (BRAIN) studying a larger patient population (Friedman et al., 2009). In this study, 167 patients with recurrent glioblastoma were randomly assigned to either treatment with bevacizumab alone (n=85) or in combination with irinotecan (n=82). Median overall survival was 9.2 months and 8.7 months, respectively, 6-month progression-free survival rates were 42.6% and 50.3%, and objective response rates were 28.2% and 37.8%, respectively.

The tumor blood supply may not only be therapeutically attacked by anti-angiogenic means inhibiting the formation of new tumor-supplying blood vessels, but also by destroying already existing tumor blood vessels. The combretastatins are small molecule microtubule-depolymerising agents which cause selective disruption of the tumor-supplying vasculature. The best studied member of this group of agents is represented by CA4P (Zybrestat™, Oxigene Inc., Lund, Sweden).

The blood supply of spontaneous and ortho- and heterotopically transplanted rodent tumors as well as human xenografted tumors was shown to be significantly reduced within 10-20 min after application of CA4P, an effect lasting for up to 24 hrs in some tumors (Kanthou & Tozer, 2007; Tozer et al., 2001). However, despite the fact that a single-dose application of CA4P was shown to induce abundant tumor necrosis within a short period of time, cells in the outer rim of the tumor survived (Dark et al., 1997; Tozer et al., 2001). The cells in this niche may continue or restart to grow causing tumor recurrence. In a heterotopic rat glioma model, blood flow in subcutaneous tumors dropped to about half of the initial tumor blood flow during the first 110 min after administration of CA4P (Eikesdal et al., 2000). However, treatment with CA4P at a dose of 50 mg/kg did not significantly affect tumor growth in comparison to controls. Remarkably, when the treatment with CA4P preceded a hyperthermic treatment by 3 hrs, tumor growth was significantly more delayed when compared to animals receiving CA4P immediately before hyperthermia or animals subjected to hyperthermic treatment alone. In conclusion, if applied at the right time, treatment with CA4P may increase thermally induced antitumor activity.

To date, there are no clinical studies examining the effects of CA4P in glioblastoma. However, CA4P was shown to diminish perfusion and blood flow in different advanced solid tumors (Dowlati et al., 2002; Rustin et al., 2003; Stevenson et al., 2003). In addition, some patients were reported to have experienced a notable clinical benefit from the treatment with CA4P. Complete response was reported for a patient with anaplastic thyroid cancer. This patient was free of disease for more than 5 years. Another patient suffering from fibrosarcoma achieved partial response.

Aiming at the elimination of viable tumor cells remaining at the periphery of the tumor despite treatment with VDAs, a therapeutic approach was attempted combining VDAs with radiotherapy or conventional chemotherapy. Eight patients with advanced non-small cell lung cancer (NSCLC) were treated with radiotherapy (27 Gy) and CA4P at a dose of 50 mg/m^2 starting after the second fraction of radiotherapy (Ng et al., 2007). The tumor blood volume was shown to be reduced by 22.9% at 4 hrs after application of CA4P and by 29.4% after 72 hrs. Moreover, the decrease in blood volume was shown to be more pronounced at the outer rim of the tumor than at its center (51.4% vs 22.8%). These findings suggest that the antivascular effect exerted by CA4P can be enhanced by radiotherapy in the setting of NSCLC. In another study, CA4P was applied for the treatment of patients with different advanced cancers refractory to standard therapy 18-22 hrs prior to a single-agent treatment with paclitaxel or carboplatin or combination therapy with paclitaxel and carboplatin in sequential order (Rustin et al., 2010). A formal response was noted in 7 of 18 patients with ovarian cancer, primary peritoneal carcinoma, or cancer of the fallopian tube. Partial remission was achieved in another 3 out of 30 patients with non-ovarian cancer. Thus, this combinatorial regimen displays antitumor activity in patients with difficult-to-treat cancers.

Overall, VDAs are promising anticancer agents and might provide an additional benefit when combined with other antineoplastic drugs. Other therapeutics administered in addition to VDAs might be trapped in the tumor tissue due to the shut-down of tumor blood flow. Thereby, tumor cells might not only die secondary to ischemia, but surviving cells in the outer rim of the tumor may also be eliminated. This way, tumor regrowth might be retarded or prevented. At this point, there is no data on the therapeutic efficacy of a combined treatment with erlotinib and VDAs for the treatment of glioblastoma. Further studies are warranted to examine the overall antineoplastic effect of a combined treatment with erlotinib and a VDA in glioblastoma.

3. Conclusion

Unfortunately, in glioblastoma, HER1/EGFR-targeted small-molecule TK inhibitors such as erlotinib did not fulfill the enthusiastic expectations derived from the promising results obtained by preclinical studies (Brown et al., 2008; van den Bent et al., 2009). Thus, the fate of patients diagnosed with glioblastoma remains dismal despite employing the currently best standard of care. New therapeutic strategies are undoubtedly needed to overcome this frustrating situation.

One such new therapeutic approach which aims at enhancing the therapeutic efficacy against glioblastoma involves the combination of erlotinib with other targeted agents in order to inhibit key regulators that are located further downstream of the signaling cascade or with agents inhibiting other signaling pathways. Several clinical studies are ongoing to evaluate this therapeutic option. In patients with recurrent glioblastoma or gliosarcoma, a phase I/II clinical trial currently evaluates the therapeutic effects of a combined treatment with erlotinib, sorafenib (BAY 54-9085, Bayer HealthCare Pharmaceuticals, Montville, NJ, U.S.A.), an inhibitor of murine leukemia viral oncogene homolog (RAF)/mitogen-activated protein kinase kinase (MEK)/extracellular signal-regulated kinase (ERK) and VEGFR-2/PDGFR-β signaling pathways, and temsirolimus (CCI-779, Wyeth Pharmaceuticals, Madison, NJ, U.S.A.), an inhibitor of mTOR. The results are awaited. A different clinical trial investigated the effects of dual therapy with erlotinib and sorafenib in patients with progressive or recurrent glioblastoma. This study has been completed, and the results are pending.

In this chapter, we emphasize the need for a continous search for new agents replenishing our armory for the fight against glioblastoma. Some of the novel agents presented herein may allow to enhance overall antitumor activity when applied together with other compounds such as erlotinib. In addition, several candidate erlotinib resistance genes have been proposed from genetic analysis of glioblastoma cell lines (Halatsch et al., 2009) and further validation is under way.

4. References

Arteaga, C. (2001). The epidermal growth factor receptor: from mutant oncogene in nonhuman cancers to therapeutic target in human neoplasia. *J Clin Oncol*, 19, pp. 32S-40S.

Blanke, C.D., Demetri, G.D., von Mehren, M., Heinrich, M.C., Eisenberg, B., Fletcher, J.A., Corless, C.L., Fletcher, C.D., Roberts, P.J., Heinz, D., Wehre, E., Nikolova, Z. & Joensuu, H. (2008a). Long-term results from a randomized phase II trial of standard- versus higher-dose imatinib mesylate for patients with unresectable or metastatic gastrointestinal stromal tumors expressing KIT. *J Clin Oncol*, 26, pp. 620-5.

Blanke, C.D., Rankin, C., Demetri, G.D., Ryan, C.W., von Mehren, M., Benjamin, R.S., Raymond, A.K., Bramwell, V.H., Baker, L.H., Maki, R.G., Tanaka, M., Hecht, J.R., Heinrich, M.C., Fletcher, C.D., Crowley, J.J. & Borden, E.C. (2008b). Phase III randomized, intergroup trial assessing imatinib mesylate at two dose levels in patients with unresectable or metastatic gastrointestinal stromal tumors expressing the kit receptor tyrosine kinase: S0033. *J Clin Oncol*, 26, pp. 626-32.

Bolden, J.E., Peart, M.J. & Johnstone, R.W. (2006). Anticancer activities of histone deacetylase inhibitors. *Nat Rev Drug Discov*, 5, pp. 769-84.

Brown, P., Krishnan, S., Sarkaria, J., Wu, W., Jaeckle, K., Uhm, J., Geoffroy, F., Arusell, R., Kitange, G., Jenkins, R., Kugler, J., Morton, R., Rowland, K., Mischel, P., Yong, W., Scheithauer, B., Schiff, D., Giannini, C. & Buckner, J. (2008). Phase I/II trial of erlotinib and temozolomide with radiation therapy in the treatment of newly diagnosed glioblastoma multiforme: north central cancer treatment group study N0177. *J Clin Oncol*, 26, pp. 5603-5609.

Busse, D., Doughty, R., Ramsey, T., Russell, W., Price, J., Flanagan, W., Shawver, L. & Arteaga, C. (2000). Reversible G_1 arrest induced by inhibition of the epidermal growth factor receptor tyrosine kinase requires up-regulation of $p27^{KIP1}$ independent of MAPK activity. *J Biol Chem*, 275, pp. 6987-6995.

Byrd, J., Marcucci, G., Parthun, M., Xiao, J., Klisovic, R., Moran, M., Lin, T., Liu, S., Sklenar, A., Davis, M., Lucas, D., Fischer, B., Shank, R., Tejaswi, S., Binkley, P., Wright, J., Chan, K. & Grever, M. (2005). A phase 1 and pharmacodynamic study of depsipeptide (FK228) in chronic lymphocytic leukemia and acute myeloid leukemia. *Blood*, 105, pp. 959-967.

Camphausen, K., Cerna, D., Scott, T., Sproull, M., Burgan, W., Cerra, M., Fine, H. & Tofilon, P. (2005). Enhancement of *in vitro* and *in vivo* tumor cell radiosensitivity by valproic acid. *Int J Cancer*, 114, pp. 380-386.

Cetin, N., Dienel, G. & Gokden, M. (2005). CD117 expression in glial tumors. *J Neurooncol*, 75, pp. 195-202.

Chu, C., Everiss, K., Wikstrand, C., Batra, S., Kung, H. & Bigner, D. (1997). Receptor dimerization is not a factor in the signaling activity of a transforming variant epidermal growth factor receptor (EGFRvIII). *Biochem J*, 324, pp. 855-861.

Dark, G.G., Hill, S.A., Prise, V.E., Tozer, G.M., Pettit, G.R. & Chaplin, D.J. (1997). Combretastatin A-4, an agent that displays potent and selective toxicity toward tumor vasculature. *Cancer Res*, 57, pp. 1829-34.

Desjardins, A., Reardon, D.A., Herndon, J.E., 2nd, Marcello, J., Quinn, J.A., Rich, J.N., Sathornsumetee, S., Gururangan, S., Sampson, J., Bailey, L., Bigner, D.D., Friedman, A.H., Friedman, H.S. & Vredenburgh, J.J. (2008). Bevacizumab plus irinotecan in recurrent WHO grade 3 malignant gliomas. *Clin Cancer Res*, 14, pp. 7068-73.

Doherty, L., Gigas, D., Kesari, S., Drappatz, J., Kim, R., Zimmermann, J., Ostrowsky, L. & Wen, P. (2006). Pilot study of the combination of EGFR and mTOR inhibitors in recurrent malignant gliomas. *Neurology*, 67, pp. 156-158.

Dowlati, A., Robertson, K., Cooney, M., Petros, W.P., Stratford, M., Jesberger, J., Rafie, N., Overmoyer, B., Makkar, V., Stambler, B., Taylor, A., Waas, J., Lewin, J.S., McCrae, K.R. & Remick, S.C. (2002). A phase I pharmacokinetic and translational study of the novel vascular targeting agent combretastatin a-4 phosphate on a single-dose intravenous schedule in patients with advanced cancer. *Cancer Res*, 62, pp. 3408-16.

Duensing, A., Medeiros, F., McConarty, B., Joseph, N.E., Panigrahy, D., Singer, S., Fletcher, C.D., Demetri, G.D. & Fletcher, J.A. (2004). Mechanisms of oncogenic KIT signal transduction in primary gastrointestinal stromal tumors (GISTs). *Oncogene*, 23, pp. 3999-4006.

Duensing, S. & Duensing, A. (2010). Targeted therapies of gastrointestinal stromal tumors (GIST) - the next frontiers. *Biochem Pharmacol*, 80, pp. 575-83.

Eikesdal, H.P., Schem, B.C., Mella, O. & Dahl, O. (2000). The new tubulin-inhibitor combretastatin A-4 enhances thermal damage in the BT4An rat glioma. *Int J Radiat Oncol Biol Phys*, 46, pp. 645-52.

Ekstrand, A., James, C., Cavenee, W., Seliger, B., Pettersson, R. & Collins, V. (1991). Genes for epidermal growth factor receptor, transforming growth factor alpha and epidermal growth factor and their expression in human gliomas in vivo. *Cancer Res*, 51, pp. 2164-2172.

Entin-Meer, M., Yang, X., Van den Berg, S., Lamborn, K., Nudelman, A., Rephaeli, A. & Haas-Kogan, D. (2007). *In vivo* efficacy of a novel histone deacetylase inhibitor in combination with radiation for the treatment of gliomas. *Neurooncol*, 9, pp. 82-88.

Fan, Q.-W., Cheng, C., Nicolaides, T., Hackett, C., Knight, Z., Shokat, K. & Weiss, W. (2007). A dual phosphoinositide-3-kinase alpha/mTOR inhibitor cooperates with blockade of epidermal growth factor receptor in PTEN-mutant glioma. *Cancer Res*, 67, pp. 7960-7965.

Friedman, H., Prados, M., Wen, P., Mikkelsen, T., Schiff, D., Abrey, L., Yung, W., Paleologos, N., Nicholas, M., Jensen, R., Vredenburgh, J., Huang, J., Zheng, M. & Cloughesy, T. (2009). Bevacizumab alone and in combination with irinotecan in recurrent glioblastoma. *J Clin Oncol*, 27, pp. 4733-4740.

Gold, J.S., van der Zwan, S.M., Gonen, M., Maki, R.G., Singer, S., Brennan, M.F., Antonescu, C.R. & De Matteo, R.P. (2007). Outcome of metastatic GIST in the era before tyrosine kinase inhibitors. *Ann Surg Oncol*, 14, pp. 134-42.

Hagerstrand, D., Hesselager, G. & Achterberg, S. (2006). Characterization of an imatinib-sensitive subset of high-grade human glioma cultures. *Oncogene*, 25, pp. 4913-4922.

Halatsch, M.-E., Gehrke, E., Vougioukas, V., Bötefür, I., Efferth, T., Gebhardt, E., Domhof, S., Schmidt, U. & Buchfelder, M. (2004). Inverse correlation of *epidermal growth factor receptor* messenger RNA induction and suppression of anchorage-independent growth by OSI-774, an epidermal growth factor receptor tyrosine kinase inhibitor, in glioblastoma multiforme cell lines. *J Neurosurg*, 100, pp. 523-533.

Halatsch, M.-E., Löw, S., Mursch, K., Hielscher, T., Schmidt, U., Unterberg, A., Vougioukas, V. & Feuerhake, F. (2009). Candidate genes for sensitivity and resistance of human glioblastoma multiforme cell lines to erlotinib. *J Neurosurg*, 111, pp. 211-218.

Heath, V.L. & Bicknell, R. (2009). Anticancer strategies involving the vasculature. *Nat Rev Clin Oncol*, 6, 395-404.

Heinrich, M.C., Blanke, C.D., Druker, B.J. & Corless, C.L. (2002). Inhibition of KIT tyrosine kinase activity: a novel molecular approach to the treatment of KIT-positive malignancies. *J Clin Oncol*, 20, pp. 1692-703.

Insinga, A., Monestiroli, S., Ronzoni, S., Gelmetti, V., Marchesi, F., Viale, A., Altucci, L., Nervi, C., Minucci, S. & Pelicci, P.G. (2005). Inhibitors of histone deacetylases induce tumor-selective apoptosis through activation of the death receptor pathway. *Nat Med*, 11, pp. 71-6.

Ishikawa, K., Komuro, T., Hirota, S. & Kitamura, Y. (1997). Ultrastructural identification of the c-kit-expressing interstitial cells in the rat stomach: a comparison of control and Ws/Ws mutant rats. *Cell Tissue Res*, 289, pp. 137-43.

Joensuu, H., Puputti, M., Sihto, H., Tynninen, O. & Nupponen, N.N. (2005). Amplification of genes encoding KIT, PDGFRalpha and VEGFR2 receptor tyrosine kinases is frequent in glioblastoma multiforme. *J Pathol*, 207, pp. 224-31.

Kanthou, C. & Tozer, G.M. (2007). Tumour targeting by microtubule-depolymerizing vascular disrupting agents. *Expert Opin Ther Targets*, 11, pp. 1443-57.

Karpel-Massler, G., Schmidt, U., Unterberg, A. & Halatsch, M. (2009). Therapeutic inhibition of the epidermal growth factor receptor in high-grade gliomas - where do we stand? *Mol Cancer Res*, 7, pp. 1000-1012.

Kovacs, J.J., Murphy, P.J., Gaillard, S., Zhao, X., Wu, J.T., Nicchitta, C.V., Yoshida, M., Toft, D.O., Pratt, W.B. & Yao, T.P. (2005). HDAC6 regulates Hsp90 acetylation and chaperone-dependent activation of glucocorticoid receptor. *Mol Cell*, 18, pp. 601-7.

Lal, A., Glazer, C., Martinson, H., Friedman, H., Archer, G., Sampson, J. & Riggins, G. (2002). Mutant epidermal growth factor receptor up-regulates molecular effectors of tumor invasion. *Cancer Res*, 62, pp. 3335-3339.

Lane, A.A. & Chabner, B.A. (2009). Histone deacetylase inhibitors in cancer therapy. *J Clin Oncol*, 27, pp. 5459-68.

Libermann, T., Nusbaum, H., Razon, N., Kris, R., Lax, I., Soreq, H., Whittle, N., Waterfield, M., Ullrich, A. & Schlessinger, J. (1985). Amplification, enhanced expression and possible rearrangement of EGF receptor gene in primary human brain tumours of glial origin. *Nature*, 313, pp. 144-147.

Lucio-Eterovic, A.K., Cortez, M.A., Valera, E.T., Motta, F.J., Queiroz, R.G., Machado, H.R., Carlotti, C.G., Jr., Neder, L., Scrideli, C.A. & Tone, L.G. (2008). Differential expression of 12 histone deacetylase (HDAC) genes in astrocytomas and normal brain tissue: class II and IV are hypoexpressed in glioblastomas. *BMC Cancer*, 8, 243.

Marsoni, S., Damia, G. & Camboni, G. (2008). A work in progress: the clinical development of histone deacetylase inhibitors. *Epigenetics*, 3, pp. 164-71.

Mol, C.D., Lim, K.B., Sridhar, V., Zou, H., Chien, E.Y., Sang, B.C., Nowakowski, J., Kassel, D.B., Cronin, C.N. & McRee, D.E. (2003). Structure of a c-kit product complex reveals the basis for kinase transactivation. *J Biol Chem*, 278, pp. 31461-4.

Nakagawa, M., Oda, Y., Eguchi, T., Aishima, S., Yao, T., Hosoi, F., Basaki, Y., Ono, M., Kuwano, M., Tanaka, M. & Tsuneyoshi, M. (2007). Expression profile of class I histone deacetylases in human cancer tissues. *Oncol Rep*, 18, pp. 769-74.

Natali, P.G., Nicotra, M.R., Sures, I., Santoro, E., Bigotti, A. & Ullrich, A. (1992). Expression of c-kit receptor in normal and transformed human nonlymphoid tissues. *Cancer Res*, 52, pp. 6139-43.

Nebbioso, A., Clarke, N., Voltz, E., Germain, E., Ambrosino, C., Bontempo, P., Alvarez, R., Schiavone, E.M., Ferrara, F., Bresciani, F., Weisz, A., de Lera, A.R., Gronemeyer, H. & Altucci, L. (2005). Tumor-selective action of HDAC inhibitors involves TRAIL induction in acute myeloid leukemia cells. *Nat Med*, 11, pp. 77-84.

Ng, Q.-S., Goh, V., Carnell, D., Meer, K., Padhani, A., Saunders, M. & Hoskins, P. (2007). Tumor antivascular effects of radiotherapy combined with combretastatin A4 phosphate in human non-small-cell lung cancer. *Int J Radiat Oncol Biol Phys*, 67, pp. 1375-1380.

Nocka, K., Buck, J., Levi, E. & Besmer, P. (1990). Candidate ligand for the c-kit transmembrane kinase receptor: KL, a fibroblast derived growth factor stimulates mast cells and erythroid progenitors. *EMBO J*, 9, pp. 3287-94.

Nocka, K., Majumder, S., Chabot, B., Ray, P., Cervone, M., Bernstein, A. & Besmer, P. (1989). Expression of c-kit gene products in known cellular targets of W mutations in normal and W mutant mice - evidence for an impaired c-kit kinase in mutant mice. *Genes Dev*, 3, pp. 816-26.

Odenike, O., Alkan, S., Sher, D., Godwin, J., Huo, D., Brandt, S., Green, M., Xie, J., Zhang, Y., Vesole, D., Stiff, P., Wright, J., Larson, R. & Stock, W. (2008). Histone deacetylase inhibitor romidepsin has differential activity in core binding factor acute myeloid leukemia. *Clin Cancer Res*, 14, pp. 7095-7101.

Oertel, S., Krempien, R., Lindel, K., Zabel, A., Milker-Zabel, S., Bischof, M., Lipson, K., Peschke, P., Debus, J., Abdollahi, A. & Huber, P. (2006). Human glioblastoma and carcinoma xenograft tumors treated by combined radiation and imatinib (Gleevec®). *Strahlenther Onkol*, 7, pp. 400-407.

Peereboom, D., Shepard, D., Ahluwalia, M., Brewer, C., Agarwal, N., Stevens, G., Suh, J., Toms, S., Vogelbaum, M., Weil, R., Elson, P. & Barnett, G. (2010). Phase II trial of erlotinib with temozolomide and radiation in patients with newly diagnosed glioblastoma multiforme. J Neurooncol, 98, pp. 93-99.

Piekarz, R., Frye, R., Turner, M., Wright, J., Allen, S., Kirschbaum, M., Zain, J., Prince, H., Leonard, J., Geskin, L., Reeder, C., Joske, D., Figg, W., Gardner, E., Steinberg, S., Jaffe, E., Stetler-Stevenson, M., Lade, S., Fojo, A. & SE, B. (2009). Phase II multi-institutional trial of the histone deacetylase inhibitor romidepsin as monotherapy for patients with cutaneous T-cell lymphoma. *J Clin Oncol*, 27, pp. 5410-5417.

Prados, M., Chang, S., Butowski, N., DeBoer, R., Parvataneni, R., Carliner, H., Kabuubi, P., Ayers-Ringler, J., Rabbitt, J., Page, M., Fedoroff, A., Sneed, P., Berger, M., McDermott, M., Parsa, A., Vandenberg, S., James, C., Lamborn, K., Stokoe, D. & Haas-Kogan, D. (2009). Phase II study of erlotinib plus temozolomide during and after radiation therapy in patients with newly diagnosed glioblastoma multiforme or gliosarcoma. *J Clin Oncol*, 27, pp. 579-584.

Prince, H.M., Bishton, M.J. & Harrison, S.J. (2009). Clinical studies of histone deacetylase inhibitors. *Clin Cancer Res*, 15, pp. 3958-69.

Puputti, M., Tynninen, O., Sihto, H., Blom, T., Maenpaa, H., Isola, J., Paetau, A., Joensuu, H. & Nupponen, N.N. (2006). Amplification of KIT, PDGFRA, VEGFR2, and EGFR in gliomas. *Mol Cancer Res*, 4, pp. 927-34.

Raizer, J., Abrey, L., Lassman, A., Chang, S., Lamborn, K., Kuhn, J., Yung, W., Gilbert, M., Aldape, K., Wen, P., Fine, H., Mehta, M., DeAngelis, L., Lieberman, F., Cloughesy, T., Robins, H., Dancey, J. & Prados, M. (2010). A phase II trial of erlotinib in patients with recurrent malignant gliomas and nonprogressive glioblastoma multiforme postradiation therapy. *Neurooncol*, 12, pp. 95-103.

Razis, E., Selviaridis, P., Labropoulos, S., Norris, J.L., Zhu, M.J., Song, D.D., Kalebic, T., Torrens, M., Kalogera-Fountzila, A., Karkavelas, G., Karanastasi, S., Fletcher, J.A. & Fountzilas, G. (2009). Phase II study of neoadjuvant imatinib in glioblastoma: evaluation of clinical and molecular effects of the treatment. *Clin Cancer Res*, 15, pp. 6258-66.

Reardon, D., Desjardins, A., Vredenburgh, J., Gururangan, S., Friedman, A., Herndon II, J., Marcello, J., Norfleet, J., McLendon, R., Sampson, J. & Friedman, H. (2010). Phase II trial of erlotinib plus sirolimus in adults with recurrent glioblastoma. *J Neurooncol*, 96, pp. 219-230.

Reardon, D., Egorin, M., Quinn, J., Rich Sr, J., Gururangan, I., Vredenburgh, J., Desjardins, A., Sathornsumetee, S., Provenzale, J., Herndon II, J., Dowell, J., Badruddoja, M., McLendon, R., Lagattuta, T., Kicielinski, K., Dresemann, G., Sampson, J., Friedman, A., Salvado, A. & Friedman, H. (2005). Phase II study of imatinib mesylate plus hydroxyurea in adults with recurrent glioblastoma multiforme. *J Clin Oncol*, 23, pp. 9359-9368.

Ritchie, D., Piekarz, R.L., Blombery, P., Karai, L.J., Pittaluga, S., Jaffe, E.S., Raffeld, M., Janik, J.E., Prince, H.M. & Bates, S.E. (2009). Reactivation of DNA viruses in association with histone deacetylase inhibitor therapy: a case series report. *Haematologica*, 94, pp. 1618-22.

Rustin, G.J., Galbraith, S.M., Anderson, H., Stratford, M., Folkes, L.K., Sena, L., Gumbrell, L. & Price, P.M. (2003). Phase I clinical trial of weekly combretastatin A4 phosphate: clinical and pharmacokinetic results. *J Clin Oncol*, 21, pp. 2815-22.

Rustin, G.J., Shreeves, G., Nathan, P.D., Gaya, A., Ganesan, T.S., Wang, D., Boxall, J., Poupard, L., Chaplin, D.J., Stratford, M.R., Balkissoon, J. & Zweifel, M. A (2010). Phase Ib trial of CA4P (combretastatin A-4 phosphate), carboplatin, and paclitaxel in patients with advanced cancer. *Br J Cancer*, 102, pp. 1355-60.

Sathornsumetee, S., Desjardins, A., Vredenburgh, J., McLendon, R., Marcello, J., Herndon II, J., Mathe, A., Hamilton, M., Rich Sr, J., Norfleet, J., Gururangan, S., Friedman, H. & Reardon, D. (2010). Phase II trial of bevacizumab and erlotinib in patients with recurrent malignant glioma. *Neurooncol*, 12, pp. 1300-1310.

Sawa, H., Murakami, H., Kumagai, M., Nakasato, M., Yamauchi, S., Matsuyama, N., Tamura, Y., Satone, A., Ide, W., Hashimoto, I. & Kamada, H. (2004). Histone deacetylase inhibitor, FK228, induces apoptosis and suppresses cell proliferation of human glioblastoma cells in vitro and in vivo. *Acta Neuropathol*, 107, pp. 523-31.

Scagliotti, G., Selvaggi, G., Novello, S. & Hirsch, F. (2004). The biology of epidermal growth factor receptor in lung cancer. *Clin Cancer Res*, 10, pp. 4227s-4232s.

Stevenson, J.P., Rosen, M., Sun, W., Gallagher, M., Haller, D.G., Vaughn, D., Giantonio, B., Zimmer, R., Petros, W.P., Stratford, M., Chaplin, D., Young, S.L., Schnall, M. & O'Dwyer, P.J. (2003). Phase I trial of the antivascular agent combretastatin A4 phosphate on a 5-day schedule to patients with cancer: magnetic resonance imaging evidence for altered tumor blood flow. *J Clin Oncol*, 21, pp. 4428-38.

Stupp, R., Mason, W., van den Bent, M., Weller, M., Fisher, B., Taphoom, M., Belanger, K., Brandes, A., Marosi, C., Bogdahn, U., Curschmann, J., Janzer, R., Ludwin, S., Gorlia, T., Allgeier, A., Lacombe, D., Cairncross, J., Eisenhauer, E. & Mirimanoff, R. (2005). Radiotherapy plus concomitant and adjuvant temozolomide for glioblastoma. *N Engl J Med*, 352, pp. 987-996.

Svechnikova, I., Almqvist, P.M. & Ekstrom, T.J. (2008). HDAC inhibitors effectively induce cell type-specific differentiation in human glioblastoma cell lines of different origin. *Int J Oncol*, 32, pp. 821-7.

Tozer, G.M., Prise, V.E., Wilson, J., Cemazar, M., Shan, S., Dewhirst, M.W., Barber, P.R., Vojnovic, B. & Chaplin, D.J. (2001). Mechanisms associated with tumor vascular shut-down induced by combretastatin A-4 phosphate: intravital microscopy and measurement of vascular permeability. *Cancer Res*, 61, pp. 6413-22.

Turner, A.M., Zsebo, K.M., Martin, F., Jacobsen, F.W., Bennett, L.G. & Broudy, V.C. (1992). Nonhematopoietic tumor cell lines express stem cell factor and display c-kit receptors. *Blood*, 80, pp. 374-81.

Ueda, H., Nakajima, H., Hori, Y., Fujita, T., Nishimura, M., Goto, T. & Okuhara, M. (1994). FR901228, a novel antitumor bicyclic depsipeptide produced by Chromobacterium violaceum No. 968. I. Taxonomy, fermentation, isolation, physico-chemical and biological properties, and antitumor activity. *J Antibiot (Tokyo)*, 47, pp. 301-10.

van den Bent, M., Brandes, A., Rampling, R., Kouwenhoven, M., Kros, J., Carpentier, A., Clement, P., Frenay, M., Campone, M., Baurain, J., Armand, J., Taphoorn, M., Tosoni, A., Kletzl, H., Klughammer, B., Lacombe, D. & Gorlia, T. (2009). Randomized phase II trial of erlotinib versus temozolomide or carmustine in recurrent glioblastoma: EORTC brain tumor group study 26034. *J Clin Oncol*, 27, pp. 1268-1274.

Vredenburgh, J.J., Desjardins, A., Herndon, J.E., 2nd, Marcello, J., Reardon, D.A., Quinn, J.A., Rich, J.N., Sathornsumetee, S., Gururangan, S., Sampson, J., Wagner, M., Bailey, L., Bigner, D.D., Friedman, A.H. & Friedman, H.S. (2007). Bevacizumab plus irinotecan in recurrent glioblastoma multiforme. *J Clin Oncol*, 25, pp. 4722-9.

Wang, M., Lu, K., Zhu, S., Dia, E., Vivanco, I., Shackleford, G., Cavenee, W., Mellinghoff, I., Cloughesy, T., Sawyers, C. & Mischel, P. (2006). Mammalian target of rapamycin inhibition promotes response to epidermal growth factor receptor kinase inhibitors in PTEN-deficient and PTEN-intact glioblastoma cells. *Cancer Res*, 66, pp. 7864-7869.

Wen, P., Yung, W., Lamborn, K., Dahia, P., Wang, Y., Peng, B., Abrey, L., Raizer, J., Cloughesy, T., Fink, K., Gilbert, M., Chang, S., Junck, L., Schiff, D., Lieberman, F., Fine, H., Mehta, M., Robins, H., DeAngelis, L., Groves, M., Puduvalli, V., Levin, V., Conrad, C., Maher, E., Aldape, K., Hayes, M., Letvak, L., Egorin, M., Capdeville, R., Kaplan, R., Murgo, A., Stiles, C. & Prados, M. (2006). Phase I/II study of imatinib mesylate for recurrent malignant gliomas: north american brain tumor consortium study 99-08. *Clin Cancer Res*, 12, pp. 4899-4907.

Whitesell, L. & Lindquist, S.L. (2005). Hsp90 and the chaperoning of cancer. *Nat Rev Cancer*, 5, pp. 761-72.

Whittaker, S., Demierre, M.-F., Kim, E., Rook, A., Lerner, A., Duvic, M., Scarisbrick, J., Reddy, S., Robak, T., Becker, J., Samtsov, A., McCulloch, W. & Kim, Y. (2010). Final results from a multicenter, international, pivotal study of romidepsin in refractory cutaneous T-cell lymphoma. *J Clin Oncol*, 28, pp. 4485-4491.

Woodman, S.E. & Davies, M.A. (2010) Targeting KIT in melanoma: a paradigm of molecular medicine and targeted therapeutics. *Biochem Pharmacol*, 80, pp. 568-74.

Yarden, Y., Kuang, W.-J., Yang-Feng, T., Coussens, L., Munemitsu, S., Dull, T., Chen, E., Schlessinger, J., Francke, U. & Ullrich, A. (1987). Human proto-oncogene c-kit: a new cell surface receptor tyrosine kinase for an unidentified ligand. *EMBO J*, 11, pp. 3341-3351.

Yoo, C.B. & Jones, P.A. (2006). Epigenetic therapy of cancer: past, present and future. *Nat Rev Drug Discov*, 5, pp. 37-50.

Zhang, Y., Adachi, M., Kawamura, R. & Imai, K. (2006). Bmf is a possible mediator in histone deacetylase inhibitors FK228 and CBHA-induced apoptosis. *Cell Death Differ*, 13, pp. 129-40.

Zhao, Y., Tan, J., Zhuang, L., Jiang, X., Liu, E.T. & Yu, Q. (2005). Inhibitors of histone deacetylases target the Rb-E2F1 pathway for apoptosis induction through activation of proapoptotic protein Bim. *Proc Natl Acad Sci U S A*, 102, pp. 16090-5.

Part 3

MicroRNAs in Treatment of Glioma

MicroRNA and Glial Tumors: Tiny Relation with Great Potential

Jiri Sana, Marian Hajduch and Ondrej Slaby*
Masaryk Memorial Cancer Institute, Brno,
Central European Institute of Technology, Brno,
Institute of Molecular and Translational Medicine, Olomouc,
Czech Republic

1. Introduction

MicroRNAs (miRNAs) are endogenously expressed small non-coding RNAs that act as post-transcriptional regulators of gene expression. Dysregulation of these molecules has been observed in many types of cancers. Altered expression levels of several miRNAs were identified also in gliomas. It was many times showed that miRNAs are involved in core signaling pathways, which play roles in crucial cellular processes, such as proliferation, apoptosis, cell cycle regulation, invasion, angiogenesis and stem cell behaviour. Therefore, miRNAs have a great potential for oncodiagnostic as well as could be promising therapeutic targets in gliomas.

2. MicroRNA: Function and biogenesis

MicroRNAs (miRNAs) comprise a numerous class of endogenous small non-coding RNAs, 18 – 25 nucleotides in length, which function as post-transcriptional regulators of gene expression. The regulation proceeds through binding of miRNAs to their mRNA targets (Bartel, 2004). Currently, the miRBase annotates over 800 verified miRNA sequences in the human genome and the number is still expanding (Griffiths-Jones et al., 2008). Bioinformatics and cloning studies have estimated that miRNAs may regulated more than 50% of all human genes and each miRNA can control hundreds of gene targets. This is possible among others due to the fact that the binding of miRNA to the mRNA doesn't require perfect complementarity. MiRNAs are highly conserved in sequence between distantly related organisms, indicating their participation in essential biological processes. It is well known today that miRNAs are involved in many signaling pathways playing crucial roles in such cellular processes as differentiation, proliferation, and apoptosis that affect biological processes including development and cancerogenesis (Alvarez-Garcia & Miska, 2005; Carthew & Sontheimer, 2009; Croce, 2009; Hatfield & Ruohola-Baker, 2008; Winter & Diederichs, 2011; Lakomy, 2011). A large fraction of miRNAs exhibits strict developmental stage-specific and tissue-specific expression patterns. Moreover, the levels of many miRNAs

* Corresponding Author

are altered in various disseses including many types of cancers (Krol et al., 2010; Siomi & Siomi, 2010; Winter et al., 2009).

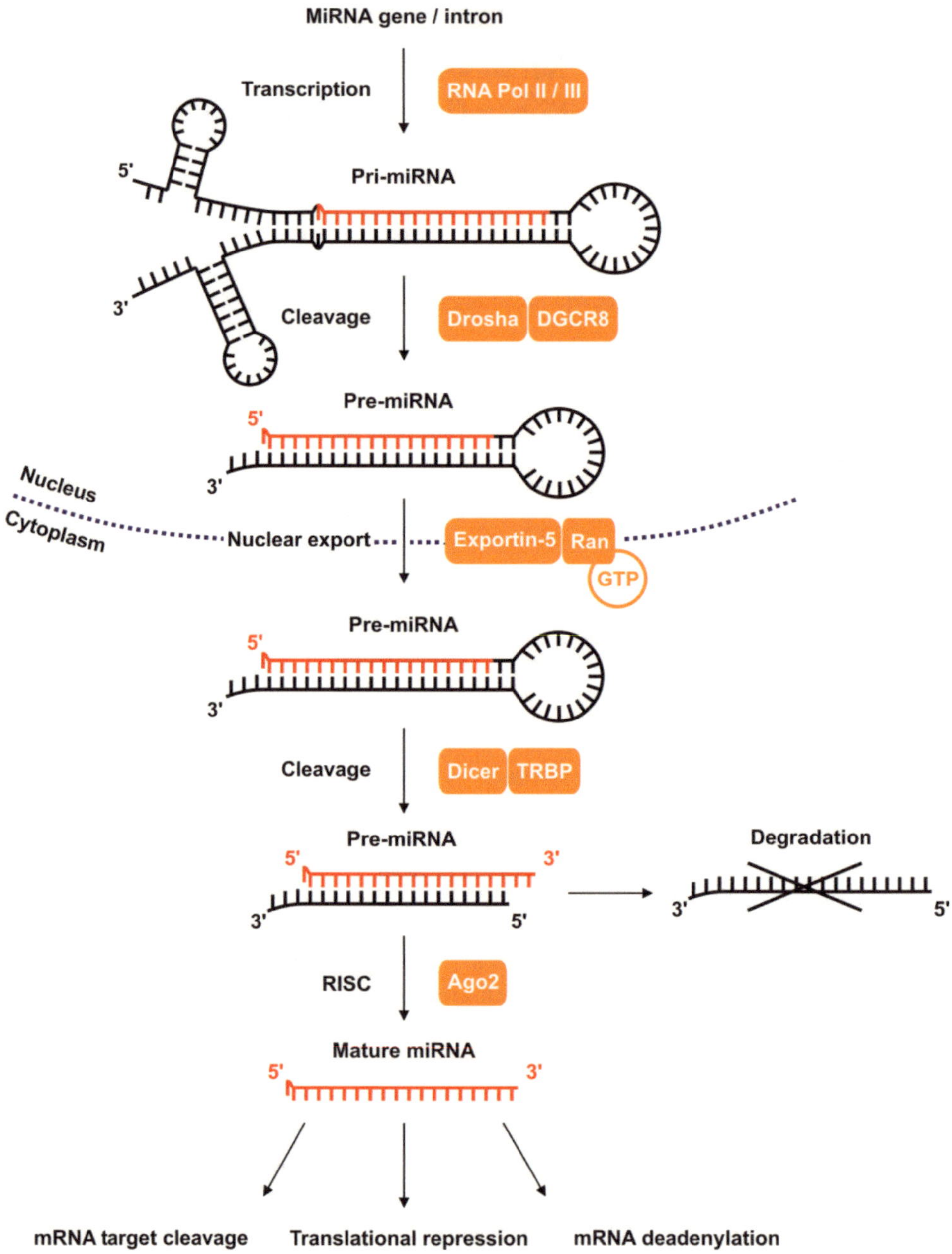

Fig. 1. Linear "canonical" pathway of miRNA processing

Most miRNA genes have own promoters and are transcribed as autonomous transcription units (Carthew & Sontheimer, 2009). Primary transcripts (pri-miRNAs) are generated by RNA polymerase II. These are processed to short 70-nucleotide stem-loop structures known as pre-miRNAs by the ribonuclease called Drosha and the double-stranded-RNA-binding protein known as Pasha. The pre-miRNAs are transported to the cytoplasm where they are processed to mature miRNA duplexes by their interaction with the endonuclease enzyme Dicer in complex with dsRNA binding protein TRBP (Siomi & Siomi, 2010). One strand of the mature miRNA duplex ultimately gets integrated into the miRNA-induced silencing complex (miRISC), whereas the second strand is released and degraded. The resulting complex of mature miRNA and miRISC exerts regulatory effect by binding to its target site in the 3′ untranslated region (3′UTR) of mRNA that controls many aspects of mRNA metabolism, such as transport, localization, efficiency of translation and stability (Chiang et al., 2010; Krol et al., 2010) (summarized in Fig. 1).

3. MicroRNAs as potential biomarkers for diagnostic, prediction of therapy response, and prognosis of patients

As described above, the expression levels of many miRNAs are altered in various types of cancers. Thus, specific tissue miRNA signature could be an useful tool for diagnostic oncology. Among all gliomas, miRNAs are the most studied in glioblastomas that is associated with the very poor prognosis. Global analysis of miRNA expression profiles of glioblastoma tissues allowed to identify a group of miRNAs with significantly altered expression levels compared to non-malignant brain tissues (Sana et al., 2011). Two independent research groups described significant up-regulation of miR-21 in glioblastomas what fully corresponds to the expression levels of miR-21 observed in other cancers (Chan et al., 2005; Esquela-Kerscher & Slack, 2006; Zhang & Farwell, 2008). Furthermore, miR-125b was over-expressed, and miR-128a and miRNA-181 family were significantly down-regulated in both studies. On the other hand, miR-221 generates conflict between these studies. Ciafré described this miRNA as up-regulated in glioblastoma, whereas, Slaby showed lower level in comparison to the adult brain tissue (Ciafre et al., 2005; Slaby et al., 2010). The last-named autor speculated this discrepancy and concluded that it is likely that the brain tissues used as control samples in their study, though excised from the margin of resection materials, contained traces of micro-capillaries from around the arteriovenous malformation. This could be responsible for the relatively low levels of miR-221 and miR-222 in glioblastomas despite their absolute levels because it is generally known that endothelial cells are characterized by highest expression levels of these miRNAs (Slaby et al., 2010) (Tab. 1). Furthermore, Ciafré performed miRNA expression analysis of several glioblastoma cell lines and has come to the conclusion that miRNAs underexpressed in glioblastoma cell lines generally confirmed primary tumour data, whereas only miR-21 and miR-221 that were overexpressed in tumours were deregulated also in the cell lines (Ciafre et al., 2005). Taken together, only miR-21 and miR-181 family were significantly and consistently altered in all three studies.

The clinical significance of miRNA expression profiles in malignant gliomas is not yet much explored. Nevertheless, Guan published a set of 16 candidate miRNAs associated with the malignant progresiion from anaplastic astrocytomas to glioblastomas. Among these miRNAs, the members of miR-196 family, indicated the highest level of significance. MiR-196 expression levels significantly correlated with poor survival by Kaplan-Meier method ($p = 0.0073$) and, moreover, multivariate analysis showed that its expression levels were an independent predictor of overall survival in glioblastoma patients (p = 0.021; HR 2.81) (Guan et al., 2010). Another research group investigated the miRNA expression profiles in four patients with primary WHO grade II gliomas that spontaneously progressed to WHO grade IV secondary glioblastomas. They identified 12 miRNAs (miR-9, miR-15a, miR-16, miR-17, miR-19a, miR-20a, miR-21, miR-25, miR-28, miR-130b, miR-140, and miR-210) showing increased expression, and two miRNAs (miR-184 and miR-328) with reduced expression upon progression (Malzkorn et al., 2010). Validation experiments on an independent series of primary low-grade and secondary high-grade astrocytomas confirmed miR-17 and miR-184 as interesting candidates contributing to glioma progression. Taken together, only miR-184 was significantly altered in all three studies. However, miR-21, which was identified in two independent studies but not confirmed by validation study, could also probably play an important role in progression of glioma tumors with respect to its oncogene function described in many other cancers.

Treatment of malignant gliomas remains one of the greatest challenges facing oncologists today through a frequent resistance to both chemo- and radiotherapeutics and short survival (Ziegler et al., 2008). Important question for management of glioblastoma patients is the possibility of predicting therapeutic outcome. MiRNA expression could have a great potential in prediction of therapeutic outcome after treatment by temozolomide (TMZ) that is an oral alkylating agent frequently used for the treatment of glioblastoma. Slaby showed that expression levels of miR-181b and miR-181c in glioblastoma tissued was successfully associated with response to concomitant chemoradiotherapy with temozolomide (RT/TMZ). MiR-181b and miR-181c were significantly down-regulated in patients who responded to RT/TMZ (p = 0.016; p = 0.047, respectively) in comparison to patients with progredient disease (Slaby et al., 2010). In other study, Ujifuku described miR-195, miR-455-3p, and miR-10a* as the three most up-regulated miRNAs in the TMZ-resistant cell lines. Moreover, knockdown of miRNA-195 in the TMZ-resistant cell line led to overcome of TMZ resistance and increase the cell killing effect of TMZ (Ujifuku et al., 2010).

4. MicroRNAs involved in drug resistance

It was many time showed that miRNAs play important role in drug resistance many cancers, including glioblastoma. Shi described that overexpression of miR-21 in glioblastoma cells could significantly reduce TMZ-induced apoptosis by decreasing Bax/Bcl-2 ratio and caspase-3 activity (Shi et al., 2010). The miR-21 inhibitor also enhances the chemosensitivity of human glioblastoma cells to paclitaxel via inhibition of STAT3 expression and phosphorylation. Moreover, the same treatment by miR-21 antisense oligonucleotides led to enhanced cytotoxicities of vepesid because miR-21 likely contributes to resistance through depression of LRRFIP1 expression, leading to the reduction of cytotoxicity of chemotherapeutic drugs through activation of the NF-κB pathway (Li et al., 2009b; Papagiannakopoulos et al., 2008; Ren et al., 2010). Li observed that miR-328 is in glioblastoma poorly expressed and contributes to tumour chemoresistance through multidrug resistance protein ABCG2 (Li et al., 2010). Finally, it was reported the possible impact on the therapeutic effect by transfection of miR-451 in combination with imatinib mesylate treatment. Up-regulation of miR-451 led to differentiation of glioblastoma stem cells (Gal et al., 2008).

	Ciafre et al., 2005		Slaby et al., 2010	
	miRNA	C/P ratio†	miRNA	Fold change (P)‡
Up-regulated	miR-9-2	1.88 - 10.16		
	miR-10b	1.97 - 13.6		
	miR-21	**1.81 - 9.3**	**miR-21**	**8.35 (<0.001)**
	miR-25	1.99 - 3.6		
	miR-123	1.9 - 2.45		
	miR-125b-1	**2.19 - 2.73**	**miR-125b**	**1.45 (0.502)**
	miR-125b-2	**1.95 - 2.88**		
	miR-130a	2.11 - 5.3		
	miR-221	1.84 - 4.8		
Down-regulated	**miR-128a**	**0.34 - 0.56**	**miR-128a**	**0.03 (<0.001)**
	miR-181a	**0.082 - 0.56**	**miR-181a**	**0.4 (0.073)**
	miR-181b	0.098 - 0.56	miR-181b	0.28 (0.036)
	miR-181c	0.096 - 0.56	miR-181c	0.29 (0.043)
			miR-221	0.25
			miR-222	0.22

Table 1. miRNAs significantly deregulated in human glioblastoma tissues

5. MicroRNAs and invasion

Invasion of malignant glioma is a highly complex phenomenon involving molecular and cellular processes, whose precise interplay is still not fully understood (Tektonidis et al., 2011). Several studies indicate that one of the possible players in this tumor feature are miRNAs (Sana et al., 2011). These observations are highlighted by the recently demonstrated relation of some miRNAs with molecules considered key in tumor invasion. Among these molecules belongs matrix metalloproteinases (MMPs). MMPs are zinc-containing endopeptidases, which degrade the extracellular matrix and basement membrane, and process bioactive mediators involved in promoting aspects of tumor growth, including gliomas (Badiga et al., 2011; Chetty et al., 2011). The activity of MMPs is regulated at several levels, including posttranscriptional regulation through miRNAs (Hadler-Olsen et al., 2011; Sana et al., 2011). Sun et al. found that miR-10b induced glioma cell invasion by modulating tumor invasion factors MMP-14 and urokinase-type plasminogen activator receptor (uPAR) espression via the direct target HOXD10 (Sun et al., 2011). Sasayama et al. came to the same conclusion in the study including 43 glioma samples of various grade and 6 glioma cell lines. Therefore, the miR-10b/HOXD10/MMP-14/uPAR signaling pathway might contribute to the invasion of glioma (Sasayama et al., 2009; Sun et al., 2011). Accordingly, glioma cells lost their invasive ability when treated with miR-10b inhibitors, suggesting that miR-10b could be used as a new bio-target to cure glioma (Sun et al., 2011). Another group established miRNA expression profile (14 positively and 31 negatively correlated miRNAs with MMP-9) in 60 GBM samples. Among them, two miRNAs: miR-885-5p and miR-491-5p,

† C/P ratio represents the range of ratio between tumour samples values (C, centre of the tumour) and the control samples values (P, peripheral brain area from the same patient)

‡ P value is presented (Mann-Whitney U-test)

were chosen for functional validation for their high positive correlation with MMP-9 expression. Both miRNAs were demonstrated to reduce the levels of MMP-9 expression and inhibit cellular invasion in glioma cells. Furthermore, miR-491-5p suppressed glioma cell invasion via targeting MMP-9 directly (Yan et al., 2011). Xia et al. observed that miR-146b overexpression by transfection with the precursor miR-146b, or knock-down by LNA-anti-miR-146b, has no effect on the growth of human glioblastoma cells. However, precursor miR-146b transfection significantly reduced the migration and invasion of these cells, while LNA-anti-miR-146b transfection generated the opposite result. Furthermore, they discovered that MMP16 is one of the downstream targets of miR-146b (Xia et al., 2009). Moreover, miR-146-5p supresses translation of EGFR and introduction of miR-146b-5p decreases cell invasion, migration, and phosphorylation of protein kinase B (AKT) (Katakowski et al., 2010). Another group described regulation of podoplanin membrane sialo-glycoprotein (PDPN) through direct targeting of PDPN gene by miR-29b and 125a in GBM. Earlier, it was demonstrated that PDPN is over-expressed and related to cellular invasion in astrocytic tumors. The similar findings, but in GBM, were published by Cortez et al. (Cortez et al., 2010). With GBM invasion are also related miR-124a and miR-34a whose targeted over-expression may be novel approach in GBM treatment (Fowler et al., 2011; Li et al., 2009a).

6. MicroRNAs involved in core signaling pathways: Possible therapeutic potential

The involvement of miRNAs in core signaling patways that regulate important cell processes of glioblastoma, led to the suggestion that miRNAs could serve as a potential therapeutic targets (Novakova et al., 2009; Sana et al., 2011). The most frequently explored miRNA is the miR-21, which has been found to act as an oncogene. It is evident that miR-21 influences multiple important components of oncogenic signaling pathways in glioblastoma. MiR-21 was revealed as post-transcriptional regulator involved in NF-κB signaling pathway. Aberrant activation of NF-κB signaling pathway has been proved to be important for invasiveness and metastatic capacity of tumors through up-regulation of matrix metalloproteinases (MMPs) and transcription factors regulating E-cadherin. Li et al. identified LRRFIP1 gene, which was remarkably up-regulated in miR-21-knockdown cells, as a candidate target gene of miR-21. Further, they found that LRRFIP1 mRNA carried a putative miR-21 binding site. Further analyses confirmed LRRFIP1 as a direct target of miR-21 (Li et al., 2009b). In connection with this signaling pathway, it was also identified miR-218 that in vitro dramatically reduced the migratory speed and invasive ability of analysed cells. Ectopic expression of miR-218 down-regulated matrix MMP-9 and reduced NF-κB transactivity at transcriptional level, whereas inhibition of miR-218 enhanced the expression of MMP-9 and transcriptional activity of NF-κB. Authors demonstrated that miR-218 could inactivate NF-kB/MMP-9 signaling by directly targeting the 3′-UTR of the IKK-κ which is a critical component in NF-κϒϒB regulation (Song et al., 2010).

PI3K/AKT and EGFR are in term of tumor biology other very important signaling pathways that are regulated by miR-21. Mechanistic studies identified mRNA targets of miR-21 among important components of the PI3K/AKT and EGFR signaling pathways. Glioblastoma cell lines U251 (mutant PTEN) and LN229 (wild-type PTEN) showed a decreased expression of EGFR, activated AKT, Cyclin D and Bcl-2 after treatment by miR-21-specific antisense oligonucleotide (Zhou et al., 2010a). Although miR-21 is known to regulate PTEN and down-regulation of miR-21 led to increased PTEN expression, the glioblastoma suppressor effect of antisense-miR-21 is most likely independent of PTEN status because U251 has mutated PTEN (Ren et al., 2010; Zhou et al., 2010a). PTEN down-regulation followed by AKT activation was described after transfection of glioblastoma cells with the primary transcript of miR-26a-2. Similarly, the miR-26a mimics decreased PTEN protein levels and increased AKT phosphorylation (Huse et al., 2009; Kim et al., 2010). Modulation of expression levels of AKT signaling cascade components such as Akt1, Cyclin D1, MMP-2, MMP-9, and Bcl-2 in glioblastoma cell lines after transfection of miR-451 mimicked was described also by Nan. By contrast, miR-451 down-regulation led to increase in p27 levels. According to phenotypic experiments, miR-451 inhibited invasive ability, induced cell cycle arrest in the G0/G1 phase, delayed the progression of cell cycle, inhibited cell proliferation and induced apoptosis in glioblastoma cells in vitro (Nan et al., 2010). Furthermore, miR-451 affects downstrem members of PI3K/AKT signaling pathway via targeting of CAB39 (MO25α), which is binding partner of LKB1. LKB1 is upstream kinase of the major energy biosensor AMPK. Godlewski published that miR-451 levels are regulated by glucose; under conditions of abundant energy miR-451 expression is high, and the suppression of AMPK signaling allows cells to maintain elevated proliferation rates via unrestrained mTOR activation. Under conditions of glucose withdrawal, miR-451 downregulation is necessary for AMPK pathway activation, leading to suppressed proliferation rates, increased cell survival and migration. Thus, miR-451 is a regulator of the LKB1/AMPK pathway, and this may represent a fundamental mechanism that contributes to cellular adaptation in response to altered energy availability (Godlewski et al., 2010a; Godlewski et al., 2010b). MiR-128 is another miRNA that significantly reduced glioma cell proliferation in vitro and glioma xenograft growth through PI3K/AKT signaling pathway. Godlewski explained this effect by binding of mentioned miRNA to the 3'UTR of Bmi-1 mRNA that is significantly up-regulated in gliomas, wheares miR-128 is down-regulated compared to normal brain. In addition, miR-128 expression leads to a decrease in H3K27 methylation and modulation of cellular pathways, especially p21CIP1 and Akt, involved in cell cycle arrest and survival (Godlewski et al., 2008). Modulation of p21 was described also in context with another miRNAs. Gabriely showed that BCL2L11/Bim, TFAP2C/AP-2gamma, CDKN2A/p16, and CDKN1A/p21 are direct targets of miR-10b. Inhibition of miR-10b reduced glioma cell growth by cell cycle arrest and apoptosis, and, furthermore, survival of glioblastoma patients expressing high levels of miR-10 family members is significantly reduced in comparison to patients with low miR-10 levels, indicating that miR-10 may contribute to glioma growth in vivo (Gabriely et al., 2011). MiR-221 and miR-222 were also revealed as potential regulators of many target genes involved in AKT signaling pathway. Up-regulation of these miRNAs resulted in remarkable increase of p-Akt and significant changes in expression of Akt-related genes in glioma cells. Consequently, miR-221 and miR-222 overexpression increased glioma cell proliferation and invasion in vitro and induced glioma growth in a subcutaneous mouse model (Zhang et al., 2010c). EGFR signaling network contributes to promotion and progression of a broad spectrum of solid tumors, and it is a promising target for anticancer therapy. Stimulation of the EGFR and, subsequently, KRAS signaling, lead to activation of numerous signal transduction molecules initiating a cascade of downstream effectors that mediate tumour growth, survival, angiogenesis and metastasis (Jancik et al., 2010). Kefas published that miR-7 directly inhibited EGFR expression via its 3'-UTR and independently suppressed the AKT pathway via targeting upstream regulators, such as IRS-1 and IRS-2. Moreover, transfection with miR-7 oligonucleotides decreased viability and invasiveness of primary glioblastoma cell lines (Kefas et al., 2008). Down-regulation of EGFR mRNA and protein expression in glioblastoma cell lines via two predicted sites of miR-7 was confirmed by Webster. This led to the induction of cell cycle arrest and apoptosis. Furthermore, the same author also described Raf1, another member of the EGFR signaling pathway, as a direct target of miR-7 in cancer cells (Webster et al., 2009). Katakowski have declared that EGFR is also direct target of miR-146b-5p. Its introduction decreased cell invasion, migration, and phosphorylation of Akt in glioma cells (Katakowski et al., 2010). Mir-21 is responsible for glioma cell invasiveness by disrupting the negative feedback circuit of EGFR components Ras/MAPK through post-transcriptional regulation of Spry2. Consistently with these results, Spry2 protein levels were significantly decreased in invasive WHO grade II-IV human glioma tissues, but not in non-invasive grade I and normal tissues (Kwak et al., 2011) (summarized in Fig. 2).

Other targets of miR-21 are p53, TGF-β, and mitochondrial apoptotic signaling networks. Papagiannakopoulos reported that these pathways are de-repressed in response to miR-21 knockdown. As direct targets of this miRNA were predicted proteins p63, JMY, TP53BP2, HNRPK, TOPORS, IGFB3, APAF1, PPIF, TGFBR2/3, DAXX, and HNRNPK. MiR-21 can also stabilize p53 protein levels by interfering with MDM2 and/or act as p53 transcriptional cofactors (Papagiannakopoulos et al., 2008). Inhibition of miR-21 increased also endogenous levels of PDCD4 in human glioma cell lines and activated caspases 9 and 3 (Chen et al., 2008; Zhou et al., 2010b). Protein PDCD4 inhibits translation by its interaction with the initiation translation factors, and proliferation via activation of $p21^{CIP1}$ (Kwak et al., 2010). In addition, specific inhibition of miR-21 led to reduced MMP activities in vitro and in model of gliomas in nude mice. Consequently, down-regulation of miR-21 decreased migratory and invasive abilities in glioma cells (Gabriely et al., 2008). Influence on glioma cell invasion by modulating MMP was observed also after treatment with miR-10b. This miRNA was overexpressed in glioma samples and directly associated with the glioma's pathological grade and malignicy. Sun found that miR-10b affected tumor invasion factors MMP-14 and uPAR expression via the direct target HOXD10 (Sun et al., 2011). Finally, it was shown that miR-221 and miR-222 directly regulated apoptotic pathway in glioblastoma through direct targeting an apoptotic gene PUMA (Zhang et al., 2010b) (summarized in Fig. 2).

Another study revealed miRNAs as possible regulators of IFN pathways. It was showed that STAT1 and STAT2 expression and phosphorylation were up-regulated in cells with silenced miR-221 and miR-222. Tyrosine phosphorylation of STAT1 and STAT2 was present in the nucleus after repression of the same miRNAs. These data illustrate a mechanism of STAT1/2 up-regulation under the transcriptional control of IFN-γ signaling after knockdown of miR-221 and miR-222 in glioma cells (Fig. 2) (Zhang et al., 2010a). Interestingly, Ohno investigated the possibility that IFN-γ may induce or down-regulate cellular miRNAs in human gliomas. They analysed the effect of IFN-γ treatment on miR-21 expression in glioma cells and intracranial glioma xenografts. Systematic delivery of IFN-γ markedly reduced the level of miR-21 in all glioma cells. The results indicate that decrease in the levels of miR-21 is the result of transcriptional suppression. In contrast, the addition of the STAT3-specific inhibitor increased the level of miR-21 and inhibited IFN-γ–mediated suppression of miR-21, suggesting that miR-21 expression is negatively regulated by STAT3 (Ohno et al., 2009).

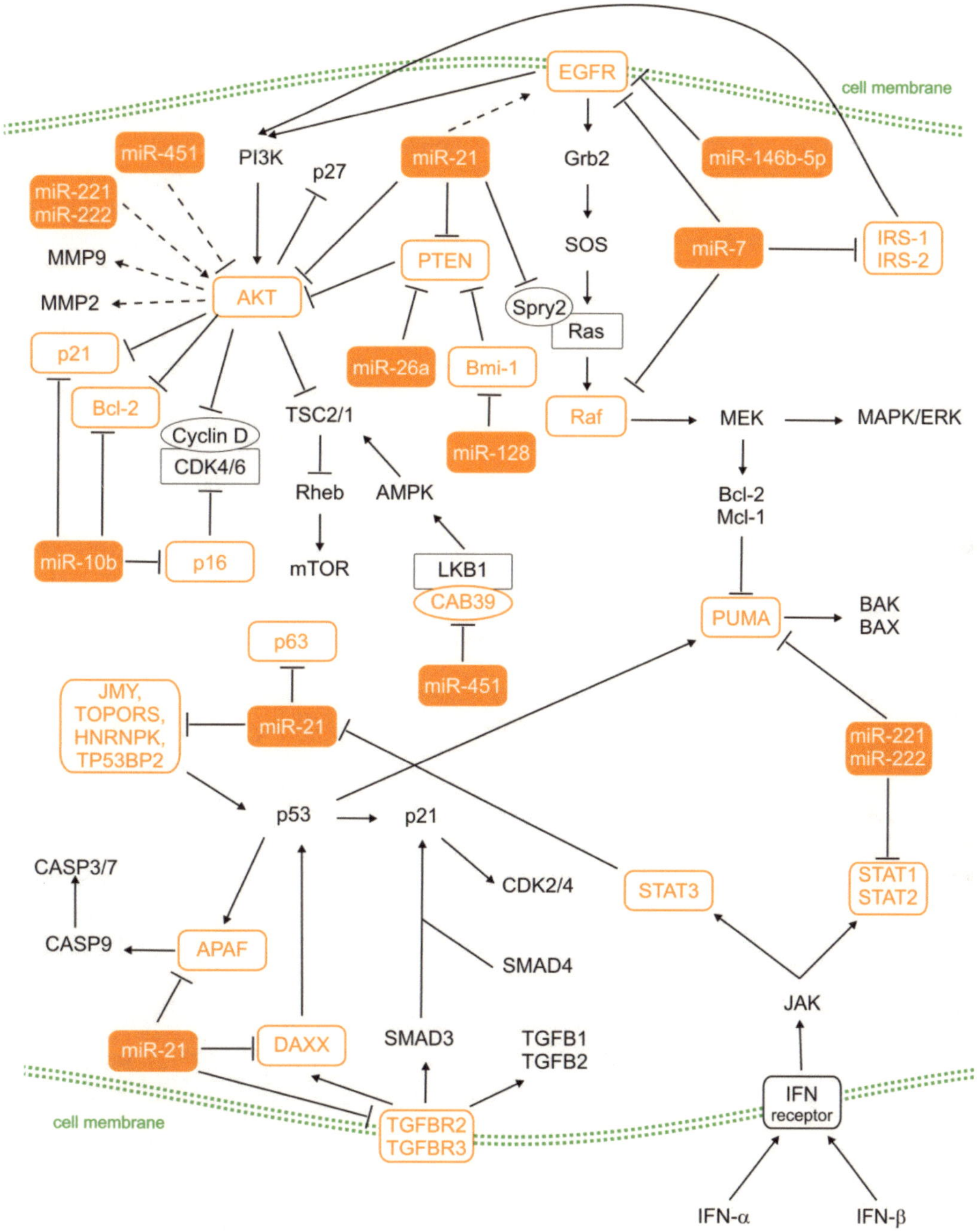

Fig. 2. MiRNAs involved in core signaling pathways

Notch signaling is critical in cell fate decisions such as neuronal versus glial fate in the developing nervous system. This pathway play also key role in stem-like phenotype maintenance and survival of normal stem cells as well as cancer stem cells that are often discussed in context with tumor initiation, progression, and metastasis. Therefore, it is not surprising that Notch pathway plays a crucial role in brain tumours, including glioblastoma (Kefas et al., 2009; Lathia et al., 2008; Sana et al., 2011). Kefas et al. performed miRNA microarray analysis of glioma tumour stem cells transfected with Notch-1 siRNA. In these Notch-1 knockdown cells, miR-326 was one of the miRNAs significantly increased. However, pre-miR-326 transfection caused substantial decrease in both Notch-1 and Notch-2 protein. Therefore, it was indicated that miR-326 is suppressed by Notch activity and regulates Notch pathway at the same time. It was observed that miR-326 induces apoptosis and decreases glioma cells proliferation, viability and invasiveness of glioblastoma stem cell-like lines. Furthermore, miR-326 transfection also reduced glioma cell tumourigenicity in vivo (Kefas et al., 2009). Another important target of miRNA-326 is pyruvate kinase type M2 (PKM2) that has recently been shown to play a key role in cancer cell metabolism (Hitosugi et al., 2009; Kefas et al., 2010). Further, it was studied the role of miR-34a in glioblastoma. MiR-34a inhibits Notch-1 and Notch-2 protein expression and 3′-UTR reporter activities as well as CDK6 and c-Met protein expression in glioma cells. In this study, Li observed for the first time that pre-miR-34a expression is down-regulated in human glioblastoma tissues compared to normal human brain (Li et al., 2009a). Other studies showed that miR-34a acts as a tumour suppressor in p53-mutant glioma cells, partially through regulating SIRT1 (Guessous et al., 2010). Transfection of miR-34a into tested glioblastoma cell lines strongly inhibited cell proliferation, cell cycle, cell survival, cell invasion and in vivo glioblastoma xenograft growth; however, the treatment did not affect human astrocyte cell survival and cell cycle (Luan et al., 2010).

At a glance

- MicroRNAs (miRNAs) are an abundant class of small non-coding RNAs able to posttranscriptionaly regulate gene expression.
- MiRNAs are involved in many signalling pathways that have been shown to control a wide range of biological processes such as cellular proliferation, differentiation and apoptosis.
- Many miRNAs are deregulated in gliomas and are associated with their biologic and clinicopathological features.
- Expression profiles of selected miRNAs could be used as novel diagnostic and prognostic biomarkers as well as possible predictors of therapy response.
- Targeted regulation of miRNAs in gliomas represents promising therapeutic approach leading to the improvement of unsatisfactory survival in glioma patients.

7. Conclusion

The discovery of miRNA function has markedly spread the view on regulation of gene expression. Its remarkable ability to regulate large number of genes, including oncogenes and tumor suppressor genes, has catapulted miRNAs into the centre of cancer molecular biology over the past few years. It is now evident that dysregulation of miRNAs is an important step in the development of many cancers, including gliomas. Some few studies based on expression profiling have proven there are significant changes of miRNA expression levels in gliomas compared to adult brain tissue; these expression levels identified groups of miRNAs with potential of prognostic stratification and prediction of responses to chemoradiotherapy in glioma patients. But much more studies have been focused on the improvement our knowledge of role of miRNAs in glioma core signaling pathways. The results of these studies suggest a great potential and relevance of miRNAs as a novel class of therapeutic targets and possibly powerful intervention tools in glioblastoma.

8. Acknowledgment

This work was supported by grant IGA NT/11214-4/2010 of the Czech Ministry of Health, Project No. MZ0MOU2005 of the Czech Ministry of Health and by the project "CEITEC - Central European Institute of Technology" (CZ.1.05/1.1.00/02.0068). Infrastructural part of this project (Institute of Molecular and Translational Medicine) was supported from the Operational Programme Research and Development for Innovations (project CZ.1.05/2.1.00/01.0030).

9. References

Alvarez-Garcia, I. & Miska, E.A. (2005). MicroRNA functions in animal development and human disease. *Development,* Vol.132, No.21, pp. 4653-4662, ISSN 0950-1991

Badiga, A.V.; Chetty, C.; Kesanakurti, D.; Are, D.; Gujrati, M.; Klopfenstein, J.D.; Dinh, D.H. & Rao, J.S. (2011). MMP-2 siRNA inhibits radiation-enhanced invasiveness in glioma cells. *PLoS One,* Vol.6, No.6, pp. e20614, ISSN 1932-6203

Bartel, D.P. (2004). MicroRNAs: genomics, biogenesis, mechanism, and function. *Cell,* Vol.116, No.2, pp. 281-297, ISSN 0092-8674

Carthew, R.W. & Sontheimer, E.J. (2009). Origins and Mechanisms of miRNAs and siRNAs. *Cell,* Vol.136, No.4, pp. 642-655, ISSN 1097-4172

Chan, J.A.; Krichevsky, A.M. & Kosik, K.S. (2005). MicroRNA-21 is an antiapoptotic factor in human glioblastoma cells. *Cancer Res,* Vol.65, No.14, pp. 6029-6033, ISSN 0008-5472

Chen, Y.; Liu, W.; Chao, T.; Zhang, Y.; Yan, X.; Gong, Y.; Qiang, B.; Yuan, J.; Sun, M. & Peng, X. (2008). MicroRNA-21 down-regulates the expression of tumor suppressor PDCD4 in human glioblastoma cell T98G. *Cancer Lett,* Vol.272, No.2, pp. 197-205, ISSN 1872-7980

Chetty, C.; Rao, J.S. & Lakka, S.S. (2011). Matrix metalloproteinase pharmacogenomics in non-small-cell lung carcinoma. *Pharmacogenomics,* Vol.12, No.4, pp. 535-546, ISSN 1744-8042

Chiang, H.R.; Schoenfeld, L.W.; Ruby, J.G.; Auyeung, V.C.; Spies, N.; Baek, D.; Johnston, W.K.; Russ, C.; Luo, S.; Babiarz, J.E.; Blelloch, R.; Schroth, G.P.; Nusbaum, C. & Bartel, D.P. (2010). Mammalian microRNAs: experimental evaluation of novel and previously annotated genes. *Genes Dev,* Vol.24, No.10, pp. 992-1009, ISSN 1549-5477

Ciafre, S.A.; Galardi, S.; Mangiola, A.; Ferracin, M.; Liu, C.G.; Sabatino, G.; Negrini, M.; Maira, G.; Croce, C.M. & Farace, M.G. (2005). Extensive modulation of a set of microRNAs in primary glioblastoma. *Biochem Biophys Res Commun,* Vol.334, No.4, pp. 1351-1358, ISSN 0006-291X

Cortez, M.A.; Nicoloso, M.S.; Shimizu, M.; Rossi, S.; Gopisetty, G.; Molina, J.R.; Carlotti, C., Jr.; Tirapelli, D.; Neder, L.; Brassesco, M.S.; Scrideli, C.A.; Tone, L.G.; Georgescu,

M.M.; Zhang, W.; Puduvalli, V. & Calin, G.A. (2010). miR-29b and miR-125a regulate podoplanin and suppress invasion in glioblastoma. *Genes Chromosomes Cancer,* Vol.49, No.11, pp. 981-990, ISSN 1098-2264

Croce, C.M. (2009). Causes and consequences of microRNA dysregulation in cancer. *Nat Rev Genet,* Vol.10, No.10, pp. 704-714, ISSN 1471-0064

Esquela-Kerscher, A. & Slack, F.J. (2006). Oncomirs - microRNAs with a role in cancer. *Nat Rev Cancer,* Vol.6, No.4, pp. 259-269, ISSN 1474-175X

Fowler, A.; Thomson, D.; Giles, K.; Maleki, S.; Mreich, E.; Wheeler, H.; Leedman, P.; Biggs, M.; Cook, R.; Little, N.; Robinson, B. & McDonald, K. (2011). miR-124a is frequently down-regulated in glioblastoma and is involved in migration and invasion. *Eur J Cancer,* Vol.47, No.6, pp. 953-963, ISSN 1879-0852

Gabriely, G.; Wurdinger, T.; Kesari, S.; Esau, C.C.; Burchard, J.; Linsley, P.S. & Krichevsky, A.M. (2008). MicroRNA 21 promotes glioma invasion by targeting matrix metalloproteinase regulators. *Mol Cell Biol,* Vol.28, No.17, pp. 5369-5380, ISSN 1098-5549

Gabriely, G.; Yi, M.; Narayan, R.S.; Niers, J.M.; Wurdinger, T.; Imitola, J.; Ligon, K.L.; Kesari, S.; Esau, C.; Stephens, R.M.; Tannous, B.A. & Krichevsky, A.M. (2011). Human glioma growth is controlled by microRNA-10b. *Cancer Res,* pp., ISSN 1538-7445

Gal, H.; Pandi, G.; Kanner, A.A.; Ram, Z.; Lithwick-Yanai, G.; Amariglio, N.; Rechavi, G. & Givol, D. (2008). MIR-451 and Imatinib mesylate inhibit tumor growth of Glioblastoma stem cells. *Biochem Biophys Res Commun,* Vol.376, No.1, pp. 86-90, ISSN 1090-2104

Godlewski, J.; Bronisz, A.; Nowicki, M.O.; Chiocca, E.A. & Lawler, S. (2010a). microRNA-451: A conditional switch controlling glioma cell proliferation and migration. *Cell Cycle,* Vol.9, No.14, pp. 2742-2748, ISSN 1551-4005

Godlewski, J.; Nowicki, M.O.; Bronisz, A.; Nuovo, G.; Palatini, J.; De Lay, M.; Van Brocklyn, J.; Ostrowski, M.C.; Chiocca, E.A. & Lawler, S.E. (2010b). MicroRNA-451 regulates LKB1/AMPK signaling and allows adaptation to metabolic stress in glioma cells. *Mol Cell,* Vol.37, No.5, pp. 620-632, ISSN 1097-4164

Godlewski, J.; Nowicki, M.O.; Bronisz, A.; Williams, S.; Otsuki, A.; Nuovo, G.; Raychaudhury, A.; Newton, H.B.; Chiocca, E.A. & Lawler, S. (2008). Targeting of the Bmi-1 oncogene/stem cell renewal factor by microRNA-128 inhibits glioma proliferation and self-renewal. *Cancer Res,* Vol.68, No.22, pp. 9125-9130, ISSN 1538-7445

Griffiths-Jones, S.; Saini, H.K.; van Dongen, S. & Enright, A.J. (2008). miRBase: tools for microRNA genomics. *Nucleic Acids Res,* Vol.36, No.Database ISSNue, pp. D154-158, ISSN 1362-4962

Guan, Y.; Mizoguchi, M.; Yoshimoto, K.; Hata, N.; Shono, T.; Suzuki, S.O.; Araki, Y.; Kuga, D.; Nakamizo, A.; Amano, T.; Ma, X.; Hayashi, K. & Sasaki, T. (2010). MiRNA-196 is upregulated in glioblastoma but not in anaplastic astrocytoma and has prognostic significance. *Clin Cancer Res,* Vol.16, No.16, pp. 4289-4297, ISSN 1078-0432

Guessous, F.; Zhang, Y.; Kofman, A.; Catania, A.; Li, Y.; Schiff, D.; Purow, B. & Abounader, R. (2010). microRNA-34a is tumor suppressive in brain tumors and glioma stem cells. *Cell Cycle,* Vol.9, No.6, pp., ISSN 1551-4005

Hadler-Olsen, E.; Fadnes, B.; Sylte, I.; Uhlin-Hansen, L. & Winberg, J.O. (2011). Regulation of matrix metalloproteinase activity in health and disease. *FEBS J*, Vol.278, No.1, pp. 28-45, ISSN 1742-4658

Hatfield, S. & Ruohola-Baker, H. (2008). microRNA and stem cell function. *Cell TISSNue Res*, Vol.331, No.1, pp. 57-66, ISSN 1432-0878

Hitosugi, T.; Kang, S.; Vander Heiden, M.G.; Chung, T.W.; Elf, S.; Lythgoe, K.; Dong, S.; Lonial, S.; Wang, X.; Chen, G.Z.; Xie, J.; Gu, T.L.; Polakiewicz, R.D.; Roesel, J.L.; Boggon, T.J.; Khuri, F.R.; Gilliland, D.G.; Cantley, L.C.; Kaufman, J. & Chen, J. (2009). Tyrosine phosphorylation inhibits PKM2 to promote the Warburg effect and tumor growth. *Sci Signal*, Vol.2, No.97, pp. ra73, ISSN 1937-9145

Huse, J.T.; Brennan, C.; Hambardzumyan, D.; Wee, B.; Pena, J.; Rouhanifard, S.H.; Sohn-Lee, C.; le Sage, C.; Agami, R.; Tuschl, T. & Holland, E.C. (2009). The PTEN-regulating microRNA miR-26a is amplified in high-grade glioma and facilitates gliomagenesis in vivo. *Genes Dev*, Vol.23, No.11, pp. 1327-1337, ISSN 1549-5477

Jancik, S.; Drabek, J.; Radzioch, D. & Hajduch, M. (2010). Clinical relevance of KRAS in human cancers. *J Biomed Biotechnol*, Vol.2010, pp. 150960, ISSN 1110-7251

Katakowski, M.; Zheng, X.; Jiang, F.; Rogers, T.; Szalad, A. & Chopp, M. (2010). MiR-146b-5p suppresses EGFR expression and reduces in vitro migration and invasion of glioma. *Cancer Invest*, Vol.28, No.10, pp. 1024-1030, ISSN 1532-4192

Kefas, B.; Comeau, L.; Erdle, N.; Montgomery, E.; Amos, S. & Purow, B. (2010). Pyruvate kinase M2 is a target of the tumor-suppressive microRNA-326 and regulates the survival of glioma cells. *Neuro Oncol*, Vol.12, No.11, pp. 1102-1112, ISSN 1523-5866

Kefas, B.; Comeau, L.; Floyd, D.H.; Seleverstov, O.; Godlewski, J.; Schmittgen, T.; Jiang, J.; diPierro, C.G.; Li, Y.; Chiocca, E.A.; Lee, J.; Fine, H.; Abounader, R.; Lawler, S. & Purow, B. (2009). The neuronal microRNA miR-326 acts in a feedback loop with notch and has therapeutic potential against brain tumors. *J Neurosci*, Vol.29, No.48, pp. 15161-15168, ISSN 1529-2401

Kefas, B.; Godlewski, J.; Comeau, L.; Li, Y.; Abounader, R.; Hawkinson, M.; Lee, J.; Fine, H.; Chiocca, E.A.; Lawler, S. & Purow, B. (2008). microRNA-7 inhibits the epidermal growth factor receptor and the Akt pathway and is down-regulated in glioblastoma. *Cancer Res*, Vol.68, No.10, pp. 3566-3572, ISSN 1538-7445

Kim, H.; Huang, W.; Jiang, X.; Pennicooke, B.; Park, P.J. & Johnson, M.D. (2010). Integrative genome analysis reveals an oncomir/oncogene cluster regulating glioblastoma survivorship. *Proc Natl Acad Sci U S A*, Vol.107, No.5, pp. 2183-2188, ISSN 1091-6490

Krol, J.; Loedige, I. & Filipowicz, W. (2010). The widespread regulation of microRNA biogenesis, function and decay. *Nat Rev Genet*, Vol.11, No.9, pp. 597-610, ISSN 1471-0064

Kwak, H.J.; Kim, Y.J.; Chun, K.R.; Woo, Y.M.; Park, S.J.; Jeong, J.A.; Jo, S.H.; Kim, T.H.; Min, H.S.; Chae, J.S.; Choi, E.J.; Kim, G.; Shin, S.H.; Gwak, H.S.; Kim, S.K.; Hong, E.K.; Lee, G.K.; Choi, K.H.; Kim, J.H.; Yoo, H.; Park, J.B. & Lee, S.H. (2011). Downregulation of Spry2 by miR-21 triggers malignancy in human gliomas. *Oncogene*, pp., ISSN 1476-5594

Kwak, P.B.; Iwasaki, S. & Tomari, Y. (2010). The microRNA pathway and cancer. *Cancer Sci*, Vol.101, No.11, pp. 2309-2315, ISSN 1349-7006

Lakomý, R.; Fadrus, P.; Slampa, P.; Svoboda, T.; Kren. L.; Lzicarová, E.; Belanová, R.; Siková, I.; Poprach, A.; Schneiderová, M.; Procházková, M.; Sána, J.; Slabý, O.; Smrcka, M.; Vyzula, R.; & Svoboda, M. (2011). Multimodal treatment of glioblastoma multiforme: results of 86 consecutive patients diagnosed in period 2003-2009. *Klin Onkol*, Vol.24, No.2, pp. 112-20, ISSN 0862 -495X

Lathia, J.D.; Mattson, M.P. & Cheng, A. (2008). Notch: from neural development to neurological disorders. *J Neurochem,* Vol.107, No.6, pp. 1471-1481, ISSN 1471-4159 (Electronic)

Li, W.Q.; Li, Y.M.; Tao, B.B.; Lu, Y.C.; Hu, G.H.; Liu, H.M.; He, J.; Xu, Y. & Yu, H.Y. (2010). Downregulation of ABCG2 expression in glioblastoma cancer stem cells with miRNA-328 may decrease their chemoresistance. *Med Sci Monit,* Vol.16, No.10, pp. HY27-30, ISSN 1643-3750

Li, Y.; Guessous, F.; Zhang, Y.; Dipierro, C.; Kefas, B.; Johnson, E.; Marcinkiewicz, L.; Jiang, J.; Yang, Y.; Schmittgen, T.D.; Lopes, B.; Schiff, D.; Purow, B. & Abounader, R. (2009a). MicroRNA-34a inhibits glioblastoma growth by targeting multiple oncogenes. *Cancer Res,* Vol.69, No.19, pp. 7569-7576, ISSN 1538-7445 (Electronic)

Li, Y.; Li, W.; Yang, Y.; Lu, Y.; He, C.; Hu, G.; Liu, H.; Chen, J.; He, J. & Yu, H. (2009b). MicroRNA-21 targets LRRFIP1 and contributes to VM-26 resistance in glioblastoma multiforme. *Brain Res,* Vol.1286, pp. 13-18, ISSN 1872-6240

Luan, S.; Sun, L. & Huang, F. (2010). MicroRNA-34a: a novel tumor suppressor in p53-mutant glioma cell line U251. *Arch Med Res,* Vol.41, No.2, pp. 67-74, ISSN 1873-5487

Malzkorn, B.; Wolter, M.; Liesenberg, F.; Grzendowski, M.; Stuhler, K.; Meyer, H.E. & Reifenberger, G. (2010). Identification and functional characterization of microRNAs involved in the malignant progression of gliomas. *Brain Pathol,* Vol.20, No.3, pp. 539-550, ISSN 1750-3639

Nan, Y.; Han, L.; Zhang, A.; Wang, G.; Jia, Z.; Yang, Y.; Yue, X.; Pu, P.; Zhong, Y. & Kang, C. (2010). MiRNA-451 plays a role as tumor suppressor in human glioma cells. *Brain Res,* Vol.1359, pp. 14-21, ISSN 1872-6240

Novakova, J.; Slaby, O.; Vyzula, R. & Michalek, J. (2009). MicroRNA involvement in glioblastoma pathogenesis. *Biochem Biophys Res Commun,* Vol.386, No.1, pp. 1-5, ISSN 1090-2104

Ohno, M.; Natsume, A.; Kondo, Y.; Iwamizu, H.; Motomura, K.; Toda, H.; Ito, M.; Kato, T. & Wakabayashi, T. (2009). The modulation of microRNAs by type I IFN through the activation of signal transducers and activators of transcription 3 in human glioma. *Mol Cancer Res,* Vol.7, No.12, pp. 2022-2030, ISSN 1557-3125

Papagiannakopoulos, T.; Shapiro, A. & Kosik, K.S. (2008). MicroRNA-21 targets a network of key tumor-suppressive pathways in glioblastoma cells. *Cancer Res,* Vol.68, No.19, pp. 8164-8172, ISSN 1538-7445

Ren, Y.; Zhou, X.; Mei, M.; Yuan, X.B.; Han, L.; Wang, G.X.; Jia, Z.F.; Xu, P.; Pu, P.Y. & Kang, C.S. (2010). MicroRNA-21 inhibitor sensitizes human glioblastoma cells U251 (PTEN-mutant) and LN229 (PTEN-wild type) to taxol. *BMC Cancer,* Vol.10, pp. 27, ISSN 1471-2407

Sana, J.; Hajduch, M.; Michalek, J.; Vyzula, R. & Slaby, O. (2011). MicroRNAs and glioblastoma: roles in core signalling pathways and potential clinical implications. *J Cell Mol Med,* Vol.15, No.8, pp. 1636-1644, ISSN 1582-4934

Sasayama, T.; Nishihara, M.; Kondoh, T.; Hosoda, K. & Kohmura, E. (2009). MicroRNA-10b is overexpressed in malignant glioma and associated with tumor invasive factors, uPAR and RhoC. *Int J Cancer,* Vol.125, No.6, pp. 1407-1413, ISSN 1097-0215

Shi, L.; Chen, J.; Yang, J.; Pan, T.; Zhang, S. & Wang, Z. (2010). MiR-21 protected human glioblastoma U87MG cells from chemotherapeutic drug temozolomide induced apoptosis by decreasing Bax/Bcl-2 ratio and caspase-3 activity. *Brain Res,* Vol.1352, pp. 255-264, ISSN 1872-6240

Siomi, H. & Siomi, M.C. (2010). Posttranscriptional regulation of microRNA biogenesis in animals. *Mol Cell,* Vol.38, No.3, pp. 323-332, ISSN 1097-4164

Slaby, O.; Lakomy, R.; Fadrus, P.; Hrstka, R.; Kren, L.; Lzicarova, E.; Smrcka, M.; Svoboda, M.; Dolezalova, H.; Novakova, J.; Valik, D.; Vyzula, R. & Michalek, J. (2010). MicroRNA-181 family predicts response to concomitant chemoradiotherapy with temozolomide in glioblastoma patients. *Neoplasma,* Vol.57, No.3, pp. 264-269, ISSN 0028-2685

Song, L.; Huang, Q.; Chen, K.; Liu, L.; Lin, C.; Dai, T.; Yu, C.; Wu, Z. & Li, J. (2010). miR-218 inhibits the invasive ability of glioma cells by direct downregulation of IKK-beta. *Biochem Biophys Res Commun,* Vol.402, No.1, pp. 135-140, ISSN 1090-2104

Sun, L.; Yan, W.; Wang, Y.; Sun, G.; Luo, H.; Zhang, J.; Wang, X.; You, Y.; Yang, Z. & Liu, N. (2011). MicroRNA-10b induces glioma cell invasion by modulating MMP-14 and uPAR expression via HOXD10. *Brain Res,* Vol.1389, pp. 9-18, ISSN 1872-6240

Tektonidis, M.; Hatzikirou, H.; Chauviere, A.; Simon, M.; Schaller, K. & Deutsch, A. (2011). Identification of intrinsic in vitro cellular mechanisms for glioma invasion. *J Theor Biol,* Vol.287C, pp. 131-147, ISSN 1095-8541

Ujifuku, K.; Mitsutake, N.; Takakura, S.; Matsuse, M.; Saenko, V.; Suzuki, K.; Hayashi, K.; Matsuo, T.; Kamada, K.; Nagata, I. & Yamashita, S. (2010). miR-195, miR-455-3p and miR-10a(*) are implicated in acquired temozolomide resistance in glioblastoma multiforme cells. *Cancer Lett,* Vol.296, No.2, pp. 241-248, ISSN 1872-7980

Webster, R.J.; Giles, K.M.; Price, K.J.; Zhang, P.M.; Mattick, J.S. & Leedman, P.J. (2009). Regulation of epidermal growth factor receptor signaling in human cancer cells by microRNA-7. *J Biol Chem,* Vol.284, No.9, pp. 5731-5741, ISSN 0021-9258

Winter, J. & Diederichs, S. (2011). MicroRNA biogenesis and cancer. *Methods Mol Biol,* Vol.676, pp. 3-22, ISSN 1940-6029 (Electronic)

1064-3745 (Linking)

Winter, J.; Jung, S.; Keller, S.; Gregory, R.I. & Diederichs, S. (2009). Many roads to maturity: microRNA biogenesis pathways and their regulation. *Nat Cell Biol,* Vol.11, No.3, pp. 228-234, ISSN 1476-4679

Xia, H.; Qi, Y.; Ng, S.S.; Chen, X.; Li, D.; Chen, S.; Ge, R.; Jiang, S.; Li, G.; Chen, Y.; He, M.L.; Kung, H.F.; Lai, L. & Lin, M.C. (2009). microRNA-146b inhibits glioma cell migration and invasion by targeting MMPs. *Brain Res,* Vol.1269, pp. 158-165, ISSN 1872-6240

Yan, W.; Zhang, W.; Sun, L.; Liu, Y.; You, G.; Wang, Y.; Kang, C.; You, Y. & Jiang, T. (2011). Identification of MMP-9 specific microRNA expression profile as potential targets of anti-invasion therapy in glioblastoma multiforme. *Brain Res,* Vol.1411, pp. 108-115, ISSN 1872-6240

Zhang, B. & Farwell, M.A. (2008). microRNAs: a new emerging class of players for disease diagnostics and gene therapy. *J Cell Mol Med,* Vol.12, No.1, pp. 3-21, ISSN 1582-1838

Zhang, C.; Han, L.; Zhang, A.; Yang, W.; Zhou, X.; Pu, P.; Du, Y.; Zeng, H. & Kang, C. (2010a). Global changes of mRNA expression reveals an increased activity of the interferon-induced signal transducer and activator of transcription (STAT) pathway by repression of miR-221/222 in glioblastoma U251 cells. *Int J Oncol,* Vol.36, No.6, pp. 1503-1512, ISSN 1791-2423

Zhang, C.Z.; Zhang, J.X.; Zhang, A.L.; Shi, Z.D.; Han, L.; Jia, Z.F.; Yang, W.D.; Wang, G.X.; Jiang, T.; You, Y.P.; Pu, P.Y.; Cheng, J.Q. & Kang, C.S. (2010b). MiR-221 and miR-222 target PUMA to induce cell survival in glioblastoma. *Mol Cancer,* Vol.9, pp. 229, ISSN 1476-4598

Zhang, J.; Han, L.; Ge, Y.; Zhou, X.; Zhang, A.; Zhang, C.; Zhong, Y.; You, Y.; Pu, P. & Kang, C. (2010c). miR-221/222 promote malignant progression of glioma through activation of the Akt pathway. *Int J Oncol,* Vol.36, No.4, pp. 913-920, ISSN 1791-2423

Zhou, X.; Ren, Y.; Moore, L.; Mei, M.; You, Y.; Xu, P.; Wang, B.; Wang, G.; Jia, Z.; Pu, P.; Zhang, W. & Kang, C. (2010a). Downregulation of miR-21 inhibits EGFR pathway and suppresses the growth of human glioblastoma cells independent of PTEN status. *Lab Invest,* Vol.90, No.2, pp. 144-155, ISSN 1530-0307

Zhou, X.; Zhang, J.; Jia, Q.; Ren, Y.; Wang, Y.; Shi, L.; Liu, N.; Wang, G.; Pu, P.; You, Y. & Kang, C. (2010b). Reduction of miR-21 induces glioma cell apoptosis via activating caspase 9 and 3. *Oncol Rep,* Vol.24, No.1, pp. 195-201, ISSN 1791-2431

Ziegler, D.S.; Wright, R.D.; Kesari, S.; Lemieux, M.E.; Tran, M.A.; Jain, M.; Zawel, L. & Kung, A.L. (2008). Resistance of human glioblastoma multiforme cells to growth factor inhibitors is overcome by blockade of inhibitor of apoptosis proteins. *J Clin Invest,* Vol.118, No.9, pp. 3109-3122, ISSN 0021-9738

5

The Role of microRNAs in Gliomas and Their Potential Applications for Diagnosis and Treatment

Iris Lavon
Leslie and Michael Gaffin Center for Neuro-Oncology and Department of Neurology, The Agnes Ginges Center for Human Neurogenetics, Hadassah Hebrew University Medical Center, Jerusalem, Israel

1. Introduction

MicroRNAs (miRNAs) are a class of single-stranded non-coding RNAs that average 22 nucleotides in length. They regulate gene expression by binding to imperfectly matched sequences in the 3'-untranslated region (3'UTR) of target mRNAs, resulting in either translational repression or destabilization/degradation of their target mRNAs[1-7]. miRNAs play an important role in nearly all cancer types, where they modulate key tumorigenesis processes, such as metastasis, apoptosis, proliferation, and angiogenesis. Each miRNA can affect several different mRNAs and, depending on the target, has the potential to function as an oncogene and/or tumor suppressor.

It has recently been shown that miRNAs play important roles in gliomas [8-19]. A number of miRNAs, such as miR-21, miR-221, miR-222, miR-10b, and the miR-26a cluster [15,19], together with the genes cyclin-dependent kinase 4 (CDK4) and CENTG1, are upregulated in gliomas and appear to act in an oncogenic fashion. Other miRNAs, such as miR-124[8], miR-137[8], miR-34a[12,13], miR-128[16], miR-326[17] and members of the let-7[18] family, are downregulated indicating a tumor suppressive nature.

Several important target mRNAs and pathways have been identified for these onco-miRNAs and tumor suppressor miRNAs. For example, miR-34a is downregulated in glioblastomas as a result of p53 dysfunction, while restoring the expression of miR-34a[12] or miR-7[18] in glioma cells can strongly inhibit oncogenic pathways, such as Ras and Akt.

In addition to the singly transcribed miRNAs, our studies demonstrated that several miRNA clusters were shown to be deregulated in gliomas and might have an important role in the disease process. These clusters comprise the miR17 family, miR183-182, and the SC-specific clusters (miR367-302 and miR371-373), which are upregulated in gliomas. Because the massive cluster of 53 miRNAs on chromosome 14q32.31 is downregulated, it may represent the largest tumor suppressive miRNA cluster[20]. Some of these clusters, such as miR17-92, which is one of the three miRNA clusters related to the miR-17 family, reportedly have a pro-oncogenic roles in other type of cancers[21].

We have recently shown that gliomas share miRNA expression profiles that are similar to neural precursor cells[20]. This result is in agreement with the finding that gliomas contain heterogeneous neoplastic cell populations that phenotypically resemble undifferentiated or immature glial cells.

The study of miRNAs is rapidly developing and could considerably change the current conception of glioma biology. Detecting and quantifying microRNAs in tissue and serum will soon be routinely used for tumor classification and grading as well as diagnostic and prognostic testing for gliomas. For example, high levels of miR-21, miR-182 and miR-196 as well as low expression of miR-181b and miR-106a are associated with poor overall survival in patients with malignant gliomas[22-24], and these miRNAs might function as biomarkers of glioma progression. Furthermore, miR-195, miR-455-3p, miR-10a[25] and the miR-181 family[26] have been linked to treatment resistance, and assessing the relative expression levels of these miRNAs may assist with the design of personalized treatments.

New knowledge regarding the involvement of miRNAs in glioma biology has provided opportunities for the use of miRNAs or their inhibitors as potential candidates for the brain tumor treatments. However, such a therapeutic approach may be considerably challenging in light of several barriers *in vivo,* such as the blood–brain barrier[27], which can prevent miRNAs or their antagonists from entering the brain.

2. MicroRNA regulation of gene expression

miRNAs regulate gene expression inhibition through several proposed mechanisms. One model suggests that there is competition between RISC and eIF4E for mRNA binding, which represses initiation. A second model has proposed that Ago recruits eIF6 and, thus, prevents the association of the 60S ribosomal subunit with the 40S preinitiation complex[28,29]. The third model suggests that miRNAs destabilize target mRNAs by de-adenylation and subsequent decapping[30-34]. It was recently observed that AGO-2, mature miRNAs and translationally repressed mRNAs can accumulate in cytoplasmic processing bodies (P-bodies)[35]. These bodies are enriched with proteins involved in translational repression and in mRNA de-adenylation, decapping and degradation. Thus, they might function not only in storage but also in the decay of repressed mRNAs. However, it remains to be established whether the accumulation of these proteins in P-bodies is the cause rather than the consequence of target mRNA silencing[36,37].

3. Mechanisms responsible for altered miRNA expression in gliomas

Aberrant miRNA expression and function has been frequently observed in gliomas. A number of mechanisms are responsible for altered miRNA expression in cancer:

a. *Altered transcription regulation or abnormalities in miRNA processing.*

For miR-7, normal pre-miRNA levels were found to be associated with reduced mature miRNA levels in glioblastomas, where it was proven that the reduction in the miR-7 processing was occurred at the pri- to pre-miRNA processing step[38]. Various members of the let-7 family are regulated post-transcriptionally during embryonic brain development, the neural differentiation of embryonic stem cells (SC) and in embryocarcinoma. In these settings, the levels of the pre-miRNAs were consistent during differentiation; however, the mature forms increased [39]. Few studies shed some light on this mechanism by showing that the let-7 targets, the RNA-binding proteins Lin28 and Lin28B, bind to the loop region of let-7 precursors, which blocks the processing of let-7 at either the Drosha or the Dicer levels[40,41]. This Lin28-mediated degradation of let-7 likely plays a key role not only in development but also in tumorigenesis.

b. *Localization of miRNAs inside or close to cancer-associated genomic regions*[42,43].

This mechanism was suggested also for gliomas based on an array study on human glioma tumors and mouse and human glioma cell lines. The study demonstrated that the majority of the differentially expressed miRNAs were located in regions susceptible to genetic alterations in cancer [20].

c. *Epigenetic regulation of miRNA expression.*

This is illustrated bychanges in chromatin structures that are induced by covalent modifications of histones and/or DNA methylation[44]. For example, the epigenetic silencing of the miR-124 loci has been observed in brain tumors [8] and precancerous lesions[45]. The epigenetic masking of miR-124 induces activation of the oncogene cyclin-dependent kinase (CDK)-6 and consequent phosphorylation of Rb, resulting in accelerated cell growth.

It has been shown that the Let-7 family is downregulated in gliomas[18]. This miRNA family is considered to be comprised of tumor suppressor miRNAs. The let-7a-3 locus is generally methylated in normal tissues, but it is hypomethylated in some types of cancers. The methylation levels of let-7a-3 correlate inversely with let-7a-3 pri-miRNA expression levels; thus, Let-7a-3 hypomethylation facilitates the epigenetic reactivation of the gene resulting in elevated expression of let-7a-3 and enhanced tumor phenotypes and oncogenic changes[39,46]. Another example is miR-128, which is not regulated by epigenetics, but has been shown to play a role in the epigenesis of glioma SCs. Its downregulation in glioma tissue causes the elevated expression of Bmi-1, one of the polycomb group of genes that function as epigenetic silencers, which enhances cancer stem cell self-renewal through chromatin remodeling[16].

4. The involvement of miRNAs in pathways that may promote gliomagenesis and tumor progression

miRNAs have been shown to act as both oncogenes or tumor suppressor genes and, thus, affect pathways that bestow nearly all hallmarks of cancer[47,48]. These miRNAs can, in turn, promote gliomagenesis and tumor progression.

a. *Sustaining proliferative signaling*

For a tumor to become independent from external growth factor signals, it requires the activation of different cell proliferation and survival pathways, such as those mediated by epidermal growth factor receptor (EGFR) and Akt, which play a central role in glioblastomas. It has been demonstrated that miR-7 directly inhibits the expression of EGFR[38,49] and its downstream effector, Raf1, and suppresses the AKT pathway by targeting upstream regulators. Indeed, transfection with "mimic" miR-7 oligonucleotides decreased viability and invasiveness and induces cell cycle arrest and apoptosis of glioblastoma cell lines[38,49].

The altered regulation/activation of RAS proteins, which process signals downstream of growth receptors, plays a key role in the deregulation of multiple proliferation pathways in most types of tumors, including gliomas. Decreased levels of let-7 in gliomas correlate inversely with overexpression of RAS proteins, while restoring let-7 expression reduces the expression of RAS in glioma cell lines resulting in tumor growth inhibition *in vitro* and *in vivo*[18]. Moreover, the activation/overexpression of RAS leads to the upregulation of miR-21 *in-vitro* and *in-vivo*. Mir-21 exerts its oncogenic effect by downregulating the phosphatase and tensin homolog (PTEN) and programmed cell death 4 (PDCD4)[50]. In a number of human glioblastoma cell lines, such as T98G, A172, U87, and U251, the expression of PDCD4 protein correlates inversely with expression of miR-21. The downregulation of miR-21 in those cell lines leads to decreased proliferation, increased apoptosis, and decreased colony formation on soft agar[51].

DNA amplification of an onco-amplicon was observed in a subset of high-grade gliomas. This onco-amplicon consists of miR26a-2 and the oncoproteins CDK4 and CENTG1, which regulate the RB1 and PI3 kinase/AKT pathways, respectively. miR-26a alone can functionally target PTEN, RB1, and MAP3K2/MEKK2 protein expression, thereby increasing AKT activation, promoting proliferation, and decreasing c-JUN N-terminal kinase-dependent apoptosis *in vitro* and *in vivo*. The overexpression of miR-26a in cells overexpressing CDK4 or CENTG1 further promotes tumor growth *in vivo*. Glioblastoma patients harboring this amplification display markedly decreased survival[15,19].

b. *Evading growth suppressors*

miRNAs may also affect cell proliferation by controlling cell cycle regulators. The E2Fs transcription factor family plays a pivotal role in cell cycle progression. In response to mitogenic signaling, pRB is sequentially phosphorylated by the CDK/cyclin complexes leading to activation of E2F-responsive genes to promote cell cycle progression[52]. This pathway can be inhibited by several miRNAs. For example, miR-137, and miR-124a inhibit CDK6 expression in different cancer cell lines, including gliomas[8], where the transfection of miR-124 or miR-137 has been shown to prevent cell cycle progression in glioblastoma cell lines, which is associated with the decreased expression of CDK6 and pRB proteins[8]. miR-34a, which is transcriptionally activated by p53, can target both CDK6 and cyclin D1 preventing the downstream pro-survival signaling of the cyclin/CDK pathway. Restoring the expression of the underexpressed miR-34a in glioma cell lines downregulates CDK6 protein expressions and inhibits cell proliferation.[12]

The negative regulators of the cyclin/CDK pathway, such as members of the Cip/Kip family (p21, p27 and p57) and the INK4a/ARF family (p14 and p16), are regulated by several miRNAs. Upregulation of these miRNAs may inhibit these negative regulators and result in the proliferation and survival of the cells.

The miRNA clusters miR-106b-25 and miR-17-92 have anti-proliferative and pro-apoptotic activities in different tumor types through the inhibition of p21 in addition to other genes. Although they are also upregulated in gliomas[20], their role in the inhibition of p21 or other negative regulators of cyclin/CDK remain to be elucidated. High levels of miR-221/222, which targets both p27 and p57, appear in glioblastomas. Functional studies showed that miR-221/222 prevents quiescence when elevated during growth factor deprivation and induces precocious S-phase entry, thereby triggering cell death[53]. In addition, the overexpression of these miRNAs increases glioma cell proliferation *in-vitro* and induces glioma growth in a subcutaneous mouse model[54]. The inhibition of miR-10b, which is strongly upregulated in gliomas, reduces glioma cell growth through cell-cycle arrest and apoptosis. These cellular responses are mediated by augmented expression of its direct targets, including p21 and CDKN2A/p16[55].

c. *Resisting cell death*

In addition to the role of miR-221/222 in cell growth and cell cycle progression, it has been demonstrated that miR-221/222 directly regulates apoptosis by targeting p53-upregulated-modulator-of-apoptosis (PUMA) in glioblastoma. PUMA binds to Bcl-2 and Bcl-XL through a BH3 domain and the exogenous expression of PUMA results in an extremely rapid and profound apoptosis[56]. Thus, the forced expression of miR-221/222 downregulates PUMA and induces cell survival, whereas the knockdown of miR-221/222 induces PUMA expression and cell apoptosis as well as decreases tumor growth in a xenograft model[57].

d. *Inducing angiogenesis*

Recent studies have revealed important roles for miRNAs such as the endothelial cell (EC)-restricted miRNA miR-126 as well as miR-378, miR-296, miR-92a and the miR-17-92 cluster in regulating angiogenesis. Thus, these have been termed angiomirs[58].

The level of the angiomir miR-296, which inhibits the degradation of the VEGF receptor, is increased in EC cells co-cultured with glioma cells or in response to angiogenic growth factors (including VEGF). When miR-296 is inhibited *in vivo*, the vascularization of tumor xenografts decreases[59]. miR-93, one of the miRNAs within the miR-106b-25 cluster, a member of the miR-17 family, enhances cell survival, promotes sphere formation and augments tumor growth. *In vivo* studies revealed that miR-93-expressing cells induced blood vessel formation, likely through targeting integrin-β8, allowing blood vessels to extend to tumor tissues in high densities. These findings show that miR-93 promotes tumor growth and angiogenesis through the suppression of integrin-β8 expression.

e. *Activating invasion and metastasis*

As mentioned above, miR-21 is overexpressed in gliomas. The metalloproteinase (MMPS) inhibitors RECK and TIMP3 are two targets of miR-21. RECK is a membrane-anchorage regulator, while TIMP3 is an extracellular matrix (ECM)-bound protease inhibitor. Treatment with antisense oligonucleotides to miR-21 in glioma cell lines and in a nude mouse model of human glioma resulted in elevated levels of RECK and TIMP3 and, therefore, reduced MMP activities. Thus, downregulation of miR-21 in glioma cells leads to a decrease in their migratory and invasion abilities[11].

miR-10b is highly expressed in many tumors, including glioblastomas. It was found that miR-10b induces glioma cell invasion by modulating the expression of the tumor invasion factors MMP-14 and uPAR through directly targeting HOXD10. Accordingly, glioma cells lost their invasive ability when they were treated with specific antisense oligonucleotides to miR-10b.

Not surprisingly, additional miRNAs are currently being identified and associated with ECM reorganization in relationship to cancer. Like miR-21 and 10b, miR-146b has also been demonstrated to play a role in glioma cell invasion[60]. However, miR-146b does not function through the suppression of ECM inhibitors; rather, its loss in gliomas allows the upregulation of MMP16, which might cause proteolysis of ECM components, such as type III collagen. Thus, low levels of miR-146b contribute to the migration and invasion of glioma[60].

f. Reprogramming energy metabolism

Pyruvate kinase type M2 (PKM2) is one of four isoenzymes of pyruvate kinase, which catalyzes the last step within glycolysis. This enzyme is normally thought to be embryonically restricted; however, it has been shown to be expressed in cancerous cells[61]. Recently, it was shown that the levels of PKM2 negatively correlate with the levels of miR-326, suggesting a regulatory relationship between PKM2 and miR-326. Furthermore, miR-326 decreased the glioma metabolic activity by decreasing ATP levels, suggesting that miR-326 could regulate glioma metabolism through the downregulation of PKM2[62].

5. The glioma microRNA expression signature

Differential miRNA expression in gliomas was first reported by Ciafre`[63] and Chan[64]. Their study revealed that miR-21[64] and miR-221 are upregulated, whereas miR-128, miR-181a, miR-181b and miR-181c are downregulated, in glioblastoma[63]. Other array-based approaches identified that the expression of miR-124, miR-128a, and miR-137 are decreased in anaplastic astrocytomas and glioblastomas[8]. In addition, miR-124 is decreased in oligodendroglial tumors[65] relative to non-neoplastic control brain tissues.

The expression levels of miR-124 and miR-137 were increased during the differentiation of mouse neural progenitor cells (NPCs) following growth factor withdrawal. Thus, the authors have suggested that these specific miRNAs display "stemness" of glioma cells and that alteration of the levels of these miRNAs may induce differentiation[8].

While these studies compared microRNA expression in gliomas relative to control tissues, other studies explored the role of miRNAs in glioma progression. One study investigated miRNA expression profiles in primary WHO grade II gliomas that spontaneously progressed to WHO grade IV secondary glioblastomas. They identified 12 miRNAs (miR-9, miR-15a, miR-16, miR-17, miR-19a, miR-20a, miR-21, miR-25, miR-28, miR-130b, miR-140 and miR-210) that were upregulated and two miRNAs (miR-184 and miR-328) that were downregulated upon glioma progression[66]. Other studies have compared the differential miRNA expression between astrocytomas and glioblastomas and revealed a 23-miRNA expression signature that can discriminate glioblastomas from anaplastic astrocytomas with an overall diagnostic accuracy of 89.7%67.

Our study compared the miRNA expression signatures of glial tumors, embryonic SCs, NPCs and normal adult brains from both human and mouse tissues. We demonstrated that all gliomas displayed NPC-like miRNA signatures. About half of the miRNAs expressed in the NPCs-glioma shared profile were clustered in seven genomic regions. These clusters comprised the miR17 family (3 clusters), miR183-182, and the SC-specific clusters miR367-302 and miR371-373, which are upregulate. They also contained the bipartite cluster of 7+46 miRNAs on chromosome 14q32.31, which is downregulated in the shared expression profile. These seven regions are particularly prone to genetic and/or epigenetic aberrations in different types of cancers (e.g., LOH on chromosome 14q32.31, or the amplification of chromosome 13q31.3). Together, these findings suggest that NPCs may be the originating cells in gliomas and that aberrations in critical regions might be necessary to maintain the stem cell nature of gliomas[20].

A recent paper analyzed microRNA expression data from The Cancer Genome Atlas (TCGA) and identified five clinically and genetically distinct glioblastoma subclasses related to a different neural precursor cell types. Thus, like us they also suggested that glioblastomas can arise from neural precursor cells but emphasized that the cell of origin could arise from multiple stages of differentiation[68].

6. microRNAs as biomarkers for the diagnosis and prognosis of gliomas

As reviewed above, a large number of recent studies have discovered that miRNAs play important regulatory roles in a variety of cellular functions in gliomas. Other papers have demonstrated that miRNAs can be used for tumor classification and grading[66,67] in addition to the diagnosis[23], prognosis[22,23] and prediction of therapeutic efficacy[69, 69] of tumors. The discovery of miRNAs in the serum of cancer patients[70] opened up the exciting possibility of using miRNAs as non-invasive biomarkers. Thus, detecting and quantifying microRNAs may soon be used in routine clinical practice for diagnostic and prognostic glioma testing.

The expression levels of miR-182[22] and miR-196[23] are significant in correlation with World Health Organization glioma grading ($P < 0.001$). Multivariate analysis showed that the expression of both these miRNAs is a predictor of overall survival in glioblastoma patients [22,23]. Analysis of miRNA expression data in glioblastoma patients ($n = 222$) derived from the TCGA dataset identified an expression signature of ten miRNAs that can predict glioblastoma (GBM) patient survival[71]. In astrocytomas, the downregulation of miR-137 has been shown to be associated with advanced clinical stages of the disease; and the low expression levels of miR-181b and miR-106a, or high expression of miR-21, are significantly associated with poor patient survival[24]. Several papers aimed to identify the miRNAs specifically involved in the acquisition of temozolomide (TMZ) resistance in glioblastoma. In one article, the authors established resistant variant U251R cells from a TMZ-sensitive glioblastoma cell line (U251MG) and performed miRNA microarray on both the resistant and sensitive cell lines. The results showed that miR-195, miR-455-3p and miR-10a* were the three most upregulated miRNAs in the resistant cells. When miR-195 was reduced, the resistant cells displayed a moderate cell killing effect, and the combination with TMZ strongly enhanced this effect[25]. Another article examined the correlation between the expression levels of selected microRNAs in 22 primary glioblastomas with response to concomitant therapy (e.g., chemoradiotherapy with TMZ). They found that miR-181b and miR-181c were significantly downregulated in patients who responded to concomitant therapy compared to patients with progredient disease[26].

Over many decades, it has been shown that cell-free DNA and RNA is present in the circulation and may represent potential biomarkers. We have demonstrated that tumor-specific DNA can be detected in the serum of glioma patients and is a potentially promising tool for brain tumor diagnosis[72]. Skog et al. was the first to demonstrate that brain microvascular endothelial cells take up exosomes, which contain mRNA, miRNA, and angiogenic proteins released by glioblastoma cells. Moreover, they showed that miR-21 is more elevated in serum microvesicles from glioblastoma patients than in healthy controls[73].

Based on their potential as prognostic and diagnostic biomarkers, circulating miRNAs are promising non-invasive tumor markers. Tumor-specific circulating miRNAs may improve cancer diagnosis and prognosis because, as described above, several promising miRNAs have already been recognized as potential biomarkers for gliomas.

7. The therapeutic potential of microRNAs in gliomas

With the increased understanding of the miRNA target genes, the cellular behaviors influenced by them and the ability of one microRNA, such as let-7 or miR-21, to target more than one gene or pathway provide exciting opportunities to use miRNAs or their inhibitors as potential candidates for the treatment of brain tumors.

There have been few pre-clinical and phase I/II studies that showed some success in using synthetic miRNA mimics or anti-miRNA oligonucleotides as therapeutic agents. Two of these studies demonstrated that delivery of the locked-nucleic-acid (LNA)-anti-miR in African green monkeys silences miR-122, decreases the total plasma cholesterol[74] and suppresses HCV viremia[75] with no evidence of hepatotoxicity. Another study showed that the silencing of miR-155 in a mouse inflammation model by LNA-anti-miR administration results in derepression of the C/EBP Beta isoforms and downregulation of granulocyte-colony stimulating factor expression in mouse splenocytes[76]. In gliomas, the silencing of miR-21 by LNA-anti-miR followed by TRAIL treatment increased caspase activity *in vitro* and reduced tumor growth *in vivo*[10]. These results support the potential of LNA-anti-miR as therapeutics for inhibition of disease-associated miRNAs.

An alternative to chemically modified antisense oligonucleotides is the "miR sponge". These competitive miR inhibitors contain multiple binding sites to an miR of interest, preventing it from binding to its natural target. In this way, a single sponge can block all miR family members containing the same seed sequences. The sponge strategy has been used to inhibit miR-31 *in vivo* in a noninvasive breast cancer cell line. miR sponges that carried miR-31 recognition motifs were introduced into a retroviral vector and reduced miR-31 function significantly[77].

Some preclinical studies have shown promising results using self-complementary adeno-associated viral (scAAV) vectors. For example, a scAAV vector containing miR-26a was administered with a single tail-vein injection into mice with established liver tumors. High miR-26a levels were found in their livers and no toxic effects were observed. While six out of eight mice treated with the control virus developed tumors, eight out of ten miR-26a-treated mice developed only small tumors or had a complete absence of tumors[78].

Although most of these therapeutic approaches appear promising for systemic tumors, they would be considerably challenging in brain tumors due to several obstacles and barriers *in vivo,* such as the blood–brain barrier[27], which might prevent the miRNAs or their antagonists from entering the brain. Thus, the development of more efficient and specific delivery systems is necessary before miRNAs can be used as therapeutic agents for the treatment of malignant gliomas.

At a glance:

- A number of miRNAs are upregulated in gliomas and appear to act as oncogenes while other miRNAs, are downregulated indicating a tumor suppressive nature. These onco-miRNAs and tumor suppressor miRNAs modulate key processes that promote gliomagenesis and tumor progression, such as sustaining proliferative signaling, evading growth suppressors, resisting cell death, inducing angiogenesis, activating invasion and metastasis and reprogramming energy metabolism
- Not only individual, but also miRNA clusters are deregulated in gliomas. Some, such the huge cluster of 53 miRNAs on chromosome 14q32.31 are downregulated in gliomas, and may act as a tumor suppressive miRNA clusters and others such as miR17-92 are upregulated and reportedly have a pro-oncogenic role in cancer.
- Gliomas display miRNA expression profile that is similar to neural precursor cells. This result is compatible with the phenotypically resemble of part of the neoplastic cell populations within glioblastomas to undifferentiated or immature glial cells.
- Detecting and quantifying microRNAs in tissue and serum will soon be routinely used for tumor classification and grading as well as diagnostic and prognostic testing for gliomas and may assist with the design of personalized treatments.
- Manipulating the expression of miRNAs that are involved in glioma biology might provide opportunities for brain tumor treatments.

8. References

[1] Eulalio A, Huntzinger E, Izaurralde E. Getting to the root of miRNA-mediated gene silencing. *Cell.* Jan 11 2008;132(1):9-14.

[2] Ambros V. MicroRNA pathways in flies and worms: growth, death, fat, stress, and timing. *Cell.* Jun 13 2003;113(6):673-676.

[3] Baek D, Villen J, Shin C, Camargo FD, Gygi SP, Bartel DP. The impact of microRNAs on protein output. *Nature.* Sep 4 2008;455(7209):64-71.

[4] Selbach M, Schwanhausser B, Thierfelder N, Fang Z, Khanin R, Rajewsky N. Widespread changes in protein synthesis induced by microRNAs. *Nature.* Sep 4 2008;455(7209):58-63.

[5] Sen GL, Blau HM. Argonaute 2/RISC resides in sites of mammalian mRNA decay known as cytoplasmic bodies. *Nat Cell Biol.* Jun 2005;7(6):633-636.

[6] Yu Z, Jian Z, Shen SH, Purisima E, Wang E. Global analysis of microRNA target gene expression reveals that miRNA targets are lower expressed in mature mouse and Drosophila tissues than in the embryos. *Nucleic Acids Res.* 2007;35(1):152-164.

[7] Filipowicz W, Bhattacharyya SN, Sonenberg N. Mechanisms of post-transcriptional regulation by microRNAs: are the answers in sight? *Nat Rev Genet.* Feb 2008;9(2):102-114.

[8] Silber J, Lim DA, Petritsch C, et al. miR-124 and miR-137 inhibit proliferation of glioblastoma multiforme cells and induce differentiation of brain tumor stem cells. *BMC Med.* 2008;6:14.

[9] Sasayama T, Nishihara M, Kondoh T, Hosoda K, Kohmura E. MicroRNA-10b is overexpressed in malignant glioma and associated with tumor invasive factors, uPAR and RhoC. *Int J Cancer.* Sep 15 2009;125(6):1407-1413.

[10] Corsten MF, Miranda R, Kasmieh R, Krichevsky AM, Weissleder R, Shah K. MicroRNA-21 knockdown disrupts glioma growth in vivo and displays synergistic cytotoxicity with neural precursor cell delivered S-TRAIL in human gliomas. *Cancer Res.* Oct 1 2007;67(19):8994-9000.

[11] Gabriely G, Wurdinger T, Kesari S, et al. MicroRNA 21 promotes glioma invasion by targeting matrix metalloproteinase regulators. *Mol Cell Biol.* Sep 2008;28(17):5369-5380.

[12] Li Y, Guessous F, Zhang Y, et al. MicroRNA-34a inhibits glioblastoma growth by targeting multiple oncogenes. *Cancer Res.* Oct 1 2009;69(19):7569-7576.

[13] Guessous F, Zhang Y, Kofman A, et al. microRNA-34a is tumor suppressive in brain tumors and glioma stem cells. *Cell Cycle.* Mar 18 2010;9(6).

[14] Gillies JK, Lorimer IA. Regulation of p27Kip1 by miRNA 221/222 in glioblastoma. *Cell Cycle.* Aug 15 2007;6(16):2005-2009.

[15] Kim H, Huang W, Jiang X, Pennicooke B, Park PJ, Johnson MD. Integrative genome analysis reveals an oncomir/oncogene cluster regulating glioblastoma survivorship. *Proc Natl Acad Sci U S A.* Feb 2 2010;107(5):2183-2188.

[16] Godlewski J, Nowicki MO, Bronisz A, et al. Targeting of the Bmi-1 oncogene/stem cell renewal factor by microRNA-128 inhibits glioma proliferation and self-renewal. *Cancer Res.* Nov 15 2008;68(22):9125-9130.

[17] Kefas B, Comeau L, Floyd DH, et al. The neuronal microRNA miR-326 acts in a feedback loop with notch and has therapeutic potential against brain tumors. *J Neurosci.* Dec 2 2009;29(48):15161-15168.

[18] Lee ST, Chu K, Oh HJ, et al. Let-7 microRNA inhibits the proliferation of human glioblastoma cells. *J Neurooncol.* Jul 7 2010.

[19] Huse JT, Brennan C, Hambardzumyan D, et al. The PTEN-regulating microRNA miR-26a is amplified in high-grade glioma and facilitates gliomagenesis in vivo. *Genes Dev.* Jun 1 2009;23(11):1327-1337.

[20] Lavon I, Zrihan D, Granit A, et al. Gliomas display a microRNA expression profile reminiscent of neural precursor cells. *Neuro Oncol.* May 2010;12(5):422-433.

[21] Olive V, Jiang I, He L. mir-17-92, a cluster of miRNAs in the midst of the cancer network. *Int J Biochem Cell Biol.* Aug 2010;42(8):1348-1354.

[22] Jiang L, Mao P, Song L, et al. miR-182 as a prognostic marker for glioma progression and patient survival. *Am J Pathol.* Jul 2010;177(1):29-38.

[23] Guan Y, Mizoguchi M, Yoshimoto K, et al. MiRNA-196 is upregulated in glioblastoma but not in anaplastic astrocytoma and has prognostic significance. *Clin Cancer Res.* Aug 15 2010;16(16):4289-4297.

[24] Zhi F, Chen X, Wang S, et al. The use of hsa-miR-21, hsa-miR-181b and hsa-miR-106a as prognostic indicators of astrocytoma. *Eur J Cancer.* Jun 2010;46(9):1640-1649.

[25] Ujifuku K, Mitsutake N, Takakura S, et al. miR-195, miR-455-3p and miR-10a(*) are implicated in acquired temozolomide resistance in glioblastoma multiforme cells. *Cancer Lett.* Oct 28 2010;296(2):241-248.

[26] Slaby O, Lakomy R, Fadrus P, et al. MicroRNA-181 family predicts response to concomitant chemoradiotherapy with temozolomide in glioblastoma patients. *Neoplasma.* 2010;57(3):264-269.

[27] Purow B. The elephant in the room: do microRNA-based therapies have a realistic chance of succeeding for brain tumors such as glioblastoma? *J Neurooncol.* Nov 17 2010.

[28] Kiriakidou M, Tan GS, Lamprinaki S, De Planell-Saguer M, Nelson PT, Mourelatos Z. An mRNA m7G cap binding-like motif within human Ago2 represses translation. *Cell.* Jun 15 2007;129(6):1141-1151.

[29] Chendrimada TP, Finn KJ, Ji X, et al. MicroRNA silencing through RISC recruitment of eIF6. *Nature.* Jun 14 2007;447(7146):823-828.

[30] Beilharz TH, Humphreys DT, Clancy JL, et al. microRNA-mediated messenger RNA deadenylation contributes to translational repression in mammalian cells. *PLoS One.* 2009;4(8):e6783.

[31] Bagga S, Bracht J, Hunter S, et al. Regulation by let-7 and lin-4 miRNAs results in target mRNA degradation. *Cell.* Aug 26 2005;122(4):553-563.

[32] Behm-Ansmant I, Rehwinkel J, Izaurralde E. MicroRNAs silence gene expression by repressing protein expression and/or by promoting mRNA decay. *Cold Spring Harb Symp Quant Biol.* 2006;71:523-530.

[33] Wu L, Belasco JG. Micro-RNA regulation of the mammalian lin-28 gene during neuronal differentiation of embryonal carcinoma cells. *Mol Cell Biol.* Nov 2005;25(21):9198-9208.

[34] Eulalio A, Huntzinger E, Nishihara T, Rehwinkel J, Fauser M, Izaurralde E. Deadenylation is a widespread effect of miRNA regulation. *RNA.* Jan 2009;15(1):21-32.

[35] Yao B, Li S, Lian SL, Fritzler MJ, Chan EK. Mapping of Ago2-GW182 functional interactions. *Methods Mol Biol.* 2011;725:45-62.

[36] Eulalio A, Rehwinkel J, Stricker M, et al. Target-specific requirements for enhancers of decapping in miRNA-mediated gene silencing. *Genes Dev.* Oct 15 2007;21(20):2558-2570.

[37] Pauley KM, Eystathioy T, Jakymiw A, Hamel JC, Fritzler MJ, Chan EK. Formation of GW bodies is a consequence of microRNA genesis. *EMBO Rep.* Sep 2006;7(9):904-910.

[38] Kefas B, Godlewski J, Comeau L, et al. microRNA-7 inhibits the epidermal growth factor receptor and the Akt pathway and is down-regulated in glioblastoma. *Cancer Res.* May 15 2008;68(10):3566-3572.

[39] Wulczyn FG, Smirnova L, Rybak A, et al. Post-transcriptional regulation of the let-7 microRNA during neural cell specification. *FASEB J.* Feb 2007;21(2):415-426.

[40] Newman MA, Thomson JM, Hammond SM. Lin-28 interaction with the Let-7 precursor loop mediates regulated microRNA processing. *RNA.* Aug 2008;14(8):1539-1549.

[41] Rybak A, Fuchs H, Smirnova L, et al. A feedback loop comprising lin-28 and let-7 controls pre-let-7 maturation during neural stem-cell commitment. *Nat Cell Biol.* Aug 2008;10(8):987-993.

[42] Calin GA, Sevignani C, Dumitru CD, et al. Human microRNA genes are frequently located at fragile sites and genomic regions involved in cancers. *Proc Natl Acad Sci U S A.* Mar 2 2004;101(9):2999-3004.

[43] Makunin IV, Pheasant M, Simons C, Mattick JS. Orthologous microRNA genes are located in cancer-associated genomic regions in human and mouse. *PLoS One.* 2007;2(11):e1133.

[44] Saito Y, Jones PA. Epigenetic activation of tumor suppressor microRNAs in human cancer cells. *Cell Cycle.* Oct 2006;5(19):2220-2222.

[45] Ando T, Yoshida T, Enomoto S, et al. DNA methylation of microRNA genes in gastric mucosae of gastric cancer patients: its possible involvement in the formation of epigenetic field defect. *Int J Cancer.* May 15 2009;124(10):2367-2374.

[46] Brueckner B, Stresemann C, Kuner R, et al. The human let-7a-3 locus contains an epigenetically regulated microRNA gene with oncogenic function. *Cancer Res.* Feb 15 2007;67(4):1419-1423.

[47] Hanahan D, Weinberg RA. The hallmarks of cancer. *Cell.* Jan 7 2000;100(1):57-70.

[48] Hanahan D, Weinberg RA. Hallmarks of cancer: the next generation. *Cell.* Mar 4 2011;144(5):646-674.

[49] Webster RJ, Giles KM, Price KJ, Zhang PM, Mattick JS, Leedman PJ. Regulation of epidermal growth factor receptor signaling in human cancer cells by microRNA-7. *J Biol Chem.* Feb 27 2009;284(9):5731-5741.

[50] Talotta F, Cimmino A, Matarazzo MR, et al. An autoregulatory loop mediated by miR-21 and PDCD4 controls the AP-1 activity in RAS transformation. *Oncogene.* Jan 8 2009;28(1):73-84.

[51] Gaur AB, Holbeck SL, Colburn NH, Israel MA. Downregulation of Pdcd4 by mir-21 facilitates glioblastoma proliferation in vivo. *Neuro Oncol.* Jun 2011;13(6):580-590.

[52] Trimarchi JM, Lees JA. Sibling rivalry in the E2F family. *Nat Rev Mol Cell Biol.* Jan 2002;3(1):11-20.

[53] Medina R, Zaidi SK, Liu CG, et al. MicroRNAs 221 and 222 bypass quiescence and compromise cell survival. *Cancer Res.* Apr 15 2008;68(8):2773-2780.

[54] Zhang J, Han L, Ge Y, et al. miR-221/222 promote malignant progression of glioma through activation of the Akt pathway. *Int J Oncol.* Apr 2011;36(4):913-920.

[55] Gabriely G, Yi M, Narayan RS, et al. Human Glioma Growth Is Controlled by MicroRNA-10b. *Cancer Res.* May 15 2011;71(10):3563-3572.

[56] Yu J, Zhang L, Hwang PM, Kinzler KW, Vogelstein B. PUMA induces the rapid apoptosis of colorectal cancer cells. *Mol Cell.* Mar 2001;7(3):673-682.

[57] Zhang CZ, Zhang JX, Zhang AL, et al. MiR-221 and miR-222 target PUMA to induce cell survival in glioblastoma. *Mol Cancer.* 2010;9:229.

[58] Wang S, Olson EN. AngiomiRs--key regulators of angiogenesis. *Curr Opin Genet Dev.* Jun 2009;19(3):205-211.

[59] Wurdinger T, Tannous BA, Saydam O, et al. miR-296 regulates growth factor receptor overexpression in angiogenic endothelial cells. *Cancer Cell.* Nov 4 2008;14(5):382-393.

[60] Xia H, Qi Y, Ng SS, et al. microRNA-146b inhibits glioma cell migration and invasion by targeting MMPs. *Brain Res.* May 7 2009;1269:158-165.

[61] Mazurek S, Boschek CB, Hugo F, Eigenbrodt E. Pyruvate kinase type M2 and its role in tumor growth and spreading. *Semin Cancer Biol.* Aug 2005;15(4):300-308.

[62] Kefas B, Comeau L, Erdle N, Montgomery E, Amos S, Purow B. Pyruvate kinase M2 is a target of the tumor-suppressive microRNA-326 and regulates the survival of glioma cells. *Neuro Oncol.* Nov 2010;12(11):1102-1112.

[63] Ciafre SA, Galardi S, Mangiola A, et al. Extensive modulation of a set of microRNAs in primary glioblastoma. *Biochem Biophys Res Commun.* Sep 9 2005;334(4):1351-1358.

[64] Chan JA, Krichevsky AM, Kosik KS. MicroRNA-21 is an antiapoptotic factor in human glioblastoma cells. *Cancer Res.* Jul 15 2005;65(14):6029-6033.

[65] Nelson PT, Baldwin DA, Kloosterman WP, Kauppinen S, Plasterk RH, Mourelatos Z. RAKE and LNA-ISH reveal microRNA expression and localization in archival human brain. *RNA.* Feb 2006;12(2):187-191.

[66] Malzkorn B, Wolter M, Liesenberg F, et al. Identification and functional characterization of microRNAs involved in the malignant progression of gliomas. *Brain Pathol.* May 2010;20(3):539-550.

[67] Rao SA, Santosh V, Somasundaram K. Genome-wide expression profiling identifies deregulated miRNAs in malignant astrocytoma. *Mod Pathol.* Oct 2010;23(10):1404-1417.

[68] Kim TM, Huang W, Park R, Park PJ, Johnson MD. A Developmental Taxonomy of Glioblastoma Defined and Maintained by MicroRNAs. *Cancer Res.* May 1 2011;71(9):3387-3399.

[69] !!! INVALID CITATION !!!

[70] Lawrie CH, Gal S, Dunlop HM, et al. Detection of elevated levels of tumour-associated microRNAs in serum of patients with diffuse large B-cell lymphoma. *Br J Haematol.* May 2008;141(5):672-675.

[71] Srinivasan S, Patric IR, Somasundaram K. A ten-microRNA expression signature predicts survival in glioblastoma. *PLoS One.* 2011;6(3):e17438.

[72] Lavon I, Refael M, Zelikovitch B, Shalom E, Siegal T. Serum DNA can define tumor-specific genetic and epigenetic markers in gliomas of various grades. *Neuro Oncol.* Feb 2010;12(2):173-180.

[73] Skog J, Wurdinger T, van Rijn S, et al. Glioblastoma microvesicles transport RNA and proteins that promote tumour growth and provide diagnostic biomarkers. *Nat Cell Biol.* Dec 2008;10(12):1470-1476.

[74] Elmen J, Lindow M, Schutz S, et al. LNA-mediated microRNA silencing in non-human primates. *Nature.* Apr 17 2008;452(7189):896-899.

[75] Lanford RE, Hildebrandt-Eriksen ES, Petri A, et al. Therapeutic silencing of microRNA-122 in primates with chronic hepatitis C virus infection. *Science.* Jan 8 2010;327(5962):198-201.

[76] Worm J, Stenvang J, Petri A, et al. Silencing of microRNA-155 in mice during acute inflammatory response leads to derepression of c/ebp Beta and down-regulation of G-CSF. *Nucleic Acids Res.* Sep 2009;37(17):5784-5792.

[77] Valastyan S, Reinhardt F, Benaich N, et al. A pleiotropically acting microRNA, miR-31, inhibits breast cancer metastasis. *Cell.* Jun 12 2009;137(6):1032-1046.

[78] Kota J, Chivukula RR, O'Donnell KA, et al. Therapeutic microRNA delivery suppresses tumorigenesis in a murine liver cancer model. *Cell.* Jun 12 2009;137(6):1005-1017.

Part 4

Inhibition of Invasion in Treatment of Glioma

6

Molecular Targets: Inhibition of Tumor Cell Invasion

Raquel Brandão Haga and Silvya Stuchi Maria-Engler*
Department of Clinical Chemistry and Toxicology, School of Pharmaceutical Sciences, University of São Paulo
Brazil

1. Introduction

Gliomas are solid brain tumors that arise from glial cells. According to World Health Organization (WHO), they are classified in four grades based in their histological features. Grades I and II are considered low-grade gliomas and grades III and IV, malignant gliomas. In the United States, each year more than 22,000 people are diagnosed with malignant glioma, representing almost 70% of all malignant primary brain tumors in adults (Wen & Kesari, 2008; CBTRUS 2010; Jones & Holland, 2010).

Despite years of research, mortality rates are still high for patients diagnosed with malignant gliomas. Glioblastoma multiforme (WHO grade IV) is the most frequent malignant brain tumor in adults. Even with heavy treatment that includes surgery, radiotherapy and adjuvant chemotherapy, the median survival remains in the range of 12-15 months for patients with this type of tumor (Minniti et al., 2009; Jones & Holland, 2010).

Glioblastomas are separated in two main subtypes: primary glioblastomas and secondary glioblastomas. Primary glioblastoma affects preferentially patients older than 50 years old and has genetic alterations as epidermal growth factor receptor (EGFR) amplification and mutation, loss of heterozygosity of chromosome 10q, deletion of the phosphatase and tensin homologue on chromosome 10 (PTEN), and p16 deletion. Secondary glioblastoma starts as low-grade or anaplastic astrocytomas in younger patients and progresses to glioblastoma over the years. Its main alterations involve mutations in *TP53*, overexpression of platelet derived growth factor receptor (PDGFR), changes in p16 and retinoblastoma pathways, and loss of heterozygosity of chromosome 10q. Even morphologically similar, primary and secondary glioblastomas may differ in their response to molecular targeted therapy (Wen & Kesari, 2008).

1.1 Current treatment

Choosing the best treatment depends on the type of tumor, position in the brain, its size and its grade. For patients newly diagnosed with brain malignancies, the current standard treatment protocols include maximally surgical resection, followed by chemotherapy concomitant to fractioned radiation therapy of the tumor. Adjuvant chemotherapy for

* Corresponding Author

glioblastomas is based on alkylating agents-based as temozolomide (TMZ) or carmusite wafers (Gliadel®), the latter being inserted in the surgery cavity during operation (Argyriou et al., 2009; Minniti et al., 2009). TMZ is a second-generation imidazotetrazine derivative and its cytotoxic effects are caused by the methylation of specific DNA site as O_6 position of guanine. In recurrent tumors some patients undergo reoperation. The chemotherapy used in this case is carmusite wafers (Gliadel®), conventional therapy as lomusite, PCV and carboplatin, bevacizumab plus irinotecan, and experimental therapies (Wen & Kesari, 2008). Although these treatments are well established, they are still just palliative and not curative in almost all cases.

The failure in malignant glioma treatment is due multiple causes that include invasive nature of glioma cells, resistance to radiotherapy and chemotherapy; and presence of the blood brain barrier (Figure 1).

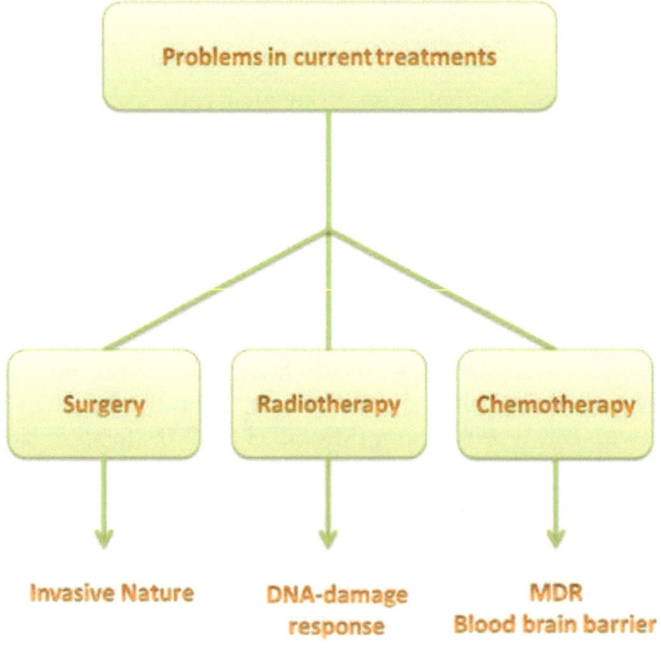

Fig. 1. Causes of resistance to current treatments. MDR = multidrug resistance.

1.2 Resistance

Resistance is a current problem in the treatment of almost all cancers, and in glioma this would not be different. Malignant gliomas have some characteristics that make them especially difficult to treat. Due to the diffuse nature of gliomas, they should not be considered a local disease. This feature limits the effectiveness of local therapeutic approaches, as surgery (Goldbrunner et al., 1999). Other important factors are the presence of the blood brain barrier (BBB) and the inter- and intratumor heterogeneity which lead to fail in radio and chemotherapies (Jones & Holland).

Combination of chemotherapy with radiation has improved a little the patient survival. However, these results are still very far from providing an effective treatment. Multidrug resistance (MDR) is one of the reasons for the poor response to standard treatments. MDR is a characteristic of cancer cells where these cells are resistant to an abroad spectrum of drugs with different modes of action. The mechanisms of chemoresistance are complex and multifactorial; and can be separated in intrinsic resistance or acquired resistance. The intrinsic resistance is present at the beginning of the treatment. The drug-resistant cells already express one or more resistance-mediating proteins or pathways. The acquired resistance is the resistance that is developed during the treatment. The three major mechanisms of drug resistance in cells are related to decreased uptake, especially for drugs that need transporters to enter the cell; changes in the cell regarding cell cycle, DNA-damage repair, apoptosis and drug metabolism, leading to alteration in the cytotoxicity of some drugs; and increase in the energy demanding to hydrophobic drugs to enter the cell caused by the activity of drug pumps as the ATP-binding cassette (ABC) transporters (Szakács et al., 2006; Lage, 2008; Lu & Shervington, 2008).

An important type of cell involved in malignant glioma resistance is the cancer stem cell. Although stem cells represent just a small part of the cells within malignant gliomas, it seems that they have an important role in the resistance to standard treatments, being radioresistant and chemoresistant (Adamson et al., 2009; Huang et al., 2010; Huse & Holland, 2010; Lamszus & Günther, 2010). Cancer stem cells are more resistant to radiation when compared to non-stem glioma cells. Radioresistance is due to the activation of pathways involved in DNA damage checkpoint response, leading to a more efficient DNA damage repair and a more rapidly recover from genotoxic stress. Radiotherapy affects tumor cells preferentially through DNA damage. For that reason, damage checkpoint responses are essential to radiosensitivity in cells. Chemoresistance in stem cells is probably caused by enhanced expression of BCRP1 and *O6*-methylguanine-DNA-methyltransferase (MGMT) as well as anti-apoptosis proteins. The ABC transporter BCRP1 has been playing an important role in drug resistance of normal and tumor stem cells while the presence of MGMT which is a DNA repair protein protects tumor cells against alkylating chemotherapeutic agents, such as TMZ (Bao et al., 2006; Liu et al., 2006; Wen & Kesari, 2008; Van Meir et al., 2010).

The use of chemotherapy is also limited due to the presence of the blood brain barrier (BBB). It restricts the action of conventional drugs that have difficulty to reach their therapeutic concentrations into the tumor and peritumor area. Only highly hydrophobic and low-molecular weight molecules are able to penetrate into the brain and reach their targets. There have been several attempts to improve drug delivery and increase its local concentration as intra-arterial delivery or opening the BBB using analogs of bradykinin (RMP-7). However, none has shown great result (Giese et al, 2003; Argyriou et al., 2009).

Apart from mechanisms of resistance described above, most of the treatments fail because of the highly invasive nature of glioma cells. Groups of cells or single cells can detach from the main tumor mass and invade long distances. The capacity of glioma cells to penetrate within the normal brain brings great clinical challenges because the remaining cells are believed to be responsible for tumor recurrence after standard treatments. The image methods available are not able to track these cells and it is not known the proportion of migratory cells affected by the current therapy (Berens & Giese, 1999; Claes et al., 2007). Another challenge in targeting the remaining cells is redundancy in the signaling pathways that lead to cell motility. Nowadays there are a lot of studies involving targets that are unique of brain ECM, cell surface receptors, and signaling molecules activated in migrating cells. These include tenascin C, brevican, Src family of non receptor tyrosine kinases, Rho family of small GTPases, glycogen synthase kinase 3 (GSK-3), and integrins. The highly complex pro-migratory signaling, the influence of microenvironment, and the unique nature of the invasive process in the brain provide an extensive area of study for the next years (Van Mer et al., 2010). This review focuses on the mechanisms involved in glioma cell migration and the potential molecular targets within these pathways.

2. Glioma invasion and microenvironment

Invasion is a characteristic not exclusive for malignant gliomas. Low-grade astrocytomas can also show extensive infiltration of normal brain, limiting resection and eventually leading to recurrence and progression of the disease. However, the dynamic of high-grade glioma invasion seems to be more rapid (Giese et al., 2003; Louis, 2006; Jones & Holland, 2010). Although this type of tumor is extremely invasive, metastasis out of the brain is rare. Invasive cells tend to follow existing anatomical structures, and migrate along myelinated fiber tracts as corpus callosum, meninges and the ventricular lining and the perivascular regions (Tysnes & Mahesparan, 2001).

The invasive nature of glioma cells is one of the major problems of this type of cancer. After resection of the main tumor, the residual pool of invasive cells gives rise to recurrent tumor. Interaction between cells and extracellular matrix (ECM) is the main factor to maintain the normal features of tissues. The loss of ECM control is a hallmark in tumor progression toward invasion. Although brain tumor cells share common invasive characteristics with other tumor cell types, the different composition of the brain ECM suggests alternative invasive mechanisms for brain tumor cells. This unique brain ECM composition may also be one of the reasons for the poorly metastatic behavior even though the cells are highly invasive (Tysnes & Mahesparan, 2001). The human brain ECM consists mainly of glycosaminoglycans (GAGs) and proteoglycans. The four main GAGs are hyaluronic acid, chondroitin sulfate, keratin sulfate and heparin sulfate. The presence of glycoproteins as fibronectin or collagen, are limited. The interaction between GAG hyaluron and the other GAGs or glycoproteins forms a loose ECM-meshwork around axons, neurons, and glial cells of the white and gray matter (Goldbrunner et al., 1998).

Invasion is a complex and dynamic process that has three basic coordinated steps: adhesion to the ECM, cytoskeleton rearrangement, and degradation of ECM components (Figure 2). Cells have to interact with their microenvironment to be able to migrate and invade. Integrins together with CD44 receptor are the receptors responsible for glioma cells-ECM adhesions. Migrating cells interact with ECM components forming transition adhesions which will have two main functions: generate signals that lead to cytoskeletal rearrangement and support cell traction. Cells also need space to migrate and ECM proteolysis is accomplished by activation of several proteases such as matrix metalloproteinases (MMPs) and plasmin secreted by glioma cells and endothelial cells. Cytoskeletal rearrangements lead to cell polarization and formation of membrane protrusion for which RhoGTPase family plays a major role. Cells invade by actively migrating into the newly created space (Goldbrunner et al., 1999; Bellail et al., 2004; Teodorczyk & Martin-Villalba, 2010).

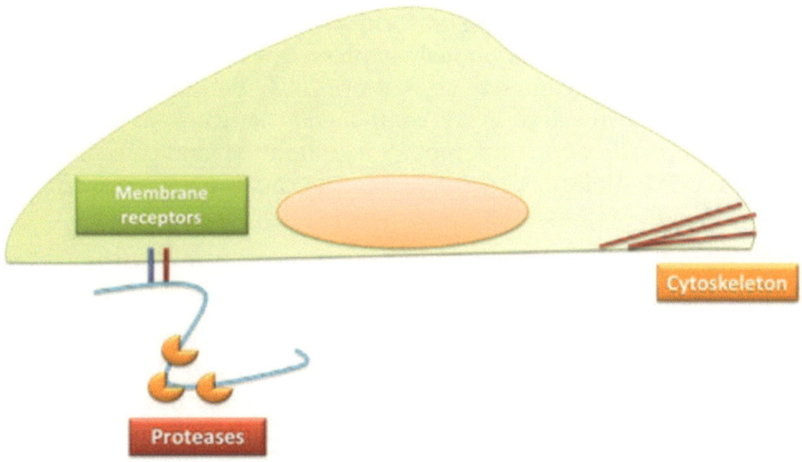

Fig. 2. The three components related to the invasion process. Membrane receptors as integrins and CD44 receptor are responsible for the cell-ECM interaction. Actin filaments are important cytoskeleton structures that rearrange to allow cell to migrate. Proteases as matrix metalloproteinases (MMPs) degrade ECM components and open space to cell migration.

2.1 ECM components

It is known that some ECM components are upregulated within tumor stroma and within brain parenchyma surrounding tumor area. Among them are hyaluronan, vitronectin, osteopontin, tenascin-C, SPARC and BEHAB (Bellail et al., 2004).

Hyaluronan (HA) is a glycosaminoglycan and the major component of brain ECM. In normal ECM, HA is responsible for tissue homeostasis, biomechanical integrity, and tissue structure. However, in malignant tumor tissue, it has been shown that HA facilitates primary brain tumor invasion *in vivo* and migration *in vitro* through its two receptors, CD44 and receptor for hyaluronan-mediatd motility (RHAMM) (Bellail et al., 2004; Park et al., 2008). The mechanisms of action are not completely elucidated but there are some evidences showing that HA induces tumor progression through pathways as PI3K/Akt/mTor/osteopontin and RhoGTPase signaling (Kim et al., 2005; Bourguignon, 2008).

Tenascin-C is a large modular glycoprotein. Tenascin-C signaling is mediated by integrin β1 via phosphorylation of focal adhesion kinase (FAK). It has been shown that tenascin-C is overexpressed in invasive glioma *in vivo* (Demuth & Berens, 2004).

BEHAB (brain-enriched hyaluronan-binding) protein, also known as brevican, is a chondroitin sulfate lectican. Its expression in the brain is very low being up-regulated in malignant gliomas. Its high expression and cleavage promote glioma invasion. Cleavage of BEHAB is mediated by metalloproteases of ADAMTs family (Gladson, 1999; Bellail et al., 2004; Viapiano et al., 2008).

2.2 Interaction with the ECM

Integrins are a family of transmembrane glycoprotein receptors. They are heterodimers and consist of α and β subunits non-covalently associated. To date there have been described 18 α subunits and 8 β subunits combining to form 24 integrins that bind to different ECM components. Some integrins are ubiquitously expressed while others depend on the tissue or stage of development (Brakebusch & Fässler, 2003; Berrier & Yamada, 2007). The interaction between integrins and ECM components activates a number of signaling pathways that control proliferation, differentiation, migration, and cell survival. Changes in both integrin and ECM molecules expression may cause important cell modifications contributing to malignant progression (Gladson, 1999).

Integrins are the main connection between ECM and cytoskeleton. When integrin binds its ligands, actin filaments and signaling proteins move to integrin´s cytoplasmic domain and form focal complexes. These complexes can grow in size and stabilize to form focal contacts or remain as focal complexes. Focal contacts are more mature and stable adhesions, usually found in the end of actin bundle called stress fibers. Focal complexes are less persistent cellular structures and suffer rapid turnover (Schoenwaelder & Burridge, 1999; Brakebusch & Fässler, 2003; Demuth & Berens, 2004).

Within Central Nervous System it has been described the presence of at least three integrin subunits. Subunits β_1 and α_v are described in a variety of cell types including neurons, glia cells, meningeal cells and endothelial cells. It has been reported differences in integrin expression in glioma cells. Subunits β_1 and α_3 are higher expressed in glioma cells when compared with normal cells and β_1 is being considered a key factor in glioma cell migration (Paulus & Tonn, 1994; Bellail et al., 2004; D´Abaco & Kaye, 2007).

CD44 receptor binds hyaluronic acid, one of the main brain ECM components. It is expressed in a variety of cells, including glial cells. Alternative mRNA splicing form several isoforms of CD44, being isoform CD44H the most important in normal brain as well as in primary brain tumor, including glioblastomas (Goldbrunner et al., 1998).

CD44 functions as both receptor and signaling molecule to induce cell migration and invasion through activation of actin reorganization pathways. As receptor, CD44 binds to HA and activates pathways described above. In tumor cells, CD44 is proteolytically cleavage at the extracellular domain by MMPs and CD44 cleavage is also important for CD44-mediated tumor cell migration. Engagement of CD44 augments CD44 cleavage by Rac activation (Murai et al., 2004; Teodorczyk & Martin-Villalba, 2010).

2.3 ECM proteolysis

Proteases are enzymes that cleave ECM components. They are secreted by glioma cells and seem to play an important role in cell migration. The most studied proteases are matrix metalloproteinases (MMPs) and the serine protease urokinase-type plasminogen activator (uPA) and its receptor. The role of these enzymes in glioma invasion is complex, since low-grade glioma invades the surrounding normal brain, even with normal level of the proteases (Louis, 2006; Drappatz et al., 2009).

MMPs are a family of zinc-dependent proteases. They are generally classified in four groups: collagenases, gelatinases, membrane-type MMPs (MT-MMPs) and stromelysins. The mechanisms that control MMP expression are not completely clear but some studies showed that MMPs can be regulated by ECM components, growth factors and cytokines. All MMPs are secreted as inactive proenzymes that need proteolytic cleavage for activation. The proteolytic effect of MMPs is balanced by MMPs inhibitors as tissue-derived inhibitors of metalloproteinases (TIMPs). TIMPs bind to the active zinc-binding site of the MMP protein, forming an inactive complex. In malignant gliomas, there is an imbalance between expression of MMPs and their corresponding inhibitors which leads to a higher activity of MMPs and consequently greater ECM proteolysis (Newton, 2004).

uPA is secreted as a soluble protein and binds to its receptor (uPAR), a GPI-anchored protein. uPA is often up-regulated in malignant brain tumors and its activity is high at the edge of these tumors. Binding between this protease and its receptor is necessary for the activation of plasmin which can degrade ECM components. In 2003, Chandrasekar et al. reported that downregulation of uPA could inhibit glioblastoma cell migration and PI3K/Akt signaling *in vitro*. These results show the important role of uPA in glioma cell migration.

2.4 Cytoskeleton rearrangement

Directional cell migration undergoes a series of cytoskeletal reorganizations to create a leading edge and a trailing edge. At the leading edge there is the formation of membrane protrusions and the establishment of new matrix contacts, while at the trailing edge cell adhesions are disassembled to allow cells to move forward. Active remodeling of actin cytoskeleton is required to form structures at the front of the cell such as filopodia and lamellipodia. These structures have several actin filaments (F-actin) that are polymerized or depolymerized by the addition of G-actin at their barbed end or the release of G-actin at their pointed end. Cytoskeleton rearrangement depends on complex signaling pathways and is controlled mainly by the activation/deactivation of proteins from the Rho family of small GTPases (Berrier & Yamada, 2007; Wehrle-Haller & Imhof, 2003).

The Rho family of small GTPases has more than 20 members, including the well known proteins Cdc42, Rac and Rho. These proteins, as all small GTPases, cycle between an active GTP-bound and an inactive GDP-bound state. The activation and deactivation of Rho proteins are mediated by guanine nucleotide-exchange factors (GEFs) and GTPase-activating proteins (GAPs), respectively. There have been more than 70 RhoGTPase effector proteins described. The temporal and spatial balance between the different RhoGTPses are very important for the cellular processes. To promote cell migration, Rho protein activation is related to formation of focal adhesion complexes and stress fiber (bundle of actin filaments), while Rac and Cdc42 are associated with lamellipodia and filopodia formation, respectively (Iden & Collard, 2008).

2.5 Growth factors and other molecules

Overexpression of growth factor receptors and their ligands is very common in gliomas. Some growth factor receptors have been involved in glioma cell migration and invasion. Among these growth factor receptors are c-Met, epidermal growth factor receptor (EGFR) and platelet-derived growth factor receptor (PDGFR) (Gladson et al., 2010).

In particular, EGFR has been shown to be important for tumor growth and invasion (Tysnes & Mahesparan, 2001). Amplification and overexpression of EGFR are observed in 50% of glioblastoma multiforme. Malignant gliomas can also express a mutant receptor that is ligand independent, EGFRvIII. This receptor is constitutively phosphorylated and is more tumorigenic than the wild-type receptor (Nakada et al., 2007). Activation of EGFR leads to signaling complex formation which initiates downstream signaling cascades, including the phosphoinositide 3-kinase (PI3K) and mitogen-activated protein kinase (MAPK). These pathways regulate several cellular responses (Huang et al., 2009).

Platelet-derived growth factor (PDGF) is another growth factor that is upregulated in gliomas. Although PDGF is more related to proliferation and angiogenesis, some works have shown the influence of PDGF in cell motility in gliomas (Hoelzinger et al., 2007).

Transforming growth factor β (TGF-β) is present in tumor microenvironment and is secreted by malignant cells. This molecule can regulate cell motility, invasion, immune surveillance and angiogenesis. In glioblastoma multiforme, it has been reported the presence of TGF-β in tumor environment (Barcellos-Hoff et al., 2009; Drappatz et al., 2009).

Chemokines are small chemoattractant cytokines. These molecules and their receptors are expressed into the central nervous system by neurons and glia cells and are mediators of cell migration. In brain tumors their expression is deregulated. Special attention is given to CXCL12/CXCR4 axis because initial reports showed that CXCL12 promotes migration of glioma cells *in vitro* and activation of MMPs (Sciumè et al., 2010).

2.6 Intracellular signal

Interaction of glioma cells with their microenvironment leads to intracellular signals that are very complex and very integrated (Figure 3). When glioma cells receive a pro-invasive signal through cell-surface growth factor receptor and cell-adhesion receptor, signaling molecules are activated to amplify and propagate the message. The signaling molecules are represented by cytoplasmic tyrosine kinases, adaptor molecules, and cytoskeletal proteins (Gladson et al., 2010).

Growth factor receptor and cell-adhesion receptor signaling can be co-ordinated to control cell proliferation, survival and migration. It has been shown that integrins regulate some receptor tyrosine kinases (RTK) such as EGFR. This cross-talk can occur in at least three mechanisms: RTK activation, propagation of ligand-mediated signaling and synergetic interaction to reach a final biological response (Cabodi et al., 2004).

Focal adhesion kinase (FAK) is a downstream effector of integrins and growth factor receptors. The phosphorylation of FAK leads to the activation of several signaling pathways through protein phosphorylation and protein-protein interaction. FAK has different domains which allow the integration of different signaling pathways. Phosphorylated FAK activates several pathways, including PI3K/Akt, MAPK and $p130^{Cas}$/DOCK180/Rac. Overexpression of FAK is related with tumor progression (Schwock et al., 2010).

MAPK pathway – Activation of MAPK signaling pathway is triggered by growth factor receptor-bound-2 (Grb2)/son-of-sevenless (SOS) or FAK/Src complex. After RTK activation, autophosphorylation of the cytoplasmic domain of the receptor leads to recruitment of Grb2 and subsequently binding to the guanine exchange factor SOS. This complex interacts with small GTPase Ras and results in its activation. The next step is the sequential recruitment and activation of Raf, mitogen-activated protein kinase kinase (MEK) and extracellular signal-regulated kinase (ERK). ERK activates the expression of several transcriptional factors that control cell proliferation. Small GTPase Ras can also be activated by FAK/Src complex when ECM components bind integrin. There is evidence that Src phosphorylates FAK, creating a binding site for the complex Grb2/SOS which leads to MAPK pathway activation (Giancotti & Ruoslahti, 1999; Ramos, 2008; Huang et al., 2009).

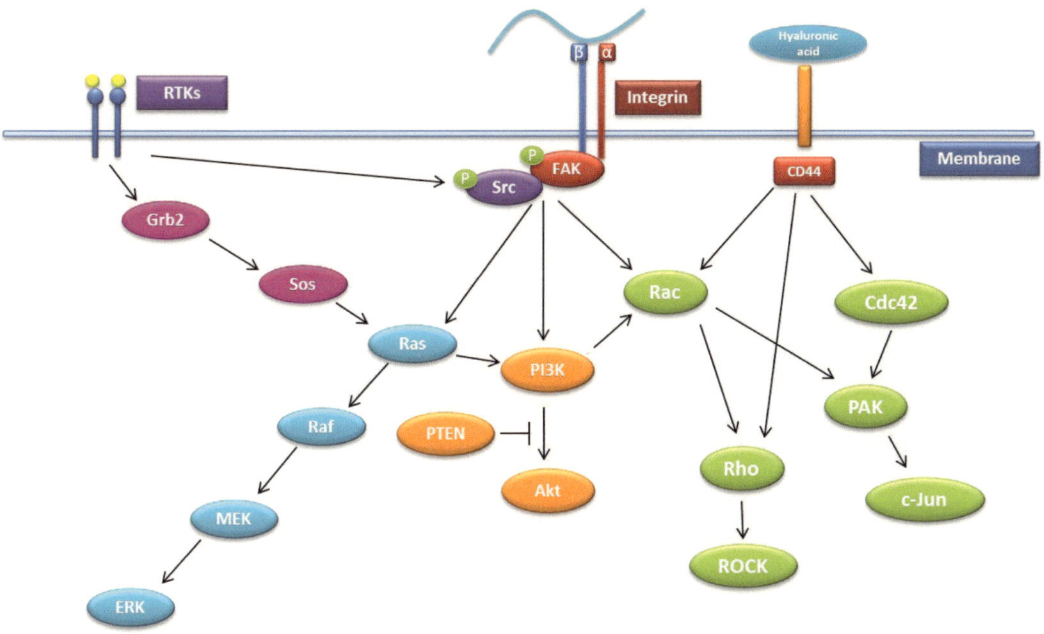

Fig. 3. Intracellular signal downstream cell-surface growth factor receptor and cell-adhesion receptor activation.

PI3K/Akt pathway - Activated PI3K converts plasma membrane phosphatidylinositol-4,5-bisphosphate (PIP_2) to phosphatidylinositol-3,4,5-triphosphate (PIP_3). PIP_3 leads to the activation of Akt that is involved in the regulation of several proteins related with cell survival. PI3K pathway is negatively regulated by phosphophoinositide phosphatases such as PTEN. PTEN acts in the opposite way of PI3K converting PIP_3 to PIP_2. Loss of PTEN leads to an imbalance of PI3K/PTEN and results in increased activation of PIP_3 and Akt (Huang et al., 2009).

ERK and Akt signaling cascades are related with proliferation and survival, respectively. However, they are also involved in the invasion process because the activation of these pathways leads to activation of MMPs as MMP-2 and MMP-9 (Park et al., 2008; Drappatz et al., 2009).

RhoGTPase pathway - Members of the Rho family of small GTPases (Rho-GTPases) are important intracellular mediators that control directional cell migration. They can be activated by several pathways, including integrin and CD44 signaling pathways. It is known that Rho-GTPases are implicated with metastasis and tumor progression, what is not so surprising since RhoGTPases are downstream pathways that are deregulated in several tumors. There are also evidences that some GEFs are up-regulated in malignant brain tumors which increase activation of RhoGTPases as Rac1 and RhoA. Rac1 and RhoA have been related to glioma cell migration and invasion (Salhia et al., 2006).

2.7 Epithelial-mesenchymal transition

Migrating cells need to detach from the tumor mass to infiltrate neighboring tissue. For that reason, other important process in glioma migration is the epithelial-mesenchymal transition (EMT). It consists on biochemical changes in polarized epithelial cells which allow the cell to assume a mesenchymal cell phenotype. This phenotype is characterized by enhanced migratory capacity, invasiveness, elevated resistance to apoptosis, and increased expression of ECM components (Kalluri & Weiberg, 2009). EMT is very important during embryogenesis but it is also present in pathological conditions such as tumorigenesis, hypoxia, and inflammation (Nieto, 2011). It is widely known that this process plays an important role in glioma migration. However, the molecules involved are still not well established.

Cadherins have an important role in EMT. Classically, expression of E-cadherin is reduced while expression of N-cadherin and cadherin-11 are increased during EMT. Nevertheless, E-cadherin expression is very low in normal brain tissue and some glioma cell lines (Lewis-Tuffin et al., 2010; Utsuki et al., 2002). The role of cadherins in gliomas is still obscure. Differences in the role of cadherins can change depending on the glioma cell line. E-cadherin is found in SF767 cells and its expression is related to more invasive phenotype. However, just N-cadherin and cadherin-11 are found in U87 cell line. Ectopic expression of E-cadherin did not show any affect in migration in the U87 cell line (Lewis-Tuffin et al., 2010).

Probably, acquisition of mesenchymal phenotype involves an E-cadherin-independent pathway in glioma. One possible candidate is the transcription factor TWIST1. Mikheeva et al., 2010 showed that TWIST1 is responsible for changes in glioma cells that correlate with the phenotype associated with carcinoma EMT.

3. Treatments involving molecular targets related to cell invasion

There are several characteristics that must be considered when choosing a therapeutic target. First of all, the target must be overexpressed in tumor cells but not in normal cells. The target must be active and contribute to the malignant phenotype. It is very important that the therapeutic agent reaches easily its pharmacological target. Usually the first approach is against secreted molecules and cell surface receptors (Rich & Bigner, 2004).

3.1 Drugs in clinical trials

Recent advances in the understanding of glioma biology and signaling pathways have provided new tools to the development of molecularly targeted agents. There are a wide variety of targeted agents being studied in preclinical and clinical trials. However, the use of these agents alone has shown limited efficacy in almost all studies. That way combined inhibition of multiple targets are being studying, using molecules against targets from the same pathway or targets of parallel pathways. Although this strategy has a great potential, it should be considered the increase in the risk of toxic effects (Clarke et al., 2010).

3.1.1 Integrins inhibitors

Integrins are highly express in gliomas. There are monoclonal antibodies and peptide-based integrin inhibitors being investigated against various tumor types. However, only cilengitide (EMD121974 - Merck KGaA, Darmstadt, Germany) is being studied in glioma. Cilengitide is a synthetic Arg-Gly-Asp (RGD) pentapeptide that recognizes RGD ligand-binding motifs on integrins $\alpha_v\beta_3$ and $\alpha_v\beta_5$, blocking ligand binding. RGD is an important motif that is present in some ECM components (Hynes, 2002). Relevant responses have been observed with cilengitide monotherapy in preclinical and clinical studies. Some combinatorial studies were carried out adding cilengitide to standard radiotherapy/TMZ in a randomized phase II trial. The results showed promising efficacy, especially in patients with MGMT promoter methylation. Phase III trial (CENTRIC) has started recruiting newly diagnosed patients with methylated promoter of MGMT to assess efficacy and safety of cilengitide in combination with standard treatment against standard treatment (Khasraw & Lassman, 2010; Onishi et al., 2010; Tabatabai et al., 2010).

3.1.2 Anti-tenascin-C

Tenascin-C is overexpress in some patients with malignant gliomas and its presence seems to increase tumor cell invasion *in vitro* (Sarkar et al., 2006). Phase II studies using tenascin-specific antibody labeled with I^{131} (Neuradiab™) showed slight increase in survival time in patients with glioblastoma multiforme. Tenascin-specific antibody was administered directly into a surgically created resection cavity followed by standard treatment. Although some questions still remain, a Phase III trial of Neuradiab has started in patients with newly diagnosed glioblastoma multiforme (Akabani et al., 2005; Drappatz et al., 2009).

3.1.3 MMP inhibitors

Since the use of MMP inhibitors have shown decrease in glioma cell invasion *in vitro*, several clinical trials were performed. However, first and second generation of MMP inhibitors showed poor bioavailability and significant side effects. Marimastat is an orally drug that can reduce MMP levels in patients with glioma but several patients were remove from phase II trial because of intolerable side effects as join pain (Newton, 2004; Nakada et al., 2007; Onishi et al., 2011). New MMP inhibitors are in development to improve selectivity and to diminish side effects. A new class of MMP inhibitors targets the MMP S_1' subsite pocket and does not interact with the zinc active site. The MMP S_1' pocket has loop residues called S_1' specificity loop that vary in size and sequence depending on the MMP. Because of that these inhibitors are more selective. However, there are no current clinical trials (Overall & Kleifeld, 2006; Devel et al., 2010).

3.1.4 Anti-EGF receptor

Tyrosine kinase inhibitors avoid phosphorylation and activation of downstream signaling. The most studied molecules are erlotinib and gefitinib. They are reversible small-molecules inhibitors for oral use. Several Phase II clinical trials showed that monotherapy using erlotinib and gefitinib did not bring any significant survival benefit when compared to control group in patients with glioblastoma multiforme. Patients that co-expressed EGFRvIII and PTEN were more responsive to erlotinib. However, this result was not reproducible in another study, showing the high complexity of individual tumors. Combination of tyrosine kinase inhibitors with standard therapy did not show also good results. Recent clinical trials are evaluating other EGFR inhibitors as irreversible EGFR inhibitors BIBW 2992 and PF-

00299804 and the humanized monoclonal antibody against EGFR, nimotuzumab (Nakada et al., 2007; Hatanpaa et al., 2010; Van Meir et al., 2010)

3.2 Potential molecules in study

3.2.1 Lithium

Studies *in vitro* using lithium potently blocked glioma cell migration. This molecule is known to activate β-catenin signaling. The treatment had little effective in cell viability and was associated with change in cell morphology with retraction of long extensions at the leading edge, suggesting an involvement of glycogen synthase kinase (GSK-3). The role of GSK-3 in cancer cell migration is not clear but it was observed an inverse correlation between GSK-3 expression and rate of glioma invasion (Barcellos-Hoff et al., 2009).

3.2.2 Emodin

Emodin is one of the active components of the *Rheum palmatum* L. and is a protein tyrosine kinase inhibitor. It has several biological activity including antiviral, antimicrobial, immunosuppressive, and anticancer effects. Studies *in vitro* and *in vivo* showed that emodin decreased MMP-2 and MMP-9 expression by blocking FAK and Akt activation. It also suppressed HA-stimulated AP1 and NFκB promoter activities (Park et al., 2008).

3.2.3 RECK

RECK (Reversion-inducing-cysteine-rich protein with Kazal motifs) is a membrane-anchored glycoprotein. RECK can be found in various normal human tissues but its expression is low or undetectable in many tumors, including gliomas. RECK was first described as a tumor and metastasis suppressor gene, inhibiting at least three different metalloproteinases; MMP-2, MMP-9 and MT1-MMP. Re-expression of RECK in some tumor cell lines leads to a strong inhibition of tumor invasion, metastasis and angiogenesis (Takahashi et al., 1998; Oh et al., 2001; Noda et al., 2003; Meng et al., 2008). Corrêa et al. (2006) showed correlation between expression of RECK and invasive potential *in vitro*. The less invasive glioma cell line had higher RECK expression when compared to the more invasive glioma cell line.

In 2010, Corrêa et al. showed that overexpression of RECK in a glioma cell line (T98G) compromises glioma cell ability to migrate and invade *in vitro*. Results demonstrated that overexpression of RECK did not alter MMP activity but was responsible for cytoskeleton rearrangement, causing changes in cell motility. It is unknown how RECK leads to changes in cell motility but the elucidation of this mechanism could bring new potential targets to inhibit cell migration.

3.3 Issues in preclinical and clinical studies

In vitro experimental system and animal models are very important to study the biology of glioma invasion and to test anti-invasive therapy. They need to be accurate, representative and valid. Monolayer cultures of permanent glioma cell lines are widely used in experimental systems. However, these cell lines suffer biological changes during cell culture and the lack of ECM-cell interaction causes changes in some gene expression, as shown by several studies (Nelson & Bissel, 2006). There are some 3D models available as spheroids but they also have some limitations because of the high complexity of tumors.

Brain tumor animal models are used to study new therapies. These models have to be accurate and reproducible to provide trustful results avoiding the exposure of patients to non-efficacious or unsafe drugs. Tumor xenografts models and transgenic models are two widely used animal models. These models have some advantages over *in vitro* models but they also have some limitations. For instance, xenografts models represent phenotypic diversity but they lack tumor environment interactions and do not reproduce invasive growth patterns. Transgenic models in the other way are good models for studying the impact of cell invasion, vascular limitations to drug delivery and interaction with the surrounding tissue. However, they do not reproduce tumor heterogeneity and genomic instability. For that reason, some drugs that have shown great anti-tumor activity fail in clinical trials (Rich & Bigner, 2004; King et al., 2005).

When studying a new drug, some parameters need to be evaluated: evaluation of dosing sequences, markers of therapeutic efficacy and intra-cerebral delivery. In clinical neuro-oncology trials there are some difficulties to measure efficacy and to obtain tumor tissue for sampling. Clinical efficacy should be based on overall survival. However, survival is not a good endpoint due to the variability of treatments that patients were submitted before and after trials. Biomarker measurement is essential to targeted therapy trials but lack of tissue sampling after experimental drug treatment is a problem (Rich & Bigner, 2004).

Chapter summary

- Failure in malignant glioma treatment is due multiple causes as local invasive nature of glioma cells, resistance to radiotherapy and chemotherapy; and presence of the blood brain barrier.
- Invasion is a major clinical problem. This process is highly complex, involving multiple pathways and relaying on a network of paracrine interactions. Contact between cells and the extracellular matrix is dynamic since it can change as cancer cells disseminate and reciprocally lead to activation of important signals for cytoskeleton rearrangement and matrix proteolyses.
- Treatment combining multiple drugs is the key to contain glioma progression, targeting not solely cancer cells but also the microenvironment. However, the discovery for new drugs is still a long process and improvement in models for preclinical tests is required.

4. Conclusion

Targeted therapy against invasion-related molecules is a promising alternative for treating malignant gliomas. Although tumor cells are widely disseminated when the patient is diagnosed, anti-invasive therapies for malignant gliomas have as its main goal to contain the disease and increase the efficacy of local treatments. Migration signaling shares common pathways with proliferation and apoptosis. That way, the use of combining therapy could increase the efficient of conventional cytotoxic treatments, improving cell death. Advances in the understanding of tumor invasion have improved the development of new therapies. However, not all questions have been answered and some challenges still remain.

5. Acknowledgment

The authors are thankful to FAPESP (Raquel Brandão Haga's Fellowship Contract Grant No.: 09/12135-2), CNPq, PRPG-USP and CAPES. We are especially grateful to Dr Mari Cleide Sogayar (Chemistry Institute, University of São Paulo) and previous members of the laboratory of Clinical Cytopathology from School of Pharmaceutical Sciences, University of São Paulo, Dr Tatiana C.S. Corrêa and Renato R. Massaro for all contribution in RECK studies in glioma model.

6. References

Adamson, C., Kanu, O.O., Mehta, A.I., Di, C., Lin, N., Mattox A.,K. & Bigner, D.D. (2009). Glioblastoma multiforme: a review of where we have been and where we are going. *Expert Opinion on Investigational Drugs*, Vol. 18, No. 8, pp. 1061-1083.

Akabani, G., Reardon, D.A., Coleman, E., Wong, T.Z., Metzler, S.D., Bowsher, J.E., Barboriak, D.P., Provenzale, J.M., Greer K.L., DeLong, D., Friedman, H.S., Friedman, A.H., Zhao, X-G., Pegram, C.N., McLendon, R.E., Bigner, D.D. & Zalutsky, M.R. (2005). Dosimetry and Radiographic Analysis of ^{131}I-Labeled Anti-Tenascin 81C6 Murine Monoclonal Antibody in Newly Diagnosed Patients with Malignant Gliomas: A Phase II Study. *The Journal of Nuclear Medicine*, Vol. 46, No. 6, pp. 1042-1051.

Argyriou, A.A., Antonacopoulou, A., Iconomou, G. & Kalofonos, H.P. (2009). Treatment options for malignant gliomas, emphasizing towards new molecularly targeted therapies. *Critical Reviews in Oncology/Hematology*, Vol. 69, pp. 199-210.

Bao, S., Qiulian, W., MacLendon, R.E., Hao, Y., Shi, Q., Hjelmeland, A.B., Dewhirst, M.W., Bigner, D.D. & Rich, J.N. (2006). Glioma stem celss promote radioresistance by preferential activation of the DNA damage response. *Nature*, Vol. 444, pp. 756-760.

Barcellos-Hoff, M.H., Newcomb, E.W., Zagzag, D. & Narayana, A. (2009). Therapeutic Targets in Malignant Glioblastoma Microenvironment. *Seminars in Radiation Oncology*, Vol. 19, pp. 163-170.

Bellail, A.C., Hunter, S.B., Brat, D.J., Tan, C., Van Meir, E.G. (2004) Microregional extracellular matrix heterogeneity in brain modulates glioma cell invasion. *The International Journal of Biochemistry & Cell Biology*, Vol. 36, pp.1046-1069.

Berens, M.E. & Giese, A. (1999). "...those left behind." Biology and Oncology of Invasive Glioma Cells. *Neoplasia*, Vol. 1, No. 3, pp. 208-219.

Berrier, A.L. & Yamada, K.M. (2007). Cell-Matrix Adhesion. *Journal of Cellular Physiology*, Vol. 213, pp.565-573.

Bourguignon, L.Y.W. (2008). Hyaluronan-mediated CD44 activation of RhoGTPase signaling and cytoskeleton function promotes tumor progression. *Seminars in Cancer Biology*, Vol. 18, No. 4, pp. 251-259.

Brakebusch, C. & Fässler, R. (2003). The integrin-actin connection, an eternal love affair. *The EMBO Journal*, Vol. 22, No. 10, pp.2324-2333.

Cabodi, S., Moro, L., Bergatto, E., Boeri Erba, E., Di Stefano, P., Turco, E. Tarone, G. & Defilippi, P. (2004). Integrin regulation of epidermal growth factor (EGF) receptor and of EGF-dependent responses. *Biochemical Society Transactions*, Vol. 32, Part 3, pp. 438-442.

Central Brain Tumor Registry of the United States (2010). CBTRUS 2010 Statistical Report: Primary Brain Tumors in the United States. Central Brain Tumor Registry of the United States, 2004-2006. http://www.cbtrus.org/2010-NPCR-SEER/CBTRUS-WEBREPORT-Final-3-2-10.pdf (acessed January 27, 2011).

Chandrasekar, N., Mohanam, S., Gujrati, M., Oliveiro, W.C., Dinh, D.H. & Rao, J.S. (2003). Downregulation of uPA inhibits migration and PI3K/Akt signaling in glioblastoma cells. *Oncogene*, Vol. 22, pp. 392-400.

Claes, A., Idema, A.J. & Wesseling, P. (2007). Diffuse glioma growth: a guerilla war. *Acta Neuropathologica*, Vol. 114, pp. 443-458.

Clarke, J., Butowski, N. & Chang, S. (2010). Recent Advances in Therapy for Glioblastoma. *Archives of Neurology*, Vol. 63, No. 3, pp. 279-283.

Corrêa, T.C.S., Brohem, C.A., Winnischofer, S.M.B., Da Silva Cardeal, L.B., Sasahara, R.M., Taboga, S.R., Sogayar, M.C., Maria-Engler, S.S. (2006). Downregulation of the RECK-tumor and metastasis suppressor gene in glioma invasiveness. *Journal of Cellular Biochemistry*, Vol. 99, p.156–167.

Corrêa, T.C.S., Massaro, R.R., Brohem, C.A., Taboga, S.R., Lamers, M.L., dos Santos, M.F., Maria-Engler, S.S. (2010). RECK-mediated inhibition of glioma migration and invasion. *Journal of Cellular Biochemistry*, Vol. 110, p. 52-61.

D´abaco, G.M. & Kaye, A.H. (2007). Integrins: Molecular determinants of glioma invasion. *Journal of Clinical Neuroscience*, Vol.14, p.1041-1048.

Demuth, T & Berens, M.E. (2004). Molecular mechanisms of glioma cell migration and invasion. *Journal of Neuro-Oncology*, Vol. 70, pp. 217-228.

Devel, L., Czarny, B., Beau, F., Georgiadis, D., Stura, E. & Dive, V. (2010). Third generation of matrix metalloprotease inhibitors: Gain in selectivity by targeting the depth of the S_1´cavity. *Biochimie*, Vol. 92, pp. 1501-1508.

Drappatz, J., Norden, A.D. & Wen, P.Y. (2009). Therapeutic strategies for inhibiting invasion in glioblastoma. *Expert Review of Neurotherapeutics*, Vol. 9, No. 4, pp. 519-534.

Giancotti, F.G. & Ruoslahti, E. (1999). Integrin Signaling. *Science*, Vol. 285, pp. 1028-1032.

Giese, A., Bjerkvig, R., Berens, M.E. & Westphal, M. (2003). Cost of Migration: Invasion of Malignant Gliomas and Implications for Treatment. *Journal of Clinical Oncology*, Vol. 21, pp. 1624-1636.

Gladson, C.L. (1999). The Extracellular Matrix of Gliomas: Modulation of Cell Function. *Journal of Neuropathology & Experimental Neurology*, Vol.58, pp. 1029-1040.

Gladson, C.L., Prayson, R.A. & Liu, W.M. (2010). The Pathobiology of Glioma Tumors. *Annual Review of Pathology: Mechanisms of Disease*, Vol. 5, pp. 33-50.

Goldbrunner, R.H, Berstein, J.J. & Tonn, J-C. (1998). ECM-Mediated Glioma Cell Invasion. *Microscopy Research and Technique*, Vol. 43, pp. 250-257.

Goldbrunner, R.H., Bernstein, J.J. & Tonn, J.-C. (1999). Cell-Extracellular Matrix Interation in Glioma Invasion. *Acta Neurochirurgica (Wien)*, Vol. 141, pp. 295-305.

Hatanpaa, K.J., Burma, S., Zhao, D. & Habib, A.A. (2010). Epidermal Growth Factor Receptor in Glioma: Signal Transduction, Neuropathology, Imaging, and Radioresistance. *Neoplasia*, Vol. 12, pp. 675-684.

Hoelzinger, D.B., Demuth, T. & Berens, M.E. (2007). Autocrine Factors That Sustain Glioma Invasion and Paracrine Biology in the Brain Microenvironment. *Journal of the National Cancer Institute*, Vol. 99, pp. 1583-1593.

Huang, P.H., Xu, A.M. & White, F.M. (2009). Oncogenic EGFR Signaling Networks in Glioma. *Science Signaling*, Vol. 2, No. 87, pp. 1-13.

Huang, Z., Cheng, L., Guryanova, O.A., Wu, Q. & Bao, S. (2010). Cancer stem cells in glioblastoma - molecular signalling and therapeutic targeting. *Protein & Cell*, Vol. 1, No. 7, pp.638-655.

Huse, J.T. & Holland, E.C. (2010). Targeting brain cancer: advances in the molecular pathology of malignant glioma and medulloblastoma. *Nature Reviews Cancer*, Vol. 10, pp. 319-331.

Hynes, R.O. (2002). Integrins: Birectional Allosteric Signaling Machines. *Cell*, Vol. 110, pp. 673-687.

Iden, S. & Collard, J.G. (2008). Crosstalk between small GTPases and polarity proteins in cell polarization. *Nature Reviews Molecular Cell Biology*, Vol. 9, pp. 846-859.

Jones, T.S. & Holland, E.C. (2010). Molecular Pathogenesis of Malignant Glial Tumors. *Toxicology Pathology,* Vol. 000, No. 00, pp. 1-9.

Kalluri, R. & Weinberg, R.A. (2009). The basics of epithelial-mesenchymal transition. *The Journal of Clinical Investigation*, Vol. 119, No. 6, pp. 1420-1428.

Khasraw, M. & Lassman, A.B. (2010). Advances in the Treatment of Malignant Gliomas. *Current Oncology Reports*, Vol. 12, pp. 26-33.

Kim, M-S., Park, M-J., Moon, E-J., Kim, S-J.,Lee, C-H., Yoo, H., Shin, S-H., Song, E-S. & Lee, S-H. (2005). Hyaluronic Acid Induces Osteopontin via the Phosphatidylinositol 3-Kinase/Akt Pathway to Enhance the Motility of Human Glioma Cells. *Cancer Research*, Vol. 65, pp.686-691.

King, G.D., Curtin, J.F., Candolfi, M., Kroeger, K., Lowenstein, P.R. & Castro, M.G. (2005). Gene therapy and targeted toxins for glioma. Current Gene Therapy, Vol. 5, No. 6, pp. 535-557.

Lage, H. (2008). An overview of cancer multidrug resistance: a still unsolved problem. *Cellular and Molecular Life Sciences*, Vol. 65, pp. 3145-3167.

Lamszus, K. & Günther, H.S. (2010). Glioma stem cells as a target for treatment. *Targeted Oncology*, Vol. 5, pp. 211-215.

Lewis-Tuffin, L.J., Rodriguez, F., Giannini, C., Scheithauer, B., Necela, B.M., Sarkaria, J.N. & Anastasiadis, P.Z. Misregulated E-Cadherin Expression Associated with and Aggressive Brain Tumor Phenotype. *PLoS ONE*, Vol. 5, No. 10, e13665. doi:10.1371/journal.pone.0013665.

Liu, G., Yuan, X., Zeng, Z., Tunici, P., Ng, H., Abdulkadir, I.R., Lu, L., Irvin, D., Black, K.L. & Yu, J.S. (2006). Analysis of gene expression and chemoresistance of $CD133^{+}$ cancer stem cells in glioblastoma. In: *Molecular Cancer*, 25.02.2011, Available from http://www.molecular-cancer.com/content/5/1/67

Louis, D.N. (2006). Molecular Pathology of Malignant Gliomas. *The Annual Review of Pathology: Mechanisms of Disease*, Vol. 1, pp. 97-117.

Lu, C. & Shervington, A. (2008). Chemoresistance in gliomas. *Molecular and Cellular Biochemistry*, Vol. 312, pp. 71-80.

Meng, N., Li, Y., Zhang, H. & Sun, X-F. (2008). RECK, a novel matrix metalloproteinase regulator. *Histology and Histopathology*, Vol. 23, p.1003-1010.

Mikheeva, S.A., Mikheev, A.M., Petit, A., Beyer, R., Oxford, R.G., Khorasani, L., Maxwell, J-P., Glackin, C.A., Wakimoto, H., Gonzáles-Herrero, I., Sánchez-García, I., Silber, J.R., Homer, P.J. & Rostomily, R.C. (2010). TWIST1 promotes invasion through mesenchymal change in human glioblastoma. In: *Molecular Cancer*. Available from http://www.molecular-cancer.com/content/9/1/194

Minniti, G., Muni, R., Lanzetta, G., Marchetti, P. & Maurizi Enrici, R. (2009). Chemotherapy for Glioblastoma: Current Treatment and Future Perspectives for Cytotoxic and Targeted Agents. *Anticancer Research*, Vol. 29, pp. 5171-5184.

Murai, T., Miyazaki, Y., Nishinakamura, H., Sugahara, K.N., Miyauchi, T., Sako, Y., Yanagida, T. & Miyasaka, M. (2004). Engagement of CD44 Promotes Rac Activation and CD44 Cleavage during Tumor Cell Migration. *The Journal of Biological Chemistry*, Vol. 279, No. 6, pp. 4541-4550.

Nakada, M., Nakada, S., Demuth, T., Tran, N.L., Hoelzinger, D.B. & Berens, M.E. (2007). Molecular targets of glioma invasion. *Cellular and Molecular Life Sciences*, Vol. 64, pp. 458-478.

Newton, H.B. (2004). Molecular neuro-oncology and the development of targeted therapeutic strategies for brain tumors - Part 3: brain tumor invasiveness. *Expert Review of Anticancer Therapy*, Vol. 4, No. 5, pp. 803-821.

Nieto, M.A. (2011). The Ins and Outs of the Epithelial to Mesenchymal Transition in Health and Disease. *Annual Review of Cell and Developmental Biology*, Vol. 27, pp. 16.1-16.30.

Noda, M., Oh, J., Takahashi, R., Kondo, S., Kitayama, H. & Takahashi, C. (2003). RECK: A novel suppressor of malignancy linking oncogenic signaling to extracellular matrix remodeling. *Cancer and Metastasis Reviews*, Vol. 22, p.167–175.

Oh, J., Takahashi, R., Kondo, S., Mizoguchi, A., Adachi, E., Sasahara, R.M., Nishimura, S., Imamura, Y., Kitayama, H., Alexander, D.B., Ide, C., Horan, T.P., Arakawa, T., Yoshida, H., Nishikawa, S., Itoh, Y, Seiki, M., Itohara, S., Takahashi, C. & Noda, M. (2001). The Membrane-Anchored MMP Inhibitor RECK Is a Key Regulator of Extracellular Matrix Integrity and Angiogenesis. *Cell*, Vol. 107, p. 789-800.

Onishi, M., Ichikawa, T., Kurozumi, K. & Date, I. (2011). Angiogenesis and invasion in glioma. *Brain Tumor Pathology*, Vol. 28, No., 1, pp. 13-24.

Overall, C.M. & Kleifeld, O. (2006). Towards third generation matrix metalloproteinase inhibitors for cancer therapy. *British Journal of Cancer*, Vol. 94, pp. 941-946.

Park, J.B., Kwak, H-J. & Lee, S-H. (2008). Role of hyaluronan in glioma invasion. *Cell Adhesion & Migration*, Vol. 2, No. 3, pp. 202-207.

Paulus, W. & Tonn, J.C. (1994). Basement membrane invasion of glioma cells mediated by integrin receptors. *Journal of Neurosurgery*, Vol. 80, p.515-519.

Ramos, J.W. (2008). The regulation of extracellular signal-regulated kinase (ERK) in mammalian cells. *The International Journal of Biochemistry & Cell Biology*, Vol. 40, pp. 2707-2719.

Rich, J.N. & Bigner, D.D. (2004). Development of Novel Targeted Therapies in the Treatment of Malignant Glioma. *Nature Reviews Drug Discovery*, Vol. 3, pp. 430-446.

Salhia, B., Tran, N.L., Symons, M., Winkles, J.A., Rutka, J.T. & Berens, M.E. (2006). Molecular pathways triggering glioma cell invasion. *Expert Review of Molecular Diagnostics*, Vol. 6, No. 4., pp. 613-626.

Sarkar, S., Nuttall, R.K., Liu, S., Edwards, D.R. & Young, V.W. (2006). Tenascin-C Stimulates Glioma Cell Invasion through Matrix Metalloproteinase-12. *Cancer Research*, Vol. 66, pp. 11771-11780.

Sciumè, G.,Santoni, A. & Bernardini, G. (2010). Chemokines and glioma: Invasion and more. *Journal of Neuroimmunology*, Vol. 224, pp. 8-12.

Schoenwaelder, S.M. & Burridge, K. (1999). Bidirectional signaling between the cytoskeleton and integrins. *Current Opinion in Cell Biology*, Vol. 11, p.274-286.

Schwock, J., Dhani, N. & Hedley, D.W. (2010). Targeting focal adhesion kinase signaling in tumor growth and metastasis. *Expert Opinion on Therapeutic Targets*, Vol. 14, No. 1, pp. 77-94.

Szakács, G., Paterson, J.K., Ludwig, J.A., Booth-Genthe, C. & Gottesman, M.M. (2006). Targeting multidrug resistance in cancer. *Nature Reviews Drug Discovery*, Vol. 5, pp. 219-234.

Tabatabai, G., Weller, M., Nabors, B., Picard, M., Reardon, D., Mikkelsen, T. Ruegg, C. & Stupp, R. (2010). Targeting integrins in malignant glioma. *Targeted Oncology*, Vol. 5, pp. 175-181.

Takahashi, C., Sheng, Z., Horan, T.P., Kitayama, H., Maki, M., Hitomi, K., Kitaura, Y., Takai, S., Sasahara, R.M., Horimoto, A., Ikawa, Y., Ratzkin, B.J., Arakawa, T. & Noda, M. (1998). Regulation of matrix metalloproteinase-9 and inhibition of tumor invasion by the membrane-anchored glycoprotein RECK. *Proceedings of the National Academy of Sciences U S A*, Vol. 95, No. 22, p. 13221-13226.

Teodorczyk, M. & Martin-Villalba, A. (2010). Sensing Invasion: Cell Surface Receptors Driving Spreading of Glioblastoma. *Journal of Cellular Physiology*, Vol. 222, pp. 1-10.

Tysnes, B.B. & Mahesparan, R. (2001). Biological mechanisms of glioma invasion and potential therapeutic targets. *Journal of Neuro-Oncology*, Vol. 53, pp. 129-147.

Utsuki, S., Sato, Y., Oka, H., Tsuchiya, B., Suzuki, S. & Fujii, K. (2002). Relationship between the expression of E-, N-cadherins and beta-catenin and tumor grade in astrocytomas. *Journal of Neuro-Oncology*, Vol. 57, pp. 187-192.

Van Meir, E.G., Hadjipanavis, C.G., Norden, A.D., Shu, H-K., Wen, P.Y. & Olson, J.J. (2010). Exciting New Advances in Neuro-Oncology - The Avenue to Cure for Malignant Glioma. *CA: A Cancer Journal for Clinicians*, Vol. 60, pp. 166-193.

Viapiano, M.S., Hockfield, S. & Matthews, R.T. (2008). BEHAB/brevican requires ADAMTS-mediated proteolytic cleavage to promote glioma invasion. *Journal of Neuro-Oncology*, Vol. 88, pp. 261-272.

Wehrle-Haller, B. & Imhof, B.A. (2003). Actin, microtubules and focal adhesion dynamics during cell migration. *The International Journal of Biochemistry & Cell Biology*, Vol. 35, pp. 39-50.

Wen, P.Y. & Kesari, S. (2008). Malignant Gliomas in Adults. *The New England Journal of Medicine*, Vol. 359, pp. 492-507.

Part 5

Blood-Brain Barrier in Glioma Therapy

7

Blood-Brain Barrier and Effectiveness of Therapy Against Brain Tumors

Yadollah Omidi and Jaleh Barar
Research Center for Pharmaceutical Nanotechnology, Faculty of Pharmacy, Tabriz University of Medical Sciences, Tabriz, Iran

1. Introduction

The challenge to comprehend the physiology as well as cell biology of the blood-brain barrier (BBB) began with Ehrlich and Goldman's experimental observations that the central nervous system (CNS) is not stained by intravascular vital dyes. These studies provided the first evidence of the presence of an obstructing barrier between blood and brain. Later on, researchers like Friedemann (1942) used basic highly lipid soluble dyes to cross the BBB in order to show the brain penetration of the dyes by direct transport across the cerebral microvasculature. In 1941, Broman presented his observations upon the existence of two different barrier systems within the brain: the BBB at the cerebral microvasculature, and the blood-CSF barrier at the choroid plexus. It is now clear that in fact three main barrier layers at the interface between blood and tissue protect the CNS: the endothelium of brain capillaries, and the epithelia of the choroid plexus (CP) and the arachnoid (Abbott, 2005; Engelhardt, 2006).

In 1941, Broman proposed that it was the cerebral capillary endothelial cells that contribute the physical barrier function of the BBB, and not the astrocytic end feet. The argument concerning whether the astrocytes or the capillary endothelium constitute the BBB was supported by electron microscopic cytochemical studies performed in 1967 by Reese and Karnovsky. They used horseradish peroxidase (HRP), ~40 kDa, to visualize the BBB by systemic injections of HRP which failed to reach the brain extracellular fluid, whereas intracerebroventricular injection into the CSF stained the brain extracellular fluid positive for HRP (Reese & Karnovsky, 1967).

It is now evident that the BBB is a unique membranous barrier, which restrictively isolates the brain parenchyma from the circulating molecules/compounds within the blood. The permeability of BBB is regulated by transport machineries of the brain capillary endothelial cells that are modulated by autocrine and paracrine secretions from several types of cells, such as the pericyte, the astrocyte, and neurons (Rubin & Staddon, 1999).

The pericyte cells share the capillary basement membrane with the endothelium and physically supports endothelial cells (Allt & Lawrenson, 2001). It has been revealed that there is approximately one pericyte for every three endothelial cells (Pardridge, 1999). It is deemed that the pericyte cells play a regulatory role in brain angiogenesis, endothelial cell tight junction formation, BBB differentiation, and also contribute to the microvascular vasodynamic capacity and structural stability.

The astrocyte cells invest approximately 99% of the abluminal surface of the brain capillary and induce endothelial cells to differentiate directly through cell to cell communication or indirectly by secreting astrocytic factors (Pardridge, 1999). Brain capillary endothelial cells display different features in comparison with peripheral endothelial cells. The BBB can be thought of brain capillary endothelial cells (BCECs) with the physical and paracrine interactions between the endothelial cells (ECs), the pericyte, and the astrocyte (Abbott et al., 2006; Pardridge, 1999).

The ability of BCECs to form a restrictive barrier between blood and brain is not completely intrinsic to the brain microvascular endothelial cells, but instead is induced by the brain environment itself. Induction of BBB may be categorized as "directive" and "impremissive" events. The latter term means that the inductor functions upon a tissue that is already determined toward its final fate but still needs an exogenous stimulus for the expression of its full phenotype. Of note, with the lack of a brain neuronal environment, the selective restrictiveness characteristics of the BCECs disappear, and as a result appropriate incitement(s) ought to be continuous at the BBB microenvironment to maintain its functionalities (Abbott, 2005).

The astrocyte inductive effects upon endothelial cell differentiation have been examined by Stewart & Wiley (1981). They transplanted avascular tissue from 3-day-old quail brain into the coelomic cavity of chick embryos, the chick endothelial cells then vascularized the quail brain grafts formed a competent BBB. In contrast preformed microvessels growing in embryonic quail muscle, which were implanted in chick brain were leaky and lacked BBB enzymes (Stewart & Wiley, 1981).

With regard to the complexity of the BBB, basically, other differentiating factors apart from astrocytes may play a role on the formation of the BBB. However, we discuss the most important features of BBB in relation to drug delivery and targeting for brain tumors. Fig. 1 represents the schematic illustration of BCECs.

2. BBB junctional complexes and cell-to-cell interactions

Stable cell-to-cell interactions are required to keep the structural integrity of tissues. Dynamic changes in cell-to-cell adhesion will participate in the morphogenesis of developing tissues. Adhesion mechanisms are highly regulated during tissue morphogenesis and related to the processes of cell motility and cell migration. Cell junctions, basically, can be classified into three functional groups, including: 1) tight junctions (TJs), 2) anchoring (adherent) junctions (AJs), and 3) gap (communication) junctions (GJs). Of these junctions, the TJs seal cells together in cell sheet, the AJs attach cells to their neighbors or to the extra-cellular matrix mechanically, and the GJs mediate the passage of chemicals or electrical signals from one interacting cell to its partner (Engelhardt, 2006; Omidi & Gumbleton, 2005). Because of crucial role of TJs in restrictive function of BBB, they are briefly discussed.

Fig. 2 shows the diagrammatic representation of TJs and its complexity with other proteins at the BBB. TJs of the BBB generate a rate-limiting restrictive barrier to paracellular diffusion of solutes between endothelial cells. They are the most apical element of the junctional complex that includes both tight and adherens junctions. In terms of morphology, TJs form a continuous network of parallel, interconnected, intra-membrane strand of various proteins arranged as a series of multiple barriers.

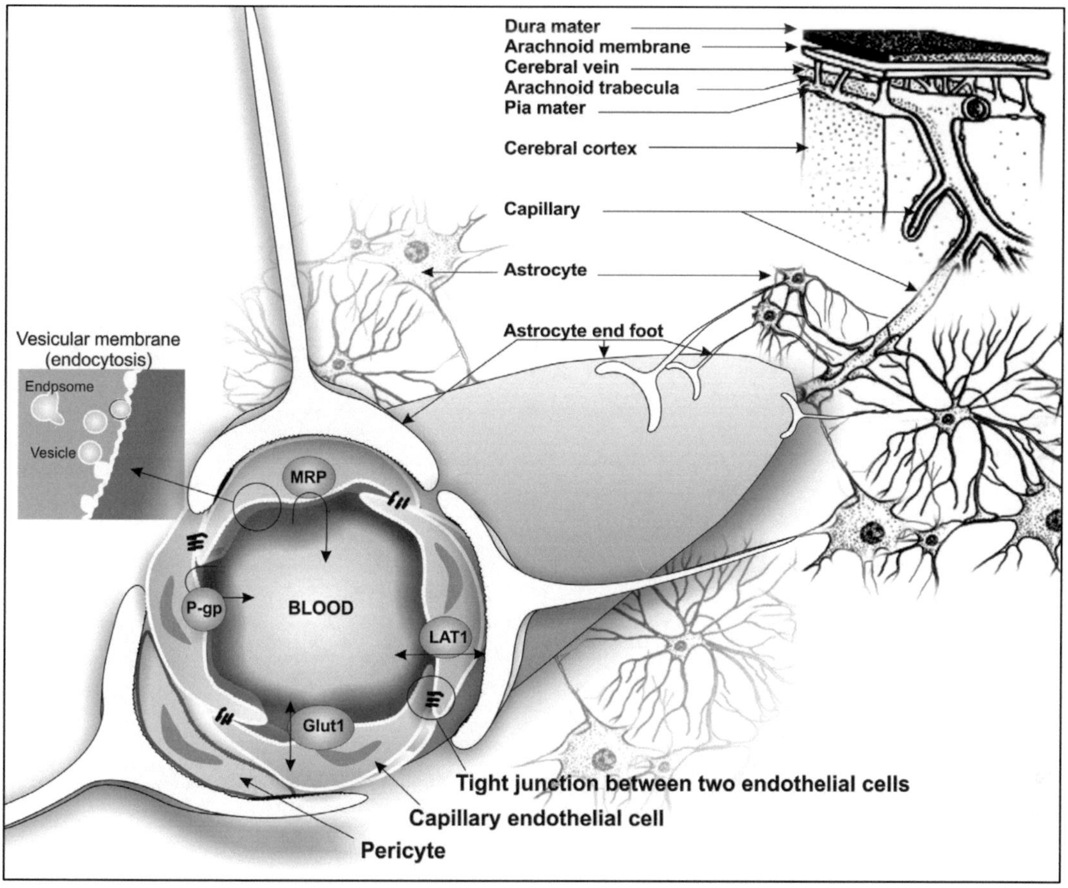

Fig. 1. Schematic demonstration of part of cortex and brain capillary endothelial cells. Star shape astrocytes are in communication with both brain capillaries and neurons via end-foot. The ultrastructural characteristics (in particular presence of tight junction) of the brain capillary endothelial cells differ them from other peripheral capillaries. Some of important specialized transporters are illustrated on luminal section which represents vesicular trafficking machineries for traverse necessary macromolecules from blood to brain, adapted with permission (Omidi & Barar, 2012).

2.1 Tight junctions of BBB

Using freeze–fracture technique, it has been shown that the tight junctions of the BBB are characterized by the highest complexity found in the vasculature, so that protoplasmic fracture face (P-face) association of the BBB compare to the peripheral endothelial cells is 55% and 10%, respectively. The altered particles distribution implies the presence of a strong interaction between TJs of the BBB and cytoskeleton. TJs of the BBB, morphologically, are more comparable to TJs of the epithelial cells than to TJs of the endothelial cells in peripheral blood vessels. Although the tight junction of BBB discloses many characteristics of epithelial TJs, there are distinctive differences between them, e.g. in terms of particle density and distribution, in relation to response to ambient factors.

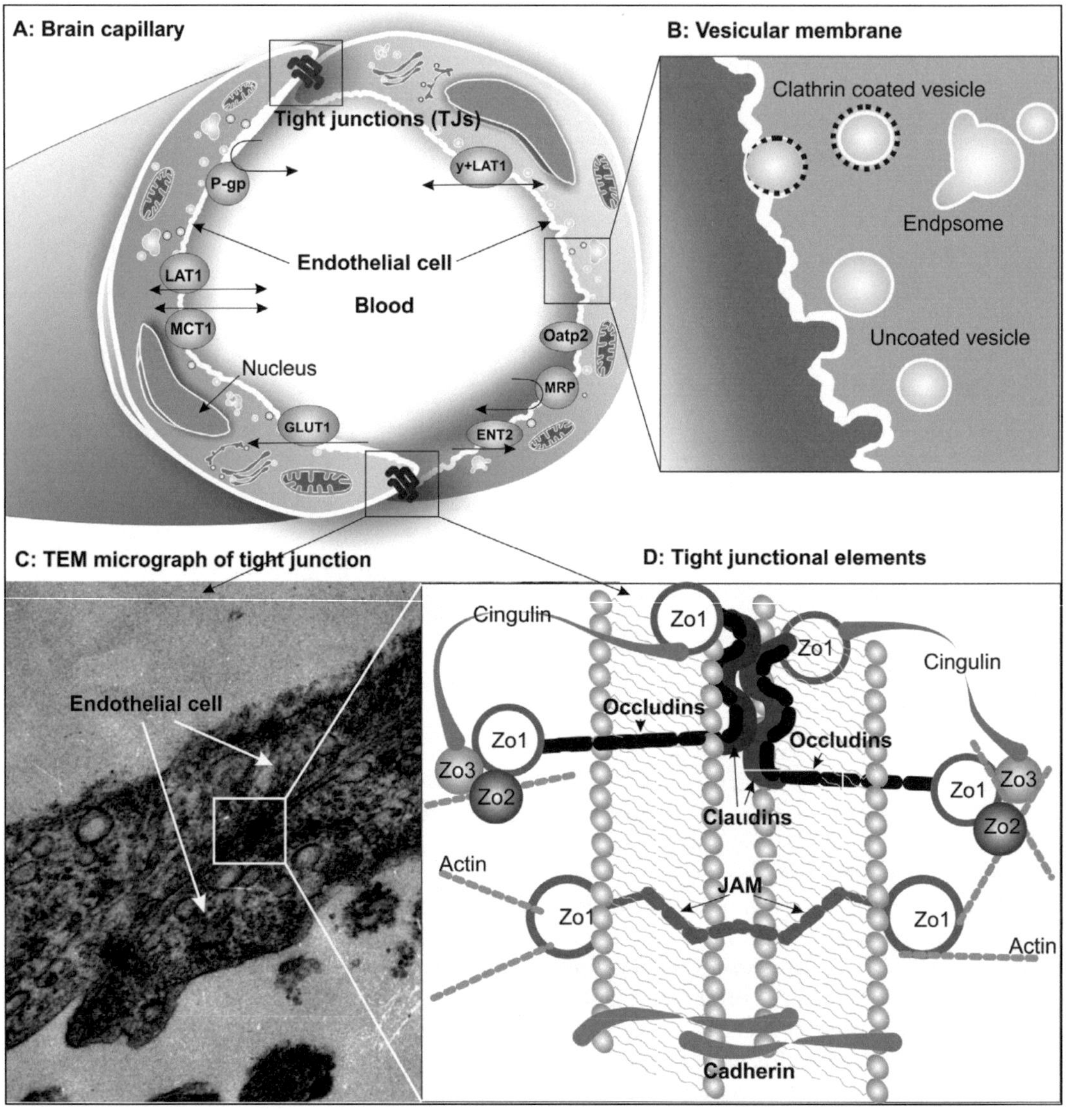

Fig. 2. Illustration of the brain capillary endothelial cells (BCECs) morphology and architecture. A) Schematic elongated two brain capillary endothelial cells with some apical transporters. B) Vesicular membrane of BCECs showing coated and uncoated vesicles. C) Transmission electron microscopy micrograph of BCECs showing tight junction (TJ). D) Tight junctional interactions of two endothelial cells. The TJ is embedded in a cholesterol-enriched region of the plasma membrane. Claudins comprise a multigene family with 20 isoforms currently identified and form the backbone of TJ strands by making dimers and binding homotypically to claudins on adjacent cells to produce the primary seal of the TJ.

Claudin 1, 3 and 5 are present at the BBB. Occludin functions as a dynamic regulatory protein causing increased electrical resistance across the membrane and decreased paracellular permeability. BBB endothelial cells in vivo reveal a P-face/E-face ratio of about 55%/45%, and as claudin-3 and claudin-5 are well expressed, it can be suggested that the degree of association with one or the other leaflet roughly reflects the stoichiometry of claudin expression in the TJs of BBB. However, in the non-BBB endothelial cells, tight junctions are almost completely associated with the E-face and claudin-3 is rarely or not expressed, adapted with permission (Omidi & Barar, 2012).

Many identified ubiquitous molecular components of junctional complexes in the epithelia such as claudins, occludins, zonula (ZO-1, ZO-2, ZO-3) , junctional adhesion molecules (JAMs), cingulin, and 7H6 have been detected at the BBB. Both tight and adherent junctions are composed of multiple protein complexes, which communicate with the actin cytoskeleton of the cells (Kniesel & Wolburg, 2000).

The TJ contains various proteins, which are necessary to form structural support for the tight junction such as zonula occludens proteins that belong to a family of membrane associated guanylate kinase-like proteins and serve as recognition proteins for tight junctional placement and as a support structure for signal transduction proteins. Junctional adherent molecules (JAMs) are localized at the TJ and are members of the immunoglobin superfamily, which can function in association with platelet-endothelial cellular adhesion molecule 1 (PECAM1) to regulate leukocyte migration. Cingulin is a double-stranded myosin-like protein that binds preferentially to ZO proteins at the globular head and to other cingulin molecules at the globular tail. The primary cytoskeletal protein, actin, has known binding sites on all of the ZO proteins, and on claudin and occludin.

In terms of TJ regulation, phosphorylation of both transmembrane and accessory proteins plays an important role in establishing and regulating the TJs. The Occludin and ZO1, as the primary regulatory proteins of the TJs, are phosphorylated on serine, threonine and tyrosine residues. The increased phosphorylation of serine/threonine correlates with decreased extractability of occludin and TJs assembly. Regulation of TJs is also dependent on tyrosine phosphorylation of proteins at cell to cell contacts. Development of TJ barrier functions has been correlated with decreased tyrosine phosphorylation of proteins at the TJ complexes. Protein kinase C (PKC) also is a major regulator of TJs formation and regulation. It plays an important role in ZO1 migration to the plasma membrane and there are PKC phosphorylation consensus sequences in the ZO1 protein, suggesting that ZO proteins serve as scaffolding for PKC signal transduction pathways on the cytoplasmic surface of intercellular junctions. It has also been shown that TJs are generally localized at cholesterol-enriched regions or rafts within the plasma membrane. Caveolin-1, an integral protein within caveolae membrane domains may associate with TJ components. Caveolin-1 itself interacts with and regulates the activity of several signal transduction pathways and downstream targets. Several cytoplasmic signaling molecules are concentrated at TJ complexes and are involved in signaling cascades that control assembly and disassembly of TJs (Krizbai & Deli, 2003).

The structure and function of TJs in primary cultures of bovine brain endothelial cells were directly analyzed, using quantitative freeze-fracture electron microscopy, and ion and inulin permeability (Wolburg et al., 1994), and it was shown that the cultured brain endothelial cells tend to lose the TJ-dependent BBB characteristics such as macromolecular impermeability and high electrical resistance with conditioned culture. The tight junction complexity index (CI), as the number of branch points per unit length of tight junctional strands, was decreased 5 hr after culturing the primary bovine brain microvessel endothelial cells. However, the association of TJ particles with the cytoplasmic leaflet of the endothelial membrane bilayer (P-face) decreased steadily during culture with a major drop between 16 hr and 24 hr. Wolburg et al. showed that the CI could be increased by elevation of intracellular cyclic adenosine monophosphate (cAMP) levels, while phorbol esters had the opposite effect - the endothelial cells P-face association of TJ particles was enhanced by elevation of cAMP levels and by astrocyte coculture (ACC) or exposure to astrocyte conditioned-medium (ACM). The authors also highlighted that astrocytes induced the latter effect on P-face association; and also showed that elevation of cAMP levels together with ACM increased trans-endothelial/epithelial electrical resistance (TEER) synergistically and decreased inulin permeability of primary cultures. They, thus, concluded that P-face association of TJ particles in brain ECs may be a critical feature of the blood-brain barrier functionality that can be specifically modulated by astrocytes and cAMP levels.

2.2 Astrocytes

Astrocytes are glial cells that envelop >99% of the BBB endothelium (Hawkins & Davis, 2005). Astrocytes and endothelial cells reciprocally affect each other's structure and/functions - their interactions induce and modulate the development of the BBB. Such interaction enhances the TJs and reduces the gap junctional area of BCECs, while increases the number of astrocytic membrane particle assemblies and astrocyte density. Astrocytes are essential for proper neuronal activities, for which the close proximity of astrocytes and BCECs appear to be essential for a functional neurovascular unit (Abbott et al., 2006). Based on *in vitro* investigations, the coculture of BCECs with astrocytes can improve the BBB functionality such as permeability and cellular transport functions (Omidi et al., 2008).

The nature of the astrocyte-derived factors (ADFs) is not fully understood, inductive effect of ADFs on brain microvascular endothelial cell differentiation and BBB formation has been well reported. Investigation upon the modulatory effects of astrocyte on BCECs have revealed that the rat astrocyte cells are able to modulate the chick peripheral ECs to make them less permeable to large molecules. On the molecular level, increased expression of barrier-relevant proteins (e.g., tight junction proteins) has so far been documented in the presence of ADFs. Many studies have shown the improvement of physiological parameters (e.g., increased TEER and decreased paracellular permeability) in different in vitro models of the BBB treated with ADFs. Moreover, it should be evoked that the interaction of BCECs and astrocytes is bidirectional and that the other cell types surrounding the brain microvasculature also contribute to BBB function or dysfunction. From many kinds of different experimental designs, it is quite clear that astrocyte factors are able to modulate TJ restrictiveness under perhaps certain defined conditions. To test the astrocytic factors effect on endothelial cells, Shivers et al. (1988) aimed to find out whether these factors can initiate development of non-CNS microvessel endothelial cells by culturing and passaging bovine aorta and pulmonary artery endothelial cells in the presence of 50% ACM. The investigators reported the endothelial cells maintained in ACM displayed complex tight junctions as well as gap junctions, but the cells plated onto plastic or fibronectin-coated substrates without

ACM showed no tight or gap junctions. This finding directed them to conclude that CNS astrocytes generate soluble factor(s), which can provoke formation of tight junction components in non-CNS endothelial cells. Astrocyte inductive effect(s) on the expression of the BBB characteristic enzymes including γ-glutamyl transpeptidase (γ-GTP) and alkaline phosphatase have been well presented (Allt & Lawrenson, 2001; Haseloff et al., 2005). Using an astrocyte coculture system with endothelial cells Rauh et al (1992) showed that a possible direct cell-to-cell contact between BCECs and astroglial cells is probably needed for astrocyte inductive effects. However this is a controversial issue as secreted ADF effects on endothelial cells are well recognized. Shivers et al (1988) and Tio et al. (1990) also reported that both ACC and ACM (isolated rat brain astrocyte cells) can induce the alkaline phosphatase activity and tight junction generation in the human umbilical cord vein endothelial cells (Shivers et al., 1988; Tio et al., 1990).

In 1999, Igarashi *et al.* examined the relationship of glial-derived neurotrophic factor (GDNF), which maintains the dopaminergic system and motor neurons *in vivo*, with BBB using isolated primary porcine brain capillary endothelial cells (PBCECs) and reported that GDNF at concentrations of 0.1 and 1 ng per ml can significantly enhance the barrier functionality (tight junction integrity) with increases in TEER values and decreases in mannitol permeability (Igarashi *et al.* 1999). It can be deduced that GDNF is able to seal tightly the paracellular pathway in addition to its homeostasis role on the CNS. Moreover, it appears that factors secreted by brain endothelial cells including leukaemia inhibitory factor (LIF) can induce astrocyte differentiation. ADFs also influence the functionality of BBB carrier-mediated transport systems (Abbott, 2005). The use of BBB transports will be discussed later in this chapter.

2.3 Pericytes

Pericytes are an imperative cellular constituent of the BBB, which also play a regulatory role in terms of brain angiogenesis and tight junction formation within BCECs. These cells also contribute to the microvascular vasodynamic capacity and structural stability. They are actively involved in the neuroimmune network operating at the BBB and confer macrophage functions. The pericyte and endothelial cell interaction occurs via cytoplasmic processes of the pericyte indenting the EC and vice versa. This contact process is called "peg and socket"-an interdigitation process (Wakui et al., 1989). Larson *et al.* (1987) studied intercellular relationship in the microvasculature using fluorescent Lucifer yellow CH dye/radiolabeled nucleotide and freeze-fracture methodology, and showed that cultured pericytes presented gap junctions in freeze-fracture replicas and extensive nucleotide and dye transfer. Observing low dye transfer and high nucleotide transfer between bovine brain microvessel endothelial cells and pericytes, they proposed a possible junctional contact between these cells that promotes their differentiation (Larson et al., 1987).

Basically, some biomolecules including adhesive glycoprotein and fibronectin have been found localized at the BCECs and pericytes junctional sites adjacent to "adhesion plaques" at the plasma membrane. The adhesion plagues implied the existence of a mechanical linkage between pericytes and ECs, i.e. a linkage that allowed mechanical contraction or relaxation of the pericyte to influence vessel diameter. This later process may assist the endothelial cells to reduce their size. Pericytes have specific and localized distribution in different tissues displaying a granular morphology reflecting lysosomal enrichment. Using an *in vivo* rat model, it has been reported that blood-brain barrier disruption, e.g. by hyperosmotic mannitol with adriamycin, causes an increase of pericyte lysosomes (Kondo et al., 1987). Pericytes are rich in plasmalemmal and cytoplasmic vesicles as well as microfilament bundles, but interestingly only about 10% of vesicles locate to the surface facing ECs. Most importantly pericytes modulate endothelial cells phenotype not only by physical action but also via secreting epidermal growth factor (EGF). Indeed, it has already been shown that EGF is an effective endothelial cell mitogen that enhances angiogenesis, and is concentrated at and during pericytes-ECs cross-talk and interdigitation processes. The expression of γ-GTP has been shown in the pericyte as well as the brain microvessel endothelial cells. Using γ-GTP as the sole marker for the primary isolated brain capillary endothelial cells seems not to be right and proper due to possible pericytic contamination. The transforming growth factor-beta (TGF-b), produced by pericytes, plays an important role in reducing lymphocyte infiltration into the CNS in inflammatory demyelinating diseases. Pericytes can stabilize capillary-like structures formed by endothelial cells in coculture with astrocytes. This latter process can be driven by TGF-b1, which is one of the TGF-b isoforms (Allt & Lawrenson, 2001; Ramsauer et al., 2002).

The cultured pericytes in the endothelial cell conditioned-medium (ECCM) allowed the cerebral pericyte aminopeptidase N (pAPN) to be re-expressed, while purified pericytes deprived of endothelial cells even in the presence of ACM showed no reexpression. This indicates that endothelial cells constitute an essential requirement for the in vitro re-expression of pAPN, but not astrocytes. Pericytes are involved in amino acid and peptide catabolism of the brain. This suggests that pericytes play a key metabolic role aside from structural role in relation to the BBB maintenance and homeostasis. In addition, based on the reciprocal pericytes-ECs interactions and cross talk, it can be suggested that the two-way interdigitations may stimulate not only the BBB endothelial cell activities but also promote pericyte functions. Pericytes may have a role in the possible cross-talk between pericytes, astrocyte and endothelial cells, a triple intercommunication process that may bring us to consider the notion of pericyte positive contribution in the physiopathology of the BBB as well as certain diseases such as Alzheimer. For example, β-amyloid peptide 42 can be uptaken by the phagocytic pericytes and astrocytes. This process helps to clear the exogenous peptide from the brain extracellular space and deliver it to the blood circulation system that shows also the contribution of pericytes in the BBB transport functionality (Allt & Lawrenson, 2001; Balabanov & Dore-Duffy, 1998; Pluta et al., 2000).

3. Bioelectrical properties and permeability

Due to the association of the TEER with permeability, TEER values commonly are exploited to describe the permeability of the BBB. The [^{14}C] sucrose permeability is used to assess the restrictiveness of BBB in relation to *in vivo* (1.2×10^{-7} cm.sec^{-1}). *In vivo* TEER values vary in the epithelial and endothelial cells. For instance human placental endothelium shows TEER 22–52 Ω.cm^2 that permits rapid paracellular exchange of nutrients and waste between the mother and fetus (Jinga *et al.* 2000), whereas urinary bladder epithelium has a very high TEER of 6000–30000 Ω.cm^2, necessary for preserving urine composition (Powell 1981). The BBB possesses TEER vales of ~2000 Ω.cm^2, which helps to maintain brain homeostasis (Engelhardt, 2006).

Efforts to generate an *in vitro* BBB model, in fact, have been based upon measurement of the TEER, assessment of the sucrose permeability and expression of the specific enzymes and markers of the BBB. The higher TEER and the lower sucrose permeability confer the better characteristics. To achieve this aim different techniques have been recruited, e.g. utilizing of the hydrocortisone and serum free medium in order to increase the TEER (up to 1000 $\Omega.cm^2$) by stimulating the formation of barrier properties (Hoheisel *et al.* 1998).

4. Modulation of BBB permeability

4.1 Extracellular matrix

The influence of extracellular matrix on the BBB properties has been investigated by several researchers using cell lines and primary isolated BCECs. Shivers *et al.* (1988) showed that the local control of tight junction biogenesis in brain capillary endothelial cells depends on astrocyte-produced factors and extracellular matrix. The ECs in general do not express their final destination-specific differentiated features until those features are induced by local environment-produced conditions including extracellular matrix. Using primary cultures of PBCECs, Tilling *et al.* (1998) examined the effect of collagen IV, fibronectin, laminin and a secreted acidic protein and rich in cysteine alone or one-to-one mixtures of them. They showed that these proteins are involved in tight junction formation between cerebral capillary endothelial cells by presenting increased TEER (Robert & Robert, 1998; Tilling et al., 1998).

4.2 The role of cyclic AMP (cAMP)

The effect of cAMP on BBB function has been studied by several researchers. Using combination of astrocyte conditioned-medium and cAMP elevators, Rubin et al (1991) reported a cell culture *in vitro* BBB model that generated high resistance tight junctions and exhibited low rates of paracellular permeability. Hurst et al (1996) showed that a coculture BBB model of the immortalized human umbilical vein endothelial cells ECV304 (reassigned later as T24 bladder epithelial carcinoma cell) with rat C6 glioma cells can generate a BBB model with high TEER (~400-600 $\Omega.cm^2$). They demonstrated bioelectrical alterations by vasoactive agonists and cAMP elevators (i.e. decreased TEER by histamine, bradykinin, and serotonin and increased TEER by cAMP, such as forskolin elevators). The researchers also showed formation of inositol triphosphates (IPs) that can induce the release of calcium ions from cellular storage sites and a subsequent rise in intracellular calcium which can activate diacylglycerol (DAG) and accordingly the PKC that could increase the permeability of the endothelial cells (Hurst & Clark, 1998). Investigation on the effects of elevated intracellular cAMP and astrocyte derived factors on the F-actin cytoskeleton and paracellular permeability of RBE4 cell monolayers have revealed that the cAMP effects on the TEER appear likely to be independent of new gene transcription (Rist et al., 1997).

The protein GDNF can activate the barrier functions of the BCECs in the presence of cAMP. It has been reported that GDNF not only can promote the barrier restrictiveness but also support the survival of neurons in the presence of cAMP. The role of other factors on brain ECs signaling and the BBB formation is uncertain (Igarashi et al., 1999). However, some other factors such as vascular endothelial growth factor (VEGF) appear to increase the permeability of BCECs because of loss of occludin and ZO-1 from the endothelial cell junctions (Wang et al., 2001), while cAMP acts against such phenomenon. All of these processes, somehow, play a role in modulating the full BBB characteristics. By means of an unpassaged primary culture of rat BCECs, it has been shown that certain cell-surface receptors may fulfill a role in BBB regulation. For example, brain endothelial regulation was shown by P2Y2 receptors coupled to phospholipase C, Ca^{2+} and MAPK; and by P2Y1-like (2MeSATP-sensitive) receptors that are linked to Ca^{2+} mobilization. It should be stated that differential MAPK coupling of these receptors appear to exert fundamentally distinct influences over brain endothelial function in terms of cAMP modulation (Albert et al., 1997).

4.3 Inflammatory mediators

Basically, the brain endothelium forming the BBB can be modulated by a range of inflammatory mediators. Given that the main routes for penetration of polar solutes across the BBB include the paracellular tight junctional pathway and vesicular machineries, inflammatory mediators appear to influence both pathways, while such impacts can also be seen in other closely associated cells such as pericytes, astrocytes, smooth muscle, microglia, mast cells, and neurons. Various inflammatory agents are able to increase both endothelial permeability and vessel diameter, and these together can result in significant leakiness of BBB and accordingly cerebral edema. Of these agents, the bradykinin (Bk) is able to increases the permeability of BBB by acting on B2 receptors, perhaps via elevation of Ca^{2+}, activation of phospholipase A2, release of arachidonic acid, and production of free radicals. Serotonin (5HT) can also increase the permeability of BBB through a calcium-dependent mechanism. Histamine as nervous system neurotransmitters possesses capability of consistent blood-brain barrier opening mediated by H2 receptors and elevation of Ca^{2+}, but the H1 receptor coupled to an elevation of cAMP can decrease the permeability of BBB. Elevation of arachidonic acid may also cause gross opening of the BBB to large molecules such as peptides/proteins. There exist a number of studies showing purposed recruitment of such mechanisms for deliberate opening of the BBB for drug delivery to the brain; readers are directed to see (Abbott, 2000).

5. BBB enzymes and other differentiation markers

Several markers are most commonly exploited and include γ-GTP and alkalin phosphatase (ALP) enzymes expression, or antigenic endothelial cell markers such as: Factor VIII , von Willebrand Factor (vWF). Additionally the uptake of acetylated low density lipoprotein (LDL) i.e. dioctadecyl-indocarbocyanine (Di-I) labeled acetylated LDL (Di-I-Ac-LDL) and the binding of lectin, i.e. biotinylated lectins (BL) *Ultex europaeus I* (UE I) and *Bandeiraea simplicifolia* isolation B_4 (BSA IB_4) have been exploited. Further, a high glucose transporter (GLUT-1) density has been shown as a marker of brain microvascular endothelia. The γ-GTP, ALP and membrane peptidases (aminopeptidase N, peptidyle dipeptidase and dipeptidyl peptidase IV) have been used as marker for the BBB. The γ-GTP is of special importance due to its high expression in the BCECs, therefore it is used as a marker for ECs of the BBB. By contrast, this marker is absent from brain ECs of paraventricular nucleus, where the BBB characteristics and properties are lacking. The induction of γ-GTP by astrocyte has been reported, even though the high expression of this enzyme in the pericytes makes it a non-specific marker of the BBB. The ALP is highly expressed in the BCECs and used as a marker. Like γ-GTP, its expression can be modulated by astrocytes. The metabolism of neuropeptides is mediated by membrane peptidases at the BBB. Three members of the membrane peptidases (dipeptidyl peptidase A; aminopeptidase N; dipeptidyl peptidase IV) have been found in the BCECs, but many more vessels are positive for them, in particular more positive for dipeptidyl peptidase A than other two. The expression of the BBB enzymes depends on the different parameters such as direct cell-to-cell communications or cell-derived factors. Enzymatic activities of the γ-GTP and ALP are taken as indicators for the expression of the BBB phenotype; reader is directed to see (Allt & Lawrenson, 2000; Allt & Lawrenson, 2001; Orte et al., 1999).

6. Transportation of exogenous/endogenous compounds across BBB

The capability of a particular substance to cross the BBB and enter the CNS is dependent upon a number of parameters, including physicochemical properties such as molecular weight (MW), lipophilicity, pKa, hydrogen bonding as well as biological factors. The BBB transportation, nevertheless, may generally be classified into different categories, including: 1) passive diffusion that depends on physicochemical properties and mainly on the lipophilicity of the molecule, 2) facilitated transport via carrier-mediated transporters (Glut1, LAT1), 3) paracellular pathway (small hydrophilic componds), 4) receptor-mediated endocytosis/transcytosis, and 4) Liquid-phase (adsorptive) endocytosis/transcytosis. Fig. 3 represents schematic illustration of BBB transport systems.

Brain drug delivery and targeting requires overcoming the limited access of drugs to the brain. Different methods have been developed to achieve BBB penetration, including: opening of BBB TJs by means of osmotic or biologically active agents (such as bradykinin and histamine); exploiting of various specific transport mechanisms. The last methodology includes: conjugation of a drug with a targeting protein, or to a monoclonal antibody that gains access to the brain by receptor-mediated transcytosis, or to a small peptide-vectors to enhance brain uptake of several therapeutic drugs. Further the use of drug delivery devices such as liposomes has also been reported. As shown in Fig. 4, the BBB carrier-mediated transporters comprise two different classes, including the efflux and the influx pump transport systems.

6.1 Efflux transporters

The BBB represents a major hindrance to the entry of many therapeutic drugs into the brain and efflux pumps are part of this protection. P-glycoprotein (P-gp; MDR1/ABCB1) is an ATP-binding cassette (ABC) drug transport protein that is predominantly found in the apical membranes of a number of epithelial cell types in the body as well as the brain microvessel endothelial cells. The putative transmembrane structural organization of human MDR1 P-gp is primarily found in the cell plasma membrane as 12 transmembrane segments that are thought to fold together and form a three-dimensional barrier like structure in the cell plasma membrane. The latter polypeptide chain consists of two similar halves. Each half contains of six putative transmembrane segments and intracellular ATP-binding site. The hydrolysis of ATP provides the energy for active drug export. Schinkel et al (1995) showed that mouse MDR1a and the human MDR1 P-glycoprotein actively transport ivermectin, dexamethasone, digoxin, and cyclosporin A and, to a lesser extent, morphine across a polarized kidney epithelial cell layer in vitro. The investigator reported that injection of the radiolabeled substrates of P-gp in MDR1a knockout and wild-type mice resulted in 20- to

50-fold higher levels of radioactivity in the MDR1a knockout mice brain for digoxin and cyclosporin A (Schinkel et al., 1995b). These researchers generated mice with a genetic disruption of the drug-transporting MDR1a P-gp and showed that the P-gp knockout mice were overall healthy but they accumulated much higher levels of substrate drugs in the brain with markedly slower elimination. For the drugs (e.g., anticancer agents) that are P-gp substrates, this can lead to dramatically increased toxicity (Schinkel et al., 1995a). Thus, drugs inhibiting the MDR1 P-gp activity should be co-administered during chemotherapy of the brain tumors. The authors concluded that P-gp is the major determinant for the pharmacology of several medically important drugs apart from anti-cancer agents, especially in the BBB.

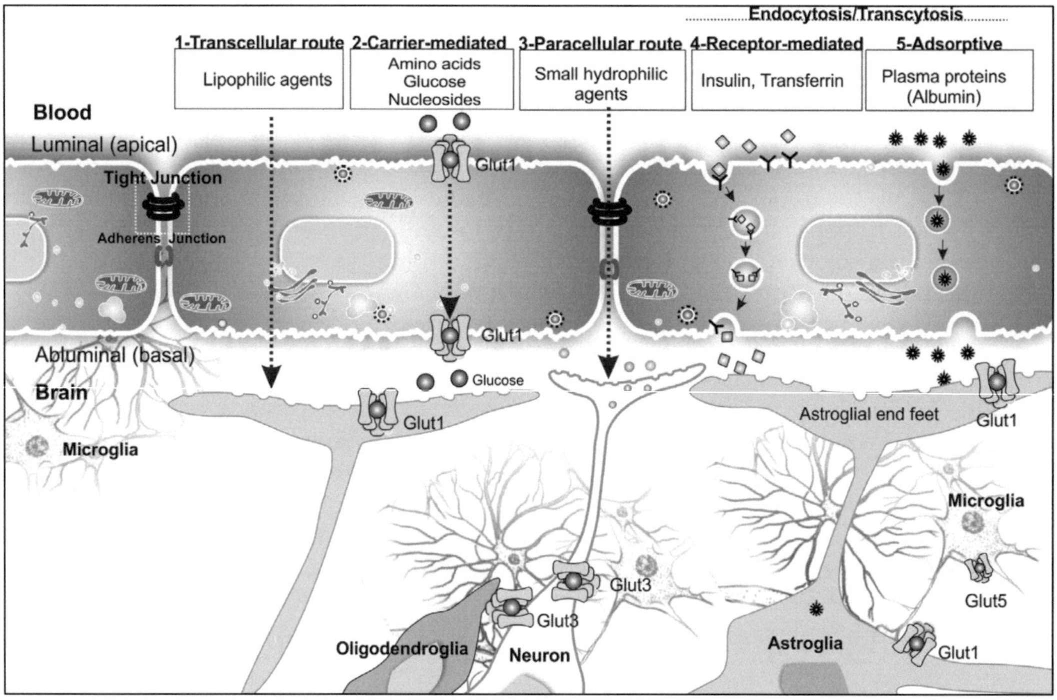

Fig. 3. Schematic illustration of transportation systems for shuttling of endogenous and/or exogenous substrates at the BBB. 1) Lipid-soluble small substrates (<500 Da) are able to diffuse across the membrane - they may be effluxed back into the blood circulation through efflux transporters (e.g., P-gp, MRP4). 2) Carrier-mediated transport machineries (e.g., Glut1, LAT1) are responsible for transport of small endogenous molecules (e.g., amino acids, nucleosides, and glucose). 3) Some small hydrophilic molecules can be transported via paracellular route. 4) Larger molecules (e.g., insulin, transferrin) are transported through receptor-mediated endpcytosis/transcytosis using vesicular trafficking towards the brain parenchyma. 5) Some large proteins (e.g., albumin) are transported across the BBB by adsorptive-mediated endocytosis/transcytosis. Of the carrier-mediated transporters, glucose transporters (Gluts) are responsible for traverse of glucose from blood to brain and btween different cells within the brain parenchyma. Adherens junctions provide a path for cell-to-cell intercommunication within endothelial cells of the BBB, adapted with permission (Omidi & Barar, 2012).

Multidrug-resistance associated protein (MRP) (Zhang *et al.* 2000) actively transports a broad range of anionic compounds out of the cell in the BBB and is known as another member of the ABC superfamily of transport proteins. It has approximately 15% amino acid sequence homology to P-gp, and the characteristics ATP binding sites that allow for the active transport of a diverse array of compounds out of the cell. In contrast to P-gp, MRP transports organic anions. Zhang et al (2000) reported that the MRP1, MRP4, MRP5, and MRP6 were consistently expressed in both the capillary-enriched fraction of the brain homogenate and the BBMEC monolayers. The expression of MRP2 has also been shown in the isolated primary porcine microvessel endothelial cells (Fricker *et al.* 2002). The presence of several different MRP homologues at the BBB highlights the MRP role in controlling the permeability of the BBB to organic anions. In the brain, MRP4 was shown to be expressed on the luminal membrane of BCECs as well as the basolateral membrane of the choroid plexus. The chemotherapeutic drug topotecan was shown to be accumulated in the brain and the CSF in an MRP4 knockout mouse model. This clearly highlights the important role that MRP4 plays in determining the CNS distribution of this drug (Leggas et al., 2004). It is likely that multiple efflux drug transporters including MRP4 govern the brain penetration and activity of this anticancer agent. Readers are directed to see (Tsuji, 2005; Urquhart & Kim, 2009).

It should be stated that most of anticancer agents are substrate to ABC transporters. Of these, the MDR1/ABCB1 can pump out a wide range of compounds (e.g., Acebutolol, Actinomycin D, Amprenavir, Azidopine, Betamethasone, Calcein-AM, Cepharanthin, Cerivastatin, Chloroquine, Cimetidine, Clarithromycin, Colchicine, Cortisol, Cyclosporin A, Daunorubicin, Dexamethasone, Digitoxin, Digoxin, Dipyridamole, Docetaxel, Domperidone, Doxorubicin, Eletriptan, Emetine, Epinastine, Erythromycin, Estradiol-17b-D-glucuronide, Estrone, Ethynyl estradiol, Etoposide, Fexofenadine, Grepafloxacin, Imatinib, Indinavir, Irinotecan, Ivermectin, Lansoprazole, Levofloxacin, Loperamide, Losartan, Lovastatin, Methylprednisolone, Mitoxantrone, Morphine, Neostigmine, Omeprazole, Pantoprazole, Prazosin, Prednisolone, Puromycin, Quinidine2, Ramosetron, Ranitidine, Reserpine, Ritonavir, Saquinavir, Somatostain, Sparfloxacin, Talinolol, Taxol, Terfenadine, Trimethoprim, Vecuronium, Verapamil, Vinblastine, Vincristine), while the MRP4/ABCC4 is able to efflux a narrower spectrum (e.g., cAMP, cGMP, Dehydroepiandrosterone-3-sulfate, Estradiol-17b-D-glucuronide, Folate, Methotrexate, Prostaglandin E1, Prostaglandin E2). The breast cancer resistance protein (BCRP/ABCG2) have been reported to be expressed as active efflux drug transporters at the BBB that can display efflux functionality similar to that of P-gp for a wide range of componds (e.g., Azidodeoxythymidine, Bisantrene, Cerivastatin, Doxorubicin, Daunorubicin, Dehydroepiandrosterone-3-sulfate, Etoposide, Estrone-3-sulfate, Estradiol-17b-D-glucuronide, Folate, Flavopiridol, Imatinib mesylate, Mitoxantrone, Methotrexate, Prazosin, Pantoprazole, Pravastatin, Rhodamine 123, Topotecan), for more details readers are directed to see (Ohtsuki & Terasaki, 2007).

Many of these chemicals are important anticancer agents (e.g., Doxorubicin, Vinblastine, Vincristine, Methotrexate, Docetaxel, Etoposide, Idarubicin, and Taxol), thus it is vital to inhibit these efflux machineries to reach suitable concentration in brain during brain tumors chemotherapy. Various compounds were reported as inhibitors for these efflux transportsers such as colchicine, phenothiazines and quinacrine.

6.2 Influx transporters

BBB influx transporters can be divided into different groups as follows:

1. the energy transport systems for transport of glucose and mannose (Glut1); lactate, short-chain fatty acids, biotin, salicylic acid and valproic acid (MCT) and creatine (CRT),
2. the amino acid transport systems such as small (LAT2/4F2hc) and large (LAT1/4F2hc) neutral amino acid transporter systems for transport of neutral amino acids and L-dopa; acidic amino acid transporter for aspartate and glutamate (ASCT2); basic amino acid transporter (BAAT) for arginine and lysine; the β-amino acid transporter for β-alanine and taurine (TAUT); System A (ATA2) for small neutral amino acids; System ASC/system B^{0+},
3. the organic anion transport system such as OATP2 for digoxin and organic anions,
4. the nucleoside transport systems such as ENT2 and CNT2,
5. the peptide transport systems such as oligopeptide transporters (PepT1, PepT2), polypeptid transport systems such as OAT3 for PAH, HVA, indoxyl sulfate; OATP14 for thyroid hormones,
6. the neurotransmitter transport systems such as GAT2/BGT1, SERT and NET respectively for transport of γ-aminobutyric acid, serotonin and norepinephrine, and
7. the choline transport system for choline and thiamine (Ohtsuki & Terasaki, 2007).

Given that the main properties of the BBB that differ the brain capillary endothelia from other blood microvessel because of the presence of restrictive high-resistance tight junctions between blood and brain parenchyma, the BBB forming BCECs almost completely prevents the uptake of potential CNS drugs via the paracellular pathway. Thus compounds passing the BBB almost exclusively have to exploit the transcellular pathway, but this is not always the case since there are increasing evidences that a broad variety of transport machineries are involved, including both carrier-mediated transport and receptor-mediated transcytosis for transporting compounds into the brain (the so called active influx) and multidrug transport pumps for actively effluxing unwanted chemicals out of brain (the so called active efflux). In the case of transport into the brain, numerous systems have been discovered, including transport proteins for amino acids, monocarboxylic acids, organic cations, hexoses, nucleotides and peptides. Several of these proteins have successfully been used in prodrug strategies to enable or at least enhance brain uptake of neurotherapeutic agents. Classic examples are l-dopa and progabide. Of these influx transport machineries, both pyrimidine and purine nucleoside analogs are currently used clinically as anti-metabolite drugs. Cytarabine, an analog of deoxycytidine (1-β-d-arabinofuranosylcytosine, araC, Cytosar-Us), is used as combination chemotherapy in the treatment of chronic myelogenous, leukemia, multiple myeloma, Hodgkin's lymphoma and non-Hodgkin's lymphomas; Gemcitabine (dFdC, 2',2'-di.uorodeoxycytidine, Gemzars), a broad spectrum agent, which is used for treatment of a variety of cancers including pancreatic and bladder cancers. Capecitabine (5'-deoxy-5-N-[(pentoxy) carbonyl]-cytidine, Xelodas) is used, as a prodrug, in treatment of metastatic colorectal cancer. Two purine nucleoside anti-metabolite drugs, Fludarabine (9-β-d-arabinofuranosyl-2-.uoroadenine), and Cladribine (2-chloro-2'-deoxyadenosine, CdA, Leustatins) are used for treatment of low-grade lymphomas and chronic lymphocytic leukemia (Omidi & Gumbleton, 2005).

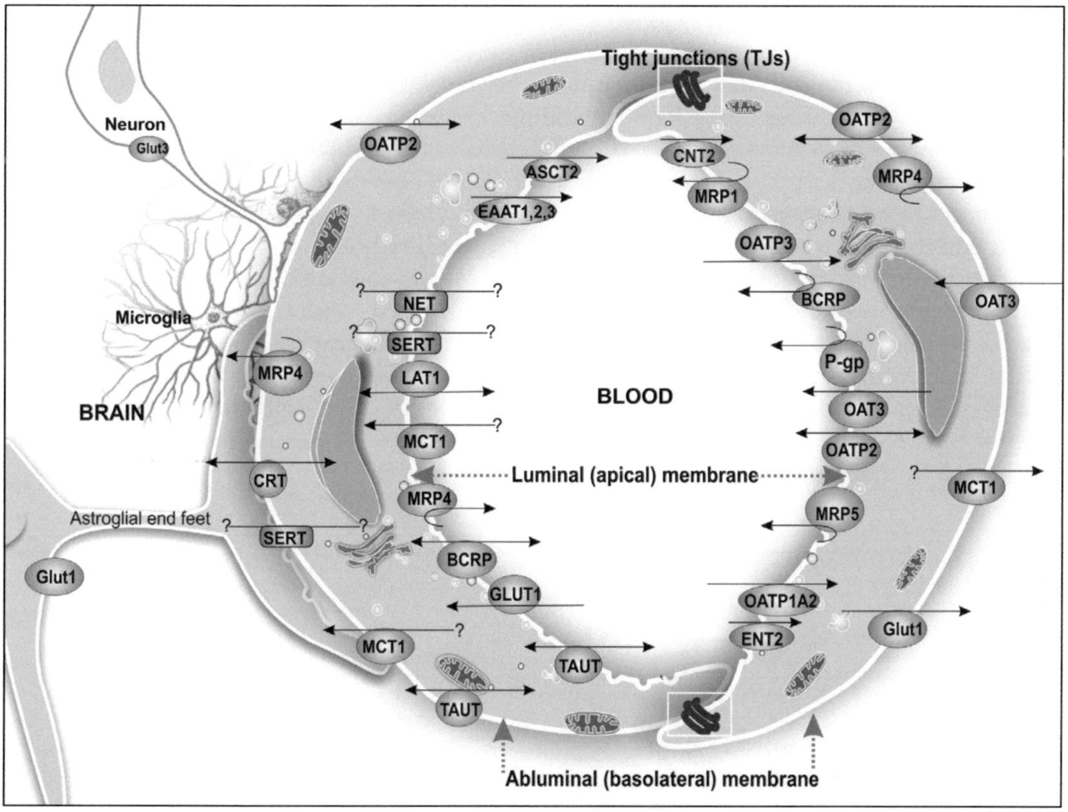

Fig. 4. Carrier-mediated transporters of the BBB (efflux and the influx transport systems) at luminal and basolateral membranes, adapted with permission from (Omidi & Barar, 2012). Astrocytes, neurons and microglial cells are intercommunication with brain capillary endotheilal cells. P-gp: P-glycoprotein. MRP1: multidrug resistance associated protein 1. MRP4: multidrug resistance associated protein 4. MRP5: multidrug resistance associated protein 5. BCRP: breast cancer resistance protein. Glut1: glucose transporter 1. MCT1: monocarboxylate transporter 1. LAT1: large neutral amino acids transporter 1. ASCT2: neutral amino acid transporter 2. EAAT: excitatory amino acid transporters. CNT2: centrative nucleoside transport 2. ENT: equilibrative nucleoside transport 2. SERT: serotonin transporter. NET: norepinephrine transporter. CRT: creatine transporter. TAUT: taurine transporter. OATP2: organic anion-transporting polypeptide. OAT3: organic anion transporter 3. OATP1A2: organic anion-transporting polypeptide. OAT2: organic anion transporter 2.

6.3 Endocytosis, transcytosis and exocytosis

Cell membranous vesicular machinery domains comprise numerous components including lipid rafts, caveolae and clathrin-coated pits. All of them appear to participate in endocytosis and probably transcytosis of macromolecules.

Caveolae are flask-shaped invaginations of the plasma membrane coated by a 22 kDa structural protein caveolin. Initially detected in endothelial cells, caveolae tend to mediate the selective uptake of molecules as small as folate to full size proteins such as albumin and lipoproteins. These micro-domains are highly enriched in glycosphingolipids, cholesterol, sphingomyelin, and lipid-anchored membrane proteins. Caveolae have been implicated in a wide range of cellular functions including transcytosis, receptor-mediated uptake, stabilization of lipid rafts and compartmentalization of a number of signaling events at the cell surface. Several studies have also shown that caveolae-mediated uptake of materials is not limited to macromolecules; in certain cell-types, viruses (e.g. simian virus 40) and even entire bacteria (e.g. specific strains of *E. Coli*) are engulfed and transferred to intracellular compartments in a caveolae-dependent fashion. Clathrin-mediated endocytosis is the most widely studied vesicular membrane internalizing system, and participation of clathrin-coated vesicles has also been investigated in terms of receptor-mediated transport in the BBB. Clathrin forms a non-covalently bound triskelion structure composed of three heavy chains (192 kDa each) and three light chains (Omidi & Gumbleton, 2005; Smith & Gumbleton, 2006). Fig. 5 represents schematic illustration of the clathrin coated vesicles (CCV) and its main protein "triskelion".

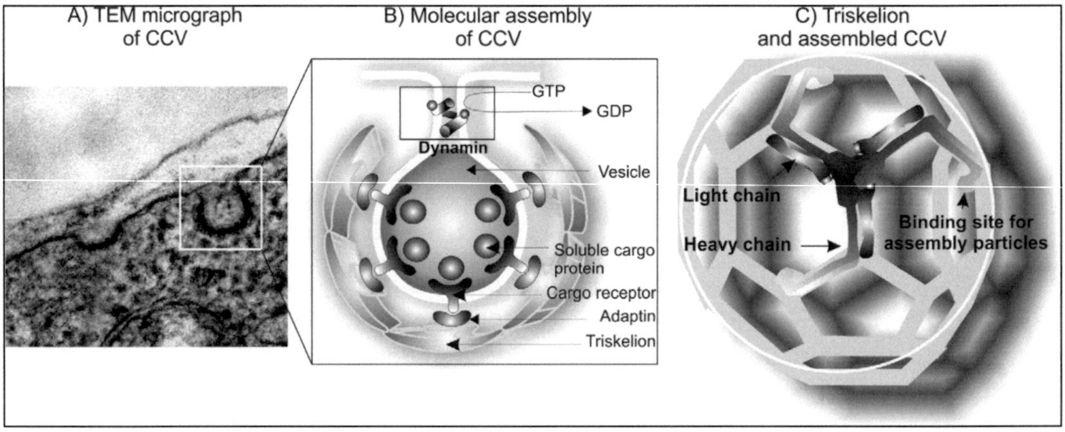

Fig. 5. TEM micrograph (A) and schematic representation of molecules involved in assembly of the clathrin coated pit (B) and its main protein triskelion (C). TEM: transmission electron microscopy; CCV: clathrin coated vesicle (Omidi & Barar, 2012).

7. BBB cell culture models

A simple, applicable, and robust *in vitro* cell based BBB model can provide a useful tool for screening of permeability to central nervous system-acting drugs. Thus, in the 1970s, techniques for isolation of brain microvessels were introduced using mechanical or enzymatic homogenization. In the late 1970's, BCECs were plated in tissue culture and this led to the early *in vitro* BBB model establishment (DeBault et al., 1979). The primary BCECs cultures are very well-characterized systems used as *in vitro* models; nevertheless they have the disadvantage of being very laborious and variable and must be repeated often to provide an adequate stock of cells. Therefore various immortalized endothelial cell lines have been developed and examined such as CR3, EC219, RBE4 b.End3, ECV304, and even epithelial cell line MDCK.

Basically, an appropriate cell culture model confers a useful platform for not only transcellular and paracellular drug diffusional processes, but also metabolism and active transport processes. Such model can be used for investigating the nondefined interactions between a drug and cellular material that may impact upon a membrane's overall permeability profile. Thus, ideally the *in vitro* BBB cell model should represent a restrictive paracellular barrier functionality, physiologically realistic cell architecture and functional expression of key transporter mechanisms. Such model should also confer ease of culture to meet the technical and time constraints of a screening program. Based upon these facts, immortalized cell based BBB models often fail to meet all these essentialities.

Despite many benefits of immortalized cell based BBB models, the lack of restrictive barrier function has limited their use for permeability screenings and therefore the primary BCECs have been isolated to be used as a cell culture BBB *in vitro* model. The main advantage from pharmaceutical perspective is that these primary models, practically the bovine and porcine models, possess a restrictive paracellular pathway. Nevertheless, BCECs grown in tissue cultures probably lack many of the characteristics of the BBB *in vivo*. In an attempt to improve such models, endothelial/astrocyte and endothelial/pericyte cocultures have been examined, even attempts to generate a 3 dimensionals (3D) model have been made. For instance aortic cells cocultured with astrocytes (C6 cells) in the presence of flow within hollow fiber tube develop a selective barrier with an estimated electrical resistance of 2,900 $\Omega.cm^2$ (Stanness et al., 1996). The same group later reported that the previously introduced 3D dynamic *in vitro* BBB model can be successfully used for the coculture of differentiated serotonergic neurons in the presence of a BBB (Stanness et al., 1999). A number of less-complicated *in vitro* coculture BBB models have also been established and developed. To produce continuous BBB *in vitro* models, several academic groups have reported the generation of immortalized brain microvessel endothelial cell lines. An immortalized human brain capillary endothelial BB19 cell line was transformed with the E6E7 genes of human papilloma virus and retained their endothelial nature. It was used to study the cytoadherence of Plasmodium falciparum-infected erythrocytes (Prudhomme et al., 1996). Human cerebral microvascular endothelial cells SV- HCEC, transfected with the plasmid pSV3-neo coding for the SV40 large T antigen, was utilized to serve as a human BBB *in vitro* model showing the expression of factor VIII-related antigen, the uptake of acetylated low-density lipoprotein, the binding of fluorescently labeled lectins, the expression of transferrin receptor, and high activities of the ALP and γ-GTP (Muruganandam et al., 1997). Immortalized brain capillary endothelial cell lines (TM-BBB1-5) were established from 3 transgenic mice harboring temperature-sensitive simian virus 40 large T-antigen gene displaying the expression of Glut-1 and P-gp. The TR-BBB cell line has also been established using same approach from a transgenic rat (Hosoya et al., 2000). An immortalized rat brain endothelial cell line, RBE4, was immortalized by transfection with a plasmid containing the E1A adenovirus gene (Roux et al., 1994). The RBE4 cell line appears to be most commonly used cell line to be exploited for investigation of different features of BBB, e.g. the transport of insulin, the expression of P-gp, the uptake of L-dopa and the expression of transferrin receptor (Balbuena et al., 2011; Hulsermann et al., 2009; Yu et al., 2007). The MBEC4 cells, established from BALB/c mouse cerebral microvessel endothelial cells, were used to investigate the high-affinity efflux transport system for glutathione conjugates (Homma et al., 1999). The CR3 cells, established by genomic introduction of the immortalizing SV40 large T gene under the control of the human vimentin promoter, displayed endothelial morphological and biochemical characteristics for up to 30 passages. The b.End3 cells was used to study the uptake and efflux of transferrin (Tf) and Fe showing the expression of Tf receptor and suggesting a receptor-mediated endocytosis for the uptake (Lechardeur et al., 1995; Lechardeur & Scherman, 1995). Given that the immortalized continuous cell lines tend not to generate a restrictive barrier property, isolated primary BCECs have been used from a variety of sources including human, bovine, porcine, monkey, rat, canine, and murine. For more details, readers are directed to see following citations (Gumbleton & Audus, 2001; Lacombe et al., 2011; Ribeiro et al., 2010).

8. BBB permeation and in-slico prediction models

Undoubtedly, the BBB is designed to protect the brain from entering of toxic compounds. As outlined above, the main underlying concept seems to be to force the compounds to take the transcellular route, where nutrients are actively transported into the brain and possibly toxic compounds are expelled via active efflux pumps. Thus, BBB permeation is a multifactorial, complex issue which requires advanced computational methods for proper modeling.

Computational models, in general, exploit two different approaches. The passive diffusion-controlled permeability is dependent upon the inherent physicochemical characteristics (e.g., logP, solubility and surface area) of the compounds, and basically molecular descriptor based methods are used to generate predictive models. The ligand-receptor (i.e., influx/efflux transporters, or receptor mediated endocytosis) active/facilitated transport can be considered for carrier/receptor mediated trafficking. Given these, predictive in-silico models suitable for both the lead identification and the lead optimization processes should include both categories. The most commonly used type of data appear to be the logBB values that are described as the ratio of the steady-state concentration of a designated compound in the brain to that of the blood which can describe by Equation (1).

$$\text{LogBB}=\text{Log}([C_{\text{Brain}}]/[C_{\text{Blood}}]) \quad (1)$$

The most commonly used in vitro model for BCECs culture is based on Transwell™ system, which consists of a porous membrane support submerged in culture media. This system is normally characterized by two direction diffusion, i.e. apical to basal (A to B) or basal to apical (B to A). Given existence of large number of drug-like compounds (e.g., ChemNavigator), a very small number of molecules have been drawn to carefully monitor the main permeation driving/limiting force (i.e. passive diffusion, active influx or active efflux), however the data available mostly represent both passive and active transport phenomena. For detailed information, reader is directed to see (Wolburg, 2006).

8.1 Passive diffusion

Having assumed that the rate of drug release from the formulation is not rate-limiting, the absorption of drug molecules across BBB depend upon: 1) the rate of drug dosing which takes into account the administered dose (mass) and the dosing interval (τ ; time), 2) the interactions of drug molecules with circulating biomolecules in blood (protein binding), 3) drug biostability and clearance, 4) the apparent absorption rate constant for the drug (K_a; time^{-1}). Clearly the stability of drug during the absorption process and importantly the intrinsic permeability of the BBB to the drug are critical factors in determining logBB.

Passive diffusion involves the movement of drug molecules down a concentration or electrochemical gradient without the expenditure of energy. Firstly, if we consider only the transport of drug molecules across BBB via passive diffusional processes then the overall flux (J) of a drug in one dimension (i.e. the net mass of drug that diffuses through a unit area per unit time) can be described by Equation (2).

$$J = -D \cdot K_p \cdot A \cdot \left({}^{dC}\!/\!_{dx} \right)_t \tag{2}$$

Where J is the flux of drug; D is the diffusion coefficient of drug across the cellular barrier; K_p is a global partition coefficient (cell membrane/aqueous fluid); A is the surface area of the barrier available for absorption; x is the thickness of the absorption barrier, and (dC/dx)t is the concentration gradient of drug across the absorption barrier. The negative sign in Equation (2) indicates that diffusion proceeds from high to low concentration and hence the flux is a positive quantity. In fact, the greater this concentration gradient, the greater the rate of diffusion of a drug across the cell membrane.

The apparent permeability coefficient (ρ) of an epithelial/endothelial barrier to a given drug approximate $D.K_p$. The processes of drug partitioning with the biomembrane (including partitioning between extracellular fluid and plasma membrane, partitioning between plasma membrane and cell cytosol, and other organelle interactions etc.) and of drug diffusion across the biomembranes (including a range of organelle and macromolecule interactions that will influence the diffusion process) are largely dependent upon the molecular properties of the drug, i.e. molecular size/shape, ionic properties (hydrogen bonding potential, pKa), and hydrophobic properties. Basically, such molecular properties will determine if passive diffusional transport across an epithelial/endothelial barrier involves either a predominantly paracellular (between cells) pathway negotiating a tortuous intercellular route via the aqueous channels formed by the anastomosing tight junctional fibrils between adjacent cells, or predominantly (but not exclusively) transcellular (across the cell) pathway requiring partitioning of drug into the plasma membrane bilayer. In fact, it should be stated that if a drug's molecular properties afford partitioning into biomembranes (i.e. nonionized form of the drug predominates and is of a sufficient hydrophobic nature) then the membrane surface area available for transcellular diffusion will be considerably greater, by many orders of magnitude, than the surface area available for diffusion via the paracellular route. As a corollary, the transcellular diffusion can potentially result in a higher permeability and a higher rate and extent of absorption. For detailed information, reader is directed to see (Omidi & Gumbleton, 2005; Wolburg, 2006)

8.2 Macromolecular permeation

With respect to in-silico methods, the passive diffusion seems to be well described by physicochemical parameters of the respective solutes (e.g., lipohilicity, H-bond acceptor/donor features, molecular weight, polar surface area, number of rotatable bonds). These descriptors can be simply calculated and are thus a versatile tool for high-throughput in-silico screening of large compound databases. Basically, small hydrophilic molecules exploit the paracellular pathway to diffuse into organs (Fig. 3).

The impact of the molecule's steric, ionic and hydrophobic properties upon passive membrane transport and epithelial/endothelial permeability are equally applicable for peptides, proteins and nucleic acids, as they are for traditional low molecular weight drugs. Nevertheless, their permeation across biological barriers will be limited by the presence of a significant number of hydrogen bond acceptor and donor groups, i.e. requiring considerable desolvation energy for the molecule to leave the aqueous environment and partition into a biological membrane. The diffusion of macromolecules (peptides, proteins and nucleic acids) across biological membranes appears to be through endocytosis/transcytosis route or in some cases via the paracellular pathway (Fig. 3). For example, to pursue the binding, uptake and transcytosis of 60 nm porous nanoparticles (NPs) differing in their surface charge and inner composition, Jallouli et al studied their trafficking at the BBB. Having used maltodextrins with/without a cationic ligand, they showed that the cationic NPs were accumulated mainly around the paracellular area, while neutral NPs were mainly on the cell surface and the dipalmitoyl phosphatidyl glycerol (DPPG) NPs were at both paracellular areas and on the surface of the cells. It was shown that filipin can increase the binding and uptake (sterols may entail in their efflux), while decrease the transcytosis of neutral NPs. They concluded that the neutral NPs, like LDL, exploit the caveolae pathway and suggested the neutral and cationic 60 nm porous NPs as potential candidates for drug delivery to the brain (Jallouli et al., 2007). It is believed that Tf receptor, as a molecular part of vesicular trafficking, can facilitate brain delivery of NPs *in vivo*. To explore the attributed mechanism of this process, Chang et al evaluated the endocytosis of poly(lactic-co-glycolic acid) (PLGA) NPs coated with transferrin using an *in vitro* coculture of BCECs and astrocytes. Using solvent diffusion method, they prepared PLGA NPs by means of DiI as a fluorescent marker and coated with Tween 20, BSA and Tf. Depending upon DiI incorporation and surface coating, the size of NPs varied from 63 to 90 nm. In comparison with BSA NPs, the Tf-NPs were found to be highly adsorbed BCECs through an energy-dependent process. Having used specific inhibition, these researchers showed that the Tf-NPs can interact with BCECs in a specific manner and enter the cells via the caveolae endocytic pathway (Chang et al., 2009). Having used a cross-reacting material 197 (CRM197) which is a non-toxic mutant of diphtheria toxin, Wang et al reported that the apical-to-basal transcytosis of CRM197 can involve the caveolae-mediated pathway in the hCMEC/D3 endothelial cells as the caveolin-1 mRNA and protein expression levels were significantly increased by CRM197. These researchers speculated that the upregulation of caveolin-1 may be mediated via a PI3K/Akt dependent pathway and reduction of the phospho-FOXO1A (forkhead box O) transcription factor. Based upon such findings, it was proposed that carrier protein CRM197-mediated delivery across the BBB is involved in the induction of FOXO1A transcriptional activity and upregulation of caveolin-1 expression (Wang et al., 2010). In fact, the BCECs exploit a variety of endocytic pathways (i.e., clathrin-mediated endocytosis, caveolar endocytosis, and macropinocytosis) for the internalization of exogenous materials. It is deemed that the properties of drug delivery vehicles can direct the intracellular processing in brain endothelial cells. Using fixed-size NPs, it has been shown that surface modifications of nanoparticles (e.g., charge and protein ligands) can affect their mode of internalization by BCECs and thereby the subcellular fate (Georgieva et al., 2011).

It should be also evoked that the diffusion coefficient of a drug is inversely proportional to its molecular weight, and while for traditional low molecular weight drugs (100-500 Da) the diffusion coefficient varies little between drugs. Further, the epithelial permeability of biotechnology products, like that of traditional low molecular drugs, are subjected to the extent of degradation occurring within the barrier itself, in which the role of proteases and nucleases will be important for biotechnology drugs, readers are directed to see (Wolburg, 2006).

9. Targeting brain tumours

The integrity of the BBB in metastatic cancerous tumors appears to be different from the normal ones. In addition to the various morphological alterations of BBB in metastatic cancerous tumors (e.g., compromised tight junction structure and increases in the perivascular space, fenestrated BCECs, increased number and activity of pinocytic vacuole), the expression of transporters has also been reported to be altered in the microvasculature of the brain tumors. This implies that the BBB is less intact in primary and metastatic brain tumors compared with the normal brain vasculature, and accordingly the pharmacotherapy of brain tumors demands specific strategies. So far, to enhance the amount of therapeutic agent to a brain tumor, a number of strategies have been exploited including: 1) increasing drug plasma concentration (e.g., intraarterial infusion), 2) physicochemical modification to increase drug permeability, 3) design of inactive drug precursors (the so-called prodrugs) that could more easily cross the blood–brain barrier before conversion to a drug with active formulation, and 4) osmotic disruption of the blood–brain barrier using osmotic-disruptive agents such as mannitol (Provenzale et al., 2005). Of these methodologies, liposomal formulations seem to be promising since they can passively target tumors in which there is disorganized vasculature. This appears to be also related to higher permeability than to disorganization *per se*; nonetheless specific features (e.g., vesicle size, chemical affinity, and thermal/pH sensitiveness) may affect the targeting potential of liposomes. The hyperthermia looms to be an important means for modifying the target environment and increasing liposome delivery to tumors. For example, in animal models, it was observed that the heating to temperatures up to 41–43°C can increase the tumor microvascular pore size and accordingly increases its permeability to various substances (e.g., ferritin, antibodies, and liposomes), perhaps hyperthermia can disaggregate the endothelial cell cytoskeleton. For instance, in a human tumor xenograft murine model (SKOV-3), the extravasation of 100 nm liposomes was not observed at 34°C, but it was seen after heating to 40°C (Kong et al., 2001). In 2010, Bellavance et al reported on development of a novel cationic liposome formulation composed of DPPC:DC-Chol:DOPE:DHPE Oregon Green, which was shown to possesses efficient internalization and intracellular delivery to F98 and U-118 glioblastoma (GBM) cells in pH-sensitive manner. At which point, they suggested such liposomal formulation as a novel potent and efficient vehicle for cytosolic delivery of intracellular therapeutics such as chemotherapy agents to the glioblastoma (Bellavance et al., 2010). So far, various liposomal and polymeric formulations have been introduced as smart (thermo-sensitive and/or pH sensitive) nanomedicines that can provide a controlled drug release in target tumors. In particular, the pH-sensitive nanosystems have been given greater attention since the pH targeting approach is regarded as a more general strategy than conventional specific tumor cell surface targeting approaches. In fact, the nanosystems display greater potential to overcome multidrug resistance of various tumors when they are combined with triggered release mechanisms by endosomal or lysosomal acidity plus endosomolytic capability – this important domain has been well reviewed recently, see (Lee et al., 2008).

In addition, little is known about impacts of metastatic disease on the BBB. Although the brain metastases respond to chemotherapy modalities, such responses are largely dependent upon condition of patients. For example, 14 patients with brain metastases from small cell lung cancer (SCLC) were treated with combination therapy of cyclophosphamide, doxorubicin, vincristine, and etoposide. Of the treated patients, 9 of 11 patients (82%) showed responses in their brain lesions, whereas 9 of 12 evaluated patients (75%) had responses in their extracranial lesions (Lee et al., 1989). In another study, patients with SCLC and brain metastases were treated with cisplatin, ifosfamide, and irinotecan with rhG-CSF support. The response rate was 50% in brain lesions and 62% in extracranial primary or metastatic lesions (Fujita et al., 2000). The most studies for assessing leakiness of the BBB in human brain tumors appear to be the T1-weighted techniques (in particular, T1-weighted dynamic contrast-enhanced imaging). In fact, researchers implement this methodology using a 3D spoiled gradient acquisition steady-state technique that monitors contrast material accumulation over a few minutes rather than observing the first-pass phenomenon. The main advantages of this technique seem to be the relatively short imaging time, a need for only a single dose of contrast material, and availability of a large number of user-friendly analysis programs (Provenzale et al., 2005).

10. Recent advancements for crossing BBB

Selective functional presence of BBB makes brain delivery and targeting very challenging issue, for which various strategies have been developed, including different classes of nanomedicines. These novel strategies are largely dependent upon biological characteristics of BBB, and accordingly nanomedicines exploit endocytic pathways. Unfortunately, patients with primary brain tumors and brain metastases have a very poor prognosis. This is often exacerbated with low responses to chemotherapy attributed to BBB selective control on permeation of cytotoxic agents. Nanomedicines represent great promise in glioma therapy as they protect therapeutic agent and allow its sustained release even though tumor specific targeting paradigms with extensive intratumoral distribution must be developed for efficient delivery.

Paclitaxel as an active agent against gliomas and various brain metastases is substrate of P-gp efflux transporter, and thus it is pumped out of brain parenchyma. To tackle this issue, Koziara et al. developed novel cetyl alcohol/polysorbate NPs for encapsulation and delivery of anticancer agents such as paclitaxel (PX) to brain. They showed significant increase of paclitaxel in brain using such NPs because of the limited binding of PX to p-gp (Koziara et al., 2004). With an effort to evaluate the characteristics of an ultrasmall superparamagnetic iron oxides (USPIO) agent in patients with brain tumors and to correlate changes on MRI with histopathologic data collected systematically in all patients, Taschner et al. examined 9 patients with brain tumors before and 24 hr after administration of a USPIO at a dose of 2.6 mg Fe/kg. They witnessed USPIO-related changes of signal intensity in gadolinium-enhancing brain tumors in 7 patients. Upon such findings, they suggested that USPIO agents can offer complementary information useful to differentiate between brain tumors and areas of radiation necrosis (Taschner et al., 2005). Interestingly, in 2006, Wu et al. reported construction of a drug delivery vehicle with ability to target the epidermal growth factor receptor (EGFR) and its mutant isoform EGFRvIII. In their work, the EGFR targeting monoclonal antibody, cetuximab, was covalently linked to a Polyamidoamine (PAMAM) dendrimer containing the cytotoxic drug methotrexate. Using the EGFR-expressing rat glioma cell line F98(EGFR), they showed that the bioconjugate retained its affinity for F98(EGFR) cells and the IC50 of the bioconjugate was 220 nmol/L. The bioconjugate in rats bearing i.c. implants of either F98(EGFR) or F98(WT) gliomas was determined 24 hr following convection enhanced delivery of (125)I-labeled complex, showing specific molecular targeting of the tumor. Based on such findings, they concluded that the antibody-drug bioconjugate is therapeutically useful approach in brain tumors (Wu et al., 2006). In 2009, Veiseh et al reported on development of an iron oxide nanoparticle coated with polyethylene glycol-grafted chitosan with ability to cross the BBB and target brain tumors in a genetically engineered mouse model. The nanoprobe was conjugated to a tumor-targeting agent, chlorotoxin, and a near-IR fluorophore. Using *in vivo* magnetic resonance, biophotonic imaging, and histologic and biodistribution analyses, they showed an innocuous toxicity profile induced by the nanoprobe, while it showed a sustained retention in tumors and suggested its application for the diagnosis and treatment of a variety of tumor types in brain (Veiseh et al., 2009). Using novel quaternary ammonium beta-cyclodextrin (QAbetaCD) NPs (with 65-88 nm diameter and controllable cationic properties), Gil et al reported successful delivery of doxorubicin (DOX) across the BBB. They showed that QAbetaCD NPs are not toxic to bovine brain microvessel endothelial cells (BBMVECs) at concentrations up to 500 µg/mL. They also showed that the DOX/QAbetaCD complexes can kill U87 cells as effectively as DOX alone, while the QAbetaCD NPs completely protect BBMVECs from cytotoxicity of DOX. And as a result, it was suggested that the QAbetaCD NPs as safe and effective delivery system for anticancer agents such as DOX for brain tumors (Gil et al., 2009). Upon the of note tropism of mesenchymal stem cells (MSCs) for brain tumors, Roger et al exploited the MSCs as NP delivery vehicles, in which they used two types of NPs loaded with coumarin-6, i.e. poly-lactic acid NPs (PLA-NPs) and lipid nanocapsules (LNCs). They showed efficient internalization of the NPs into MSCs that were able to migrate toward an experimental human glioma model. They suggested MSCs as potential cellular carriers for delivery of NPs into brain tumors (Roger et al., 2010). In 2011, A dual-targeting drug carrier (PAMAM-PEG-WGA-Tf) was developed based on the PEGylated fourth generation PAMAM dendrimer with Tf and wheat germ agglutinin (WGA) on the periphery and DOX loaded in the interior (He et al., 2011). Having nanoscaled size (~ 20 nm), the PAMAM-PEG-WGA-Tf efficiently inhibited the growth rate of the C6 glioma cells, while it reduced the cytotoxicity of DOX to the normal cells. These researchers reported significantly increase and accumulation of DOX in the tumor site (due to the targeting effects of both Tf and WGA) and suggested that it could be used as a BBB penetrating agent with tumor targeting properties (He et al., 2011).

11. Chapter summary

Entry of blood circulating agents into brain is highly controlled by selectively functional presence of BBB. This makes brain drug delivery and targeting very intricate. Owing to unique biology of brain capillary endothelial cells, carrier and/or receptor mediated transport machineries of BBB can be exploited using smart pharmaceuticals. In the case of tumors such as glioma, use of intelligent molecular Trajan horses appears to provide a combined imaging-therapy as "theranostic" to ease brain drug delivery and targeting by simultaneous imaging techniques such as positron emission tomography (PET). In near future, it is expected new multifunctional "all in one" therapeutic to be translated into clinic to cure brain tumors in much more efficient manner. Such therapeutics may consist of homing device for targeting, imaging moiety for sensing/imaging, and therapeutic itself in a vehicle that could be activated by outside/inside stimulation (pH, temperature, enzyme). To translate such fascinating molecular therapy into clinical use, however, we need to recruit several disciplines such as nanotechnology, biotechnology, biophotonics, engineering, biopharmaceutics and clinical expertise.

12. References

Abbott, N.J. (2000). Inflammatory mediators and modulation of blood-brain barrier permeability. *Cell Mol.Neurobiol.*, Vol.20, No.2, (April 2000), pp. 131-147, ISSN 0272-4340

Abbott, N.J. (2005). Dynamics of CNS barriers: evolution, differentiation, and modulation. *Cell Mol.Neurobiol.*, Vol.25, No.1, (February 2005), pp. 5-23, ISSN 0272-4340

Abbott, N.J.; Ronnback, L. & Hansson, E. (2006). Astrocyte-endothelial interactions at the blood-brain barrier. *Nat.Rev.Neurosci.*, Vol.7, No.1, (January 2006), pp. 41-53, ISSN 1471-003X

Albert, J.L.; Boyle, J.P.; Roberts, J.A.; Challiss, R.A.; Gubby, S.E. & Boarder, M.R. (1997). Regulation of brain capillary endothelial cells by P2Y receptors coupled to Ca2+, phospholipase C and mitogen-activated protein kinase. *Br.J.Pharmacol.*, Vol.122, No.5, (November 1997), pp. 935-941, ISSN 0007-1188

Allt, G. & Lawrenson, J.G. (2000). The blood-nerve barrier: enzymes, transporters and receptors--a comparison with the blood-brain barrier. *Brain Res.Bull.*, Vol.52, No.1, (May 2000), pp. 1-12, ISSN 0361-9230

Allt, G. & Lawrenson, J.G. (2001). Pericytes: cell biology and pathology. *Cells Tissues.Organs*, Vol.169, No.1, (2001), pp. 1-11, ISSN 1422-6405

Balabanov, R. & Dore-Duffy, P. (1998). Role of the CNS microvascular pericyte in the blood-brain barrier. *J.Neurosci.Res.*, Vol.53, No.6, (September 1998), pp. 637-644, ISSN 0360-4012

Balbuena, P.; Li, W. & Ehrich, M. (2011). Assessments of tight junction proteins occludin, claudin 5 and scaffold proteins ZO1 and ZO2 in endothelial cells of the rat blood-brain barrier: cellular responses to neurotoxicants malathion and lead acetate. *Neurotoxicology*, Vol.32, No.1, (January 2011), pp. 58-67, ISSN 0161-813X

Bellavance, M.A.; Poirier, M.B. & Fortin, D. (2010). Uptake and intracellular release kinetics of liposome formulations in glioma cells. *Int.J.Pharm.*, Vol.395, No.1-2, (August 2010), pp. 251-259, ISSN 0378-5173

Chang, J.; Jallouli, Y.; Kroubi, M.; Yuan, X.B.; Feng, W.; Kang, C.S.; Pu, P.Y. & Betbeder, D. (2009). Characterization of endocytosis of transferrin-coated PLGA nanoparticles by the blood-brain barrier. *Int.J.Pharm.*, Vol.379, No.2, (September 2009), pp. 285-292, ISSN 0378-5173

DeBault, L.E.; Kahn, L.E.; Frommes, S.P. & Cancilla, P.A. (1979). Cerebral microvessels and derived cells in tissue culture: isolation and preliminary characterization. *In Vitro*, Vol.15, No.7, (July 1979), pp. 473-487, ISSN 0073-5655

Engelhardt, B. (2006). Development of the Blood-Brain Interface, In: *Blood-Brain Barriers*, Dermietzel, R., Spray, D. C., and Nedergaard, M., pp. 11-40, WILEY-VCH Verlag GmbH & Co. KGaA, ISBN 3-527-31088-6, Weinheim

Fujita, A.; Fukuoka, S.; Takabatake, H.; Tagaki, S. & Sekine, K. (2000). Combination chemotherapy of cisplatin, ifosfamide, and irinotecan with rhG-CSF support in patients with brain metastases from non-small cell lung cancer. *Oncology*, Vol.59, No.4, (November 2000), pp. 291-295, ISSN 0030-2414

Georgieva, J.V.; Kalicharan, D.; Couraud, P.O.; Romero, I.A.; Weksler, B.; Hoekstra, D. & Zuhorn, I.S. (2011). Surface characteristics of nanoparticles determine their intracellular fate in and processing by human blood-brain barrier endothelial cells in vitro. *Mol.Ther.*, Vol.19, No.2, (February 2011), pp. 318-325, ISSN 1525-0016

Gil, E.S.; Li, J.; Xiao, H. & Lowe, T.L. (2009). Quaternary ammonium beta-cyclodextrin nanoparticles for enhancing doxorubicin permeability across the in vitro blood-brain barrier. *Biomacromolecules.*, Vol.10, No.3, (March 2009), pp. 505-516, ISSN 1525-7797

Gumbleton, M. & Audus, K.L. (2001). Progress and limitations in the use of in vitro cell cultures to serve as a permeability screen for the blood-brain barrier. *J.Pharm.Sci.*, Vol.90, No.11, (November 2001), pp. 1681-1698, ISSN 0022-3549

Haseloff, R.F.; Blasig, I.E.; Bauer, H.C. & Bauer, H. (2005). In search of the astrocytic factor(s) modulating blood-brain barrier functions in brain capillary endothelial cells in vitro. *Cell Mol.Neurobiol.*, Vol.25, No.1, (February 2005), pp. 25-39, ISSN 0272-4340

Hawkins, B.T. & Davis, T.P. (2005). The blood-brain barrier/neurovascular unit in health and disease. *Pharmacol.Rev.*, Vol.57, No.2, (June 2005), pp. 173-185, ISSN 0031-6997

He, H.; Li, Y.; Jia, X.R.; Du, J.; Ying, X.; Lu, W.L.; Lou, J.N. & Wei, Y. (2011). PEGylated Poly(amidoamine) dendrimer-based dual-targeting carrier for treating brain tumors. *Biomaterials*, Vol.32, No.2, (January 2011), pp. 478-487, ISSN 0142-9612

Homma, M.; Suzuki, H.; Kusuhara, H.; Naito, M.; Tsuruo, T. & Sugiyama, Y. (1999). High-affinity efflux transport system for glutathione conjugates on the luminal membrane of a mouse brain capillary endothelial cell line (MBEC4). *J.Pharmacol.Exp.Ther.*, Vol.288, No.1, (January 1999), pp. 198-203, ISSN 0022-3565

Hosoya, K.I.; Takashima, T.; Tetsuka, K.; Nagura, T.; Ohtsuki, S.; Takanaga, H.; Ueda, M.; Yanai, N.; Obinata, M. & Terasaki, T. (2000). mRna expression and transport characterization of conditionally immortalized rat brain capillary endothelial cell lines; a new in vitro BBB model for drug targeting. *J.Drug Target*, Vol.8, No.6, (2000), pp. 357-370, ISSN 1061-186X

Hulsermann, U.; Hoffmann, M.M.; Massing, U. & Fricker, G. (2009). Uptake of apolipoprotein E fragment coupled liposomes by cultured brain microvessel endothelial cells and intact brain capillaries. *J.Drug Target*, Vol.17, No.8, (September 2009), pp. 610-618, ISSN 1061-186X

Hurst, R.D. & Clark, J.B. (1998). Alterations in transendothelial electrical resistance by vasoactive agonists and cyclic AMP in a blood-brain barrier model system. *Neurochem.Res.*, Vol.23, No.2, (February 1998), pp. 149-154, ISSN 0364-3190

Igarashi, Y.; Utsumi, H.; Chiba, H.; Yamada-Sasamori, Y.; Tobioka, H.; Kamimura, Y.; Furuuchi, K.; Kokai, Y.; Nakagawa, T.; Mori, M. & Sawada, N. (1999). Glial cell line-derived neurotrophic factor induces barrier function of endothelial cells forming the blood-brain barrier. *Biochem.Biophys.Res.Commun.*, Vol.261, No.1, (July 1999), pp. 108-112, ISSN 0006-291X

Jallouli, Y.; Paillard, A.; Chang, J.; Sevin, E. & Betbeder, D. (2007). Influence of surface charge and inner composition of porous nanoparticles to cross blood-brain barrier in vitro. *Int.J.Pharm.*, Vol.344, No.1-2, (November 2007), pp. 103-109, ISSN 0378-5173

Kniesel, U. & Wolburg, H. (2000). Tight junctions of the blood-brain barrier. *Cell Mol.Neurobiol.*, Vol.20, No.1, (February 2000), pp. 57-76, ISSN 0272-4340

Kondo, A.; Inoue, T.; Nagara, H.; Tateishi, J. & Fukui, M. (1987). Neurotoxicity of adriamycin passed through the transiently disrupted blood-brain barrier by mannitol in the rat brain. *Brain Res.*, Vol.412, No.1, (May 1987), pp. 73-83, ISSN 0006-8993

Kong, G.; Braun, R.D. & Dewhirst, M.W. (2001). Characterization of the effect of hyperthermia on nanoparticle extravasation from tumor vasculature. *Cancer Res.*, Vol.61, No.7, (April 2001), pp. 3027-3032, ISSN 0008-5472

Koziara, J.M.; Lockman, P.R.; Allen, D.D. & Mumper, R.J. (2004). Paclitaxel nanoparticles for the potential treatment of brain tumors. *J.Control Release*, Vol.99, No.2, (September 2004), pp. 259-269, ISSN 0168-3659

Krizbai, I.A. & Deli, M.A. (2003). Signalling pathways regulating the tight junction permeability in the blood-brain barrier. *Cell Mol.Biol.(Noisy.-le-grand)*, Vol.49, No.1, (February 2003), pp. 23-31, ISSN 0145-5680

Lacombe, O.; Videau, O.; Chevillon, D.; Guyot, A.C.; Contreras, C.; Blondel, S.; Nicolas, L.; Ghettas, A.; Benech, H.; Thevenot, E.; Pruvost, A.; Bolze, S.; Kraczkowski, L.; Prevost, C. & Mabondzo, A. (2011). In-Vitro Primary Human and Animal Cell-Based Blood-Brain Barrier Models as a Screening Tool in Drug Discovery. *Mol.Pharm.* (March 2011), ISSN 1543-8384

Larson, D.M.; Carson, M.P. & Haudenschild, C.C. (1987). Junctional transfer of small molecules in cultured bovine brain microvascular endothelial cells and pericytes. *Microvasc.Res.*, Vol.34, No.2, (September 1987), pp. 184-199, ISSN 0026-2862

Lechardeur, D. & Scherman, D. (1995). Functional expression of the P-glycoprotein mdr in primary cultures of bovine cerebral capillary endothelial cells. *Cell Biol.Toxicol.*, Vol.11, No.5, (October 1995), pp. 283-293, ISSN 0742-2091

Lechardeur, D.; Schwartz, B.; Paulin, D. & Scherman, D. (1995). Induction of blood-brain barrier differentiation in a rat brain-derived endothelial cell line. *Exp.Cell Res.*, Vol.220, No.1, (September 1995), pp. 161-170, ISSN 0014-4827

Lee, E.S.; Gao, Z. & Bae, Y.H. (2008). Recent progress in tumor pH targeting nanotechnology. *J.Control Release*, Vol.132, No.3, (December 2008), pp. 164-170, ISSN 0168-3659

Lee, J.S.; Murphy, W.K.; Glisson, B.S.; Dhingra, H.M.; Holoye, P.Y. & Hong, W.K. (1989). Primary chemotherapy of brain metastasis in small-cell lung cancer. *J.Clin.Oncol.*, Vol.7, No.7, (July 1989), pp. 916-922,

Leggas, M.; Adachi, M.; Scheffer, G.L.; Sun, D.; Wielinga, P.; Du, G.; Mercer, K.E.; Zhuang, Y.; Panetta, J.C.; Johnston, B.; Scheper, R.J.; Stewart, C.F. & Schuetz, J.D. (2004). Mrp4 confers resistance to topotecan and protects the brain from chemotherapy. *Mol.Cell Biol.*, Vol.24, No.17, (September 2004), pp. 7612-7621, ISSN 0270-7306

Muruganandam, A.; Herx, L.M.; Monette, R.; Durkin, J.P. & Stanimirovic, D.B. (1997). Development of immortalized human cerebromicrovascular endothelial cell line as an in vitro model of the human blood-brain barrier. *FASEB J.*, Vol.11, No.13, (November 1997), pp. 1187-1197, ISSN 0892-6638

Ohtsuki, S. & Terasaki, T. (2007). Contribution of carrier-mediated transport systems to the blood-brain barrier as a supporting and protecting interface for the brain; importance for CNS drug discovery and development. *Pharm.Res.*, Vol.24, No.9, (September 2007), pp. 1745-1758, ISSN 0253-6269

Omidi, Y. & Barar, J. (2012). Impacts of blood-brain barrier in drug delivery and targeting of brain tumours. *BioImpacts*, Vol.2, No.1, (2012), pp. in press, ISSN 2228-5652

Omidi, Y.; Barar, J.; Ahmadian, S.; Heidari, H.R. & Gumbleton, M. (2008). Characterisation and astrocytic modulation of system L transporters in brain microvasculature endothelial cells. *Cell Biochem.Funct.*, Vol.26, No.3, (2008), pp. 381-391, ISSN 0263-6484

Omidi, Y. and Gumbleton, M. (2005). Biological Membranes and Barriers, In: *Biomaterials for Delivery and Targeting of Proteins Nucleic Acids,* Mahato, R. I., pp. 232-274, CRC Press, ISBN 9-780-84932334-8, New York

Orte, C.; Lawrenson, J.G.; Finn, T.M.; Reid, A.R. & Allt, G. (1999). A comparison of blood-brain barrier and blood-nerve barrier endothelial cell markers. *Anat.Embryol.(Berl)*, Vol.199, No.6, (June 1999), pp. 509-517, ISSN 0340-2061

Pardridge, W.M. (1999). Blood-brain barrier biology and methodology. *J.Neurovirol.*, Vol.5, No.6, (December 1999), pp. 556-569, ISSN 1355-0284

Pluta, R.; Misicka, A.; Barcikowska, M.; Spisacka, S.; Lipkowski, A.W. & Januszewski, S. (2000). Possible reverse transport of beta-amyloid peptide across the blood-brain barrier. *Acta Neurochir.Suppl*, Vol.76 (2000), pp. 73-77, ISSN 0001-6268

Provenzale, J.M.; Mukundan, S. & Dewhirst, M. (2005). The role of blood-brain barrier permeability in brain tumor imaging and therapeutics. *AJR Am.J.Roentgenol.*, Vol.185, No.3, (September 2005), pp. 763-767, ISSN 0361-803X

Prudhomme, J.G.; Sherman, I.W.; Land, K.M.; Moses, A.V.; Stenglein, S. & Nelson, J.A. (1996). Studies of Plasmodium falciparum cytoadherence using immortalized human brain capillary endothelial cells. *Int.J.Parasitol.*, Vol.26, No.6, (June 1996), pp. 647-655, ISSN 0020-7519

Ramsauer, M.; Krause, D. & Dermietzel, R. (2002). Angiogenesis of the blood-brain barrier in vitro and the function of cerebral pericytes. *FASEB J.*, Vol.16, No.10, (August 2002), pp. 1274-1276, ISSN 0892-6638

Reese, T.S. & Karnovsky, M.J. (1967). Fine structural localization of a blood-brain barrier to exogenous peroxidase. *J.Cell Biol.*, Vol.34, No.1, (July 1967), pp. 207-217, ISSN 0021-9525

Ribeiro, M.M.; Castanho, M.A. & Serrano, I. (2010). In vitro blood-brain barrier models--latest advances and therapeutic applications in a chronological perspective. *Mini.Rev.Med.Chem.*, Vol.10, No.3, (March 2010), pp. 262-270, ISSN 1389-5575

Rist, R.J.; Romero, I.A.; Chan, M.W.; Couraud, P.O.; Roux, F. & Abbott, N.J. (1997). F-actin cytoskeleton and sucrose permeability of immortalised rat brain microvascular endothelial cell monolayers: effects of cyclic AMP and astrocytic factors. *Brain Res.*, Vol.768, No.1-2, (September 1997), pp. 10-18, ISSN 0006-8993

Robert, A.M. & Robert, L. (1998). Extracellular matrix and blood-brain barrier function. *Pathol.Biol.(Paris)*, Vol.46, No.7, (September 1998), pp. 535-542, ISSN 0369-8114

Roger, M.; Clavreul, A.; Venier-Julienne, M.C.; Passirani, C.; Sindji, L.; Schiller, P.; Montero-Menei, C. & Menei, P. (2010). Mesenchymal stem cells as cellular vehicles for delivery of nanoparticles to brain tumors. *Biomaterials*, Vol.31, No.32, (November 2010), pp. 8393-8401, ISSN 0142-9612

Roux, F.; Durieu-Trautmann, O.; Chaverot, N.; Claire, M.; Mailly, P.; Bourre, J.M.; Strosberg, A.D. & Couraud, P.O. (1994). Regulation of gamma-glutamyl transpeptidase and alkaline phosphatase activities in immortalized rat brain microvessel endothelial cells. *J.Cell Physiol*, Vol.159, No.1, (April 1994), pp. 101-113, ISSN 0021-9541

Rubin, L.L. & Staddon, J.M. (1999). The cell biology of the blood-brain barrier. *Annu.Rev.Neurosci.*, Vol.22 (1999), pp. 11-28, ISSN 0147-006X

Schinkel, A.H.; Mol, C.A.; Wagenaar, E.; van, D.L.; Smit, J.J. & Borst, P. (1995a). Multidrug resistance and the role of P-glycoprotein knockout mice. *Eur.J.Cancer*, Vol.31A, No.7-8, (July 1995a), pp. 1295-1298, ISSN 0959-8049

Schinkel, A.H.; Wagenaar, E.; van, D.L.; Mol, C.A. & Borst, P. (1995b). Absence of the mdr1a P-Glycoprotein in mice affects tissue distribution and pharmacokinetics of dexamethasone, digoxin, and cyclosporin A. *J.Clin.Invest*, Vol.96, No.4, (October 1995b), pp. 1698-1705, ISSN 0021-9738

Shivers, R.R.; Arthur, F.E. & Bowman, P.D. (1988). Induction of gap junctions and brain endothelium-like tight junctions in cultured bovine endothelial cells: local control of cell specialization. *J.Submicrosc.Cytol.Pathol.*, Vol.20, No.1, (January 1988), pp. 1-14, ISSN 1122-9497

Smith, M.W. & Gumbleton, M. (2006). Endocytosis at the blood-brain barrier: from basic understanding to drug delivery strategies. *J.Drug Target*, Vol.14, No.4, (May 2006), pp. 191-214, ISSN 1061-186X

Stanness, K.A.; Guatteo, E. & Janigro, D. (1996). A dynamic model of the blood-brain barrier "in vitro". *Neurotoxicology*, Vol.17, No.2, (1996), pp. 481-496, ISSN 0161-813X

Stanness, K.A.; Neumaier, J.F.; Sexton, T.J.; Grant, G.A.; Emmi, A.; Maris, D.O. & Janigro, D. (1999). A new model of the blood--brain barrier: co-culture of neuronal, endothelial and glial cells under dynamic conditions. *Neuroreport*, Vol.10, No.18, (December 1999), pp. 3725-3731, ISSN 0959-4965

Stewart, P.A. & Wiley, M.J. (1981). Developing nervous tissue induces formation of blood-brain barrier characteristics in invading endothelial cells: a study using quail--chick transplantation chimeras. *Dev.Biol.*, Vol.84, No.1, (May 1981), pp. 183-192, ISSN 0012-1606

Taschner, C.A.; Wetzel, S.G.; Tolnay, M.; Froehlich, J.; Merlo, A. & Radue, E.W. (2005). Characteristics of ultrasmall superparamagnetic iron oxides in patients with brain tumors. *AJR Am.J.Roentgenol.*, Vol.185, No.6, (December 2005), pp. 1477-1486, ISSN 0361-803X

Tilling, T.; Korte, D.; Hoheisel, D. & Galla, H.J. (1998). Basement membrane proteins influence brain capillary endothelial barrier function in vitro. *J.Neurochem.*, Vol.71, No.3, (September 1998), pp. 1151-1157, ISSN 0022-3042

Tio, S.; Deenen, M. & Marani, E. (1990). Astrocyte-mediated induction of alkaline phosphatase activity in human umbilical cord vein endothelium: an in vitro model. *Eur.J.Morphol.*, Vol.28, No.2-4, (1990), pp. 289-300, ISSN 0924-3860

Tsuji, A. (2005). Small molecular drug transfer across the blood-brain barrier via carrier-mediated transport systems. *NeuroRx.*, Vol.2, No.1, (January 2005), pp. 54-62, ISSN 1545-5343

Urquhart, B.L. & Kim, R.B. (2009). Blood-brain barrier transporters and response to CNS-active drugs. *Eur.J.Clin.Pharmacol.*, Vol.65, No.11, (November 2009), pp. 1063-1070, ISSN 0031-6970

Veiseh, O.; Sun, C.; Fang, C.; Bhattarai, N.; Gunn, J.; Kievit, F.; Du, K.; Pullar, B.; Lee, D.; Ellenbogen, R.G.; Olson, J. & Zhang, M. (2009). Specific targeting of brain tumors with an optical/magnetic resonance imaging nanoprobe across the blood-brain barrier. *Cancer Res.*, Vol.69, No.15, (August 2009), pp. 6200-6207, ISSN 0008-5472

Wakui, S.; Furusato, M.; Hasumura, M.; Hori, M.; Takahashi, H.; Kano, Y. & Ushigome, S. (1989). Two- and three-dimensional ultrastructure of endothelium and pericyte interdigitations in capillary of human granulation tissue. *J.Electron Microsc.(Tokyo)*, Vol.38, No.2, (1989), pp. 136-142, ISSN 0022-0744

Wang, P.; Xue, Y.; Shang, X. & Liu, Y. (2010). Diphtheria toxin mutant CRM197-mediated transcytosis across blood-brain barrier in vitro. *Cell Mol.Neurobiol.*, Vol.30, No.5, (July 2010), pp. 717-725, ISSN 1044-7431

Wang, W.; Dentler, W.L. & Borchardt, R.T. (2001). VEGF increases BMEC monolayer permeability by affecting occludin expression and tight junction assembly. *Am.J.Physiol Heart Circ.Physiol*, Vol.280, No.1, (January 2001), pp. H434-H440, ISSN 0363-6135

Wolburg, H. (2006). The Endothelial Frontier, In: *Blood-Brain Barriers,* Dermietzel, R., Spray, D. C., and Nedergaard, M., pp. 77-108, WILEY-VCH Verlag GmbH & Co. KGaA, ISBN 3-527-31088-6, Weinheim

Wolburg, H.; Neuhaus, J.; Kniesel, U.; Krauss, B.; Schmid, E.M.; Ocalan, M.; Farrell, C. & Risau, W. (1994). Modulation of tight junction structure in blood-brain barrier endothelial cells. Effects of tissue culture, second messengers and cocultured astrocytes. *J.Cell Sci.*, Vol.107 (Pt 5) (May 1994), pp. 1347-1357, ISSN 0021-9533

Wu, G.; Barth, R.F.; Yang, W.; Kawabata, S.; Zhang, L. & Green-Church, K. (2006). Targeted delivery of methotrexate to epidermal growth factor receptor-positive brain tumors by means of cetuximab (IMC-C225) dendrimer bioconjugates. *Mol.Cancer Ther.*, Vol.5, No.1, (January 2006), pp. 52-59, ISSN 1535-7163

Yu, C.; Kastin, A.J.; Tu, H.; Waters, S. & Pan, W. (2007). TNF activates P-glycoprotein in cerebral microvascular endothelial cells. *Cell Physiol Biochem.*, Vol.20, No.6, (2007), pp. 853-858, ISSN 1015-8987

Part 6

Gene Therapy of Glioma

8

Glioma-Parvovirus Interactions: Molecular Insights and Therapeutic Potential

Jon Gil-Ranedo, Marina Mendiburu-Eliçabe,
Marta Izquierdo and José M. Almendral
Centro de Biología Molecular "Severo Ochoa"
Consejo Superior de Investigaciones Científicas (CSIC)
Universidad Autónoma de Madrid (UAM)
Departamento de Biología Molecular, Cantoblanco, Madrid
Spain

1. Introduction

Brain tumours remain one of the most devastating diseases of modern medicine. Although they only represent approximately 1.9% of primary tumours in Europe, their mortality is around 70% and they are within the group of the 10 cancer types causing the highest yearly mortality rate. Gliomas are malignancies of neuroepithelial origin and represent 40-60% of brain tumours. In particular, glioblastoma multiforme (GBM, astrocytic tumours of type IV) is the most aggressive and frequent of primary brain tumours, representing 60% of gliomas. Despite clinical practice advances, the mean survival time of GBM patients has not improved significantly within the last few decades, and it remains around 12-15 months. Current standard of care includes maximal safe surgical resection, and a combination of radio- and chemotherapy with concomitant and adjuvant temozolomide or carmustine wafers (Wen and Kesari 2008). At the moment, the clinical improvement reached is modest, with a 5-year survival rate of less than 5% (Mangiola et al. 2010). The poor results obtained with conventional therapies may be explained by their relatively unspecific nature (Newton 2010), the inefficient delivery of many drugs to the tumoral tissue due to the blood-brain and blood-tumour barriers, as well as by the intrinsic radio- and chemo-resistance of GBM (Newton 2010).

In light of the limitations of conventional treatment strategies, the necessity of new approaches that would be more effective against GBM became evident. The current understanding of the molecular biology of GBM has set researchers on the path of more targeted and specific therapies exploiting the molecular properties of the tumour. Most targeted agents are tyrosine kinase inhibitors, or monoclonal antibodies directed against either cell surface growth factor receptors or intercellular signaling molecules (angiogenesis) (Van Meir et al. 2010). The overall experience of the monotherapy with targeted agents has shown limited efficacy, with response rates of less than 10-15% and no prolongation of survival (Clarke et al. 2010; Van Meir et al. 2010). Other promising therapies for GBM are also currently being investigated, including combined therapy with targeted agents, immunotherapy, gene therapy, or oncolytic virotherapy (Clarke et al. 2010; Van Meir et al. 2010).

Virus-mediated therapy, or virotherapy, is emerging as a promising biological approach to complement or potentiate physical and chemical anti-cancer conventional treatments (reviewed in Eager and Nemunaitis 2011). The increasing knowledge on molecular mechanisms underlying cancer development, and on the host-virus interphase regulating viral infections, is allowing the rational design of virotherapies against some human tumours. Ideally, the infection of a clinically competent oncolytic virus candidate should specifically target, replicate in, and destroy the tumour cells, but sparing surrounding non-transformed cells. Multiple restrictions and uncertainties operating at different levels, such as at cellular (specificity of tumour markers in non-transformed cells, tumour microenvironment), anatomical (accessibility, vascular barriers), or physiological (innate and specific immune responses) levels, constitute important challenges against effective virotherapy. In spite of them, intensive research efforts being conducted in many laboratories are developing or using RNA and DNA oncolytic viruses for glioma therapy (see other chapters of this book). Indeed, clinical trials were performed (Haseley et al. 2009; Kroeger et al. 2010) or are currently in progress against glioblastoma using different virotherapeutic approaches. For the first time H-1, a member of the *Parvoviridae*, is within the ongoing clinical trial protocols (http://clinicaltrials.gov/). Some general features of this virus family, as well as molecular bases of the anti-glioma activities of the parvoviruses, are reviewed below.

2. The Parvoviruses: General features and anti-cancer properties

2.1 Parvovirus capsid structure and genome organization

The *Parvoviridae* is a family of spherical, non-enveloped icosahedral viruses (Berns and Parrish 2007). The number of viruses being identified as members of this family is rapidly increasing in the recent years. Current classification from the International Committee of Taxonomy of Viruses (ICTV) for the *Parvoviridae* includes two subfamilies and nine geni (see Figure 1A). The parvoviral capsids are ~260 Å in diameter, and encapsidate a ssDNA genome of ~5000 nucleotides. The number of capsid protein species per virion varies among parvoviruses, but are generally composed by three polypeptides, VP1, VP2 and VP3 (molecular weights in the range of 60-84 kDa). Capsids contain 60 copies (in total) of VP protein subunits in a T=1 icosahedral capsid arrangement. The three-dimensional structure of the capsid, which has been determined to high resolution by X-ray crystallography for many members (Tsao et al. 1991; reviewed in Chapman and Agbandje-McKenna 2006), shows a conserved overall topology of eight-stranded antiparallel beta-barrel core motif that forms the contiguous capsid shell, and large loop insertions between the beta-strands. The surface features include small protrusions (spike-like) commonly at the icosahedral three-fold axes, and depressions that may be located at the icosahedral two-fold (dimple-like) and/or around the five-fold (canyon-like) axes.

Virus members of the autonomously replicating Parvovirus genus infect mammals and have a wide range of natural hosts, including humans, monkeys, dogs, livestock, felines and rodents. A main molecular model of this genus is the mouse parvovirus Minute Virus of Mice (MVM), which genome is organized as two overlapping transcription units (see Figure 1B) timely regulated (Clemens and Pintel 1988). The left-hand gene driven by the P4 promoter encodes the NS1 and NS2 nonstructural proteins, and the right-hand gene driven by the P38 promoter encodes the VP1 and VP2 structural proteins. In spite of its small size (only 5 Kb), the use of alternate splicing, extensive postranslational modifications and proteolytic processings, maximize the coding capacity of the parvovirus genome. The two NS polypeptides play multiple roles in virus life cycle. The smaller NS2 protein (28 kDa) contains three isoforms arising from alternate splicings that can bind several cellular proteins and shuttle from the nucleus to the cytoplasm via the CRM1 export pathway. Functions assigned to NS2 include assisting capsid assembly, messenger translation, DNA replication, and virus production in a cell type specific manner. The larger NS1 (82 kDa), is a multifunctional nuclear phosphoprotein, highly toxic for most cells, and performing crucial activities in the MVM unique rolling-hairpin mode of DNA synthesis (see below).

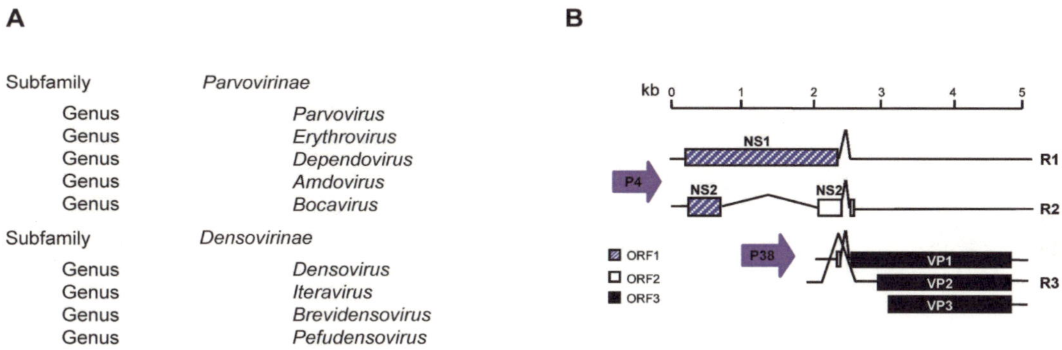

Fig. 1. Outline of the *Parvoviridae*. (A) Taxonomic structure of the *Parvoviridae* (from Tijssen et al. 2011, *in press*). (B) Organization of the MVM genome. The position of the two promoters (P4, P38) are designated by arrows. Splicing sites, and virus coded main non-structural (NS1, NS2), and structural (VP1, VP2) polypeptides are illustrated in their respective reading frame (based on Cotmore and Tattersall 1987).

2.2 Parvoviruses as oncolytic agents

Many of the members of the *Parvoviridae* were initially isolated from tumours or from transformed cell lines in culture, corresponding with the requirement of these viruses for multiple functions provided by proliferative cells. This unique biological feature, together with requirements for diverse factors that are linked to the neoplastic growth, account for the capacity of the parvoviruses to infect and lyse preferentially cells transformed by a high diversity of physico-chemical and biological agents (Mousset and Rommelaere 1982; Cornelis et al. 1988), and to interfere with tumour formation in animal models (Toolan and Ledinko 1965; Dupressoir et al. 1989; reviewed in Rommelaere et al. 2010). These studies validated, at least for some parvoviruses, many of the requirements that oncolytic viruses should fulfill to be used in the clinic, such as oncotropism, no genomic integration, low toxicity of structural components, or apathogenicity for humans.

This review is focused on the interactions of glioma cells with two parvoviruses which oncolytic properties have been best evaluated, the rat parvovirus H-1, and the p and i *wild-type* strains of the mouse parvovirus Minute Virus of Mice (MVM). Over the past decade, the characteristics of the infection of these viruses in rodent and human glioma cell lines, primary human glioblastoma cultures, and preclinical xenotransplanted animal models, have been extensively studied (see Table 1).

Infectious Parvovirus	Human GBM	Infection/Mechanism	Reference
MVMp	U373MG	Cytotoxic and productive infection/ Postencapsidation restriction	(Rubio et al. 2001)
MVMi	U87MG	Cytotoxic non-productive/ Viral DNA replication blockade	(Rubio et al. 2001)
H-1	U373MG and primary cultures	Productive cytotoxic infection/ Viral replication and maduration	(Herrero et al. 2004)
MVMp, MVMi	M059J, U87MG	Limited virus spread and cell death/ Not reported	(Wollmann et al. 2005)
H-1	U373MG, U138MG, NCH82, NCH89, NCH125 and NCH149	Death in cells resistant to TRAIL and cisplatin/ Cytosolic accumulation of lysosomal cathepsins B, L and reduction of the levels of cystatin B and C	(Di Piazza et al. 2007)
MVMp	U373MG	Productive and nuclear capsid assembly/ Raf-1 phosphorylation of capsid subunits	(Riolobos et al. 2010)
H-1	NCH82, NCH89, NCH125 and NCH149	Cytotoxic in radioresistant gliomas/ combination of ionizating radiation and H-1	(Geletneky et al. 2010a)
MVMp	U373MG	Productive gene expression/ PKR translational control	(Ventoso et al. 2010)
H-1	U87MG	Regression of glioma in immunodeficient rats/ Viral oncolysis in the tumor	(Geletneky et al. 2010b) (Kiprianova et al. 2011)

Table 1. Contributions on human Glioma-Parvovirus interactions.

The first report about cytotoxicity of a parvovirus against transformed neural cells was on the MVMp and MVMi infection of rat C6 glioma and several human glioblastoma and astrocytoma cells (Rubio et al. 2001). The MVM infections of human cells were cytotoxic but poorly productive, as found some years afterwards by an independent study (Wollmann et al. 2005). Although a parallel study with the MVM and H-1 viruses has not being carefully addressed, several subsequent reports suggested that H-1 is a more powerful oncolytic agent against human glioblastoma, regarding the levels of both cytotoxicity and virus yield in culture (Herrero et al. 2004; Di Piazza et al. 2007). Further recent preclinical studies have convincingly supported H-1 as anti-glioblastoma agent for clinical purposes, as its infection synergized with radiation (Geletneky et al. 2010a), and moreover it improved survival and remission of advanced intracranial U87MG human glioblastoma in rat models (Geletneky et al. 2010b; Kiprianova et al. 2011). However, as discussed below for MVM, there are particularly interesting aspects in the non-productive glioma-parvovirus interaction, as they may uncover molecular processes altered in glioma and helping to identify cellular targets for cancer treatments.

3. Parvovirus genome replication may be restricted in human glioblastoma

The two best characterized strains (p and i) of the MVM, exhibiting distinct tropism in spite of their sequence and capsid structure similarity (reviewed in Cotmore and Tattersall 2007), conform a valuable system to explore molecular aspects of virus-host interactions in human gliomas (Rubio et al. 2001). MVMp infection of U373MG was cytotoxic and productive, whereas U87MG and SW1088 astrocytoma cells were resistant to this virus. The MVMi infections were more interesting, as they uncovered novel insights on parvovirus-tumour cells interactions. Although this virus did not complete its life cycle, it efficiently killed the U373MG, U87MG, and SW1088 astrocytic tumour cells. The abortive infection was not restricted at the transcription or gene expression steps, as the viral messenger RNAs, as well as both non-structural (NS1) and structural (VP1, VP2) proteins, accumulated to normal levels. However, in the U87MG glioblastoma, MVMi failed to amplify its DNA genome. All these analyses consistently showed that only the non-availability of multimeric replicative DNA forms to be encapsidated hampered MVMi virions maturation in the U87MG cells.

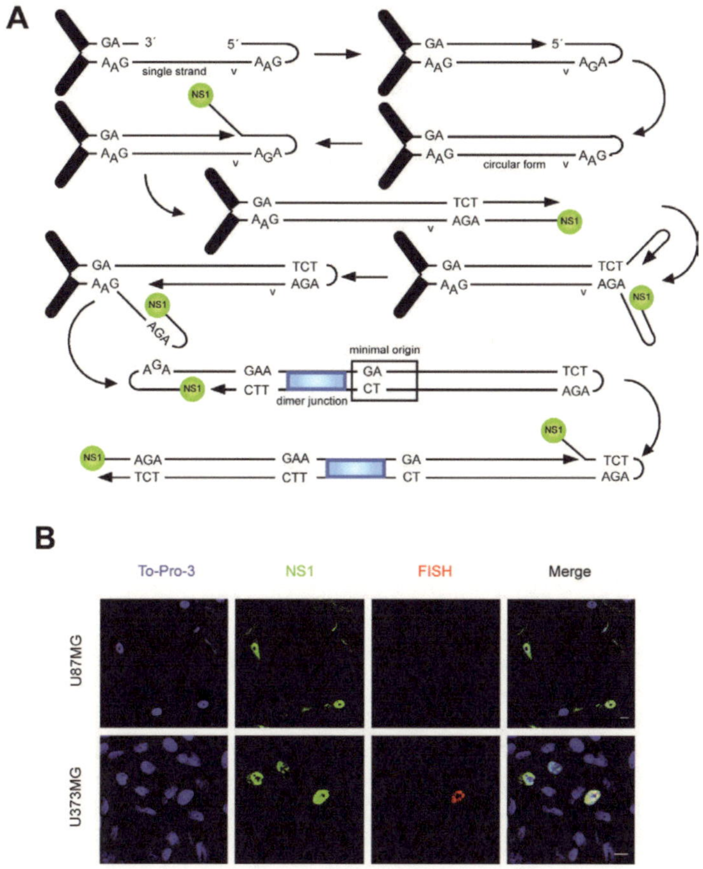

Fig. 2. Distinct genome replication capacity of parvovirus MVM in human glioblastomas. (A) Model of MVM genome replication (based on Cotmore and Tattersall 1995). The ssDNA virus genome is illustrated showing the particular structure of the 3´ left and 5´ right termini and their base mispairing. Only the initial steps of the model leading to the configuration of the dsDNA monomeric (mRF) and dimeric (dRF) intermediates, are outlined. (B) DNA replication of MVMi in human U87MG and U373MG cells. The glioblastomas were infected by MVMi, fixed and proceeded for immunofluorescence at 48hpi. Staining was with an anti-NS1 antibody and FISH using MVM specific TxR-oligonucleotides. NS1 protein accumulated into the nucleus in both glioblastoma cells, but MVM replication occurring only in U373MG, are shown (scale bar, 10 μm).

The molecular mechanisms underlying the failed DNA amplification of MVMi in U87MG glioblastoma remain unclear, although some clues can be drawn. As shown in Figure 2B, the U87MG, as the fully permissive U373MG cells, expressed high amounts of NS1 protein (the major viral replicative factor) that translocated normally into the nucleus, although viral DNA was not synthesized to detectable levels (Gil-Ranedo et al., in preparation). When the viral DNA replicative intermediates accumulated in U87MG were resolved in agarose gels (Rubio et al. 2001), a conversion of the incoming viral genome (ssDNA) to the monomeric replicative form (mRF) occurred. However, the subsequent synthesis of the dimeric form (dRF) was not observed. These findings are next interpreted under a current MVM replication model (Figure 2A). The conversion reaction (ssDNA to mRF) is exclusively accomplished by cellular factors S-phase dependent, involving elongation by the δ and other cellular polymerases (Bashir et al. 2000), which are apparently functional in U87MG cells. For several of the following steps of the replication model, the NS1 endonuclease and helicase activities are essential to provide 3´OH ends for the replication fork to proceed (Nuesch et al. 1995). It seems therefore likely that these NS1 activities, or the interaction with cellular factor recruited to the MVM origin of replication to assist NS1 activities (Christensen et al. 1997; Christensen et al. 2001), are not functional in infected U87MG cells.

It is worth mentioning that the infection of human glioblastomas by other parvoviruses may be not restricted at the DNA replication level. The also autonomous H-1 rat parvovirus, closely related to MVM, productively infected the U373MG human glioblastoma cell line, as well as human short-term cultures derived from histologically and immunologically confirmed glioblastomas (NCH82, NCH89, NCH125, NCH149) and gliosarcoma (NCH37). Cell killing, viral DNA amplification, protein expressions and infectious virus particles production was demonstrated in all of these cultures (Herrero et al. 2004). The broader host range of H-1 than MVM toward human glioblastomas may suggest that subtle genetic changes between parvovirus genomes may result in drastically different infection outcomes.

4. Translational control of parvovirus gene expression in glioblastoma

The degree of permissiveness of many host cells to a particular virus infection is regulated, to a great extent, at the level of the accessibility of the translational machinery to the viral messenger RNAs. The complexity of virus-host interaction at this level is exemplified by the multiple mechanisms evolved by viruses (e.g. affinity of viral messengers for the ribosome, or dependence on initiation factors) to overcome the also evolving cellular barriers (Bushell and Sarnow 2002; Schneider and Mohr 2003). A major role at this interface is played by the Protein Kinase R (PKR), which is activated by the dsRNA species generated by the replication of RNA and some DNA viruses (Balachandran and Barber 2000; Elde et al. 2009). Upon activation, PKR phosphorylates the Ser51 residue of the alpha subunit of the initiation factor 2 (eIF2α), preventing eIF2 from forming the ternary complex with GTP and the initiator Met-tRNA (Dever 2002; Dey et al. 2005), leading to the inhibition of translation initiation and thus aborting virus multiplication. The multiple strategies evolved by viruses to inhibit or bypass PKR activation include for example binding to PKR (Kitajewski et al. 1986; Gale et al. 1998), sequestering the dsRNA (Lu et al. 1995), or recruiting a host phosphatase that dephosphorylates eIF2α (He et al. 1997).

Cell transformation is often associated to reduction or complete suppression of the antiviral defense mechanisms, including PKR responsiveness. For example, some leukemia-derived

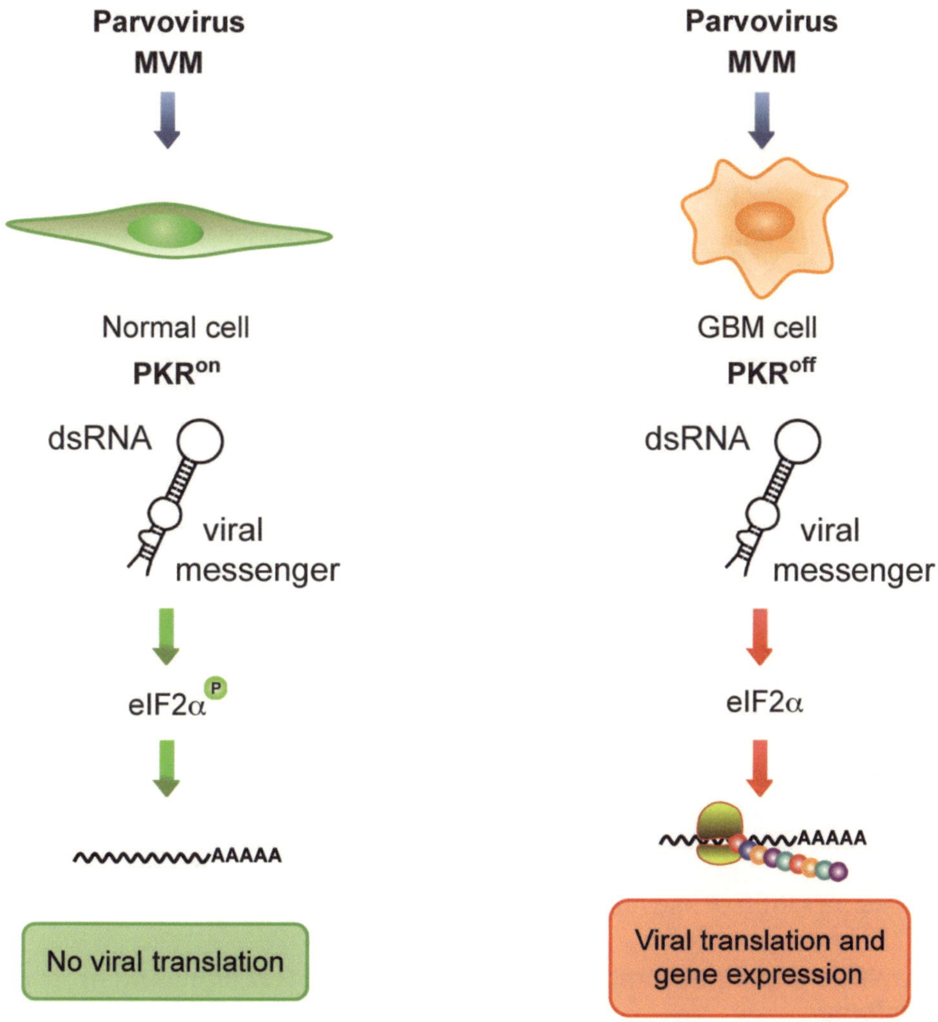

Fig. 3. Translational control of MVM gene expression in GBM based on PKR activity. Virus entry and traffic into the nucleus is followed by transcription of the early NS gene. Folding of viral messenger RNAs produces regions of dsRNA secondary structure with variable length and complexity. In most normal cells (left), the presence of dsRNA in the cytoplasm leads to PKR activation and eIF2α phosphorylation, which inhibits cap-dependent mRNA translation. In GBM (right), the failure of PKR activation in response to infection allows viral mRNA translation and replication to proceed (based on Ventoso et al. 2010).

cell lines have lost the PKR gene (Beretta et al. 1996), whereas PKR activation, but not expression, was hampered in H-Ras transformed fibroblasts (Mundschau and Faller 1992), and PKR plays a role in the tumour-suppressor function of p53 (Yoon et al. 2009). Other transformed cells however, as some human glioblastoma cells, harbor functional PKR that can be activated by specific dsRNA to promote selective killing (Shir and Levitzki 2002; Friedrich et al. 2005). Therefore, in most cell transformation processes viruses find a favoured environment for messenger translation and gene expression. The defective translational control in cancer cells have been exploited by different virotherapy systems (reviewed in Parato et al. 2005), as those conducted with naturally oncotropic VSV and Reovirus (Strong et al. 1998; Balachandran and Barber 2004), or with genetically engineered oncolytic Adenovirus and Herpesvirus (Farassati et al. 2001; Cascallo et al. 2003), which replicate inefficiently in cells with intact PKR pathways, but may complete gene expression and replication in malignant gliomas (Shah et al. 2007).

In recent years, the important role that translational control plays in the gene expression and natural oncotropism of the ssDNA virus members of the *Parvoviridae* has been recognized. In the Adeno-Associated Virus type 5 (AAV5), a member of the Dependovirus genus, viral replication and protein synthesis was highly enhanced by the co-expression of an adenovirus VA I RNA (Nayak and Pintel 2007a) that, by binding to PKR, prevents its otherwise activation by a short RNA sequence of AAV5 messengers (Nayak and Pintel 2007b). The infection of untransformed fibroblast cells by MVM of the Parvovirus genus, activated PKR and subsequently phosphorylated eIF2α (Ventoso et al. 2010). This mechanism drastically inhibited the synthesis of the NS1 protein, which controls the expression of the viral late messengers and genome replication, leading to a drastic inhibition of virus gene expression and multiplication in culture (see Figure 3, left). In support of this phenomenon observed in cells, purified PKR was highly activated by the R1 genomic messenger of MVM *in vitro*, leading to phosphorylation of the eIF2α translation initiation factor. In contrast, the human glioblastoma U373MG cells showed basal levels of eIF2α phosphorylation, and moreover failed to increase PKR-mediated eIF2α phosphorylation in response to MVM infection, thereby allowing viral gene expression to proceed (Figure 3, right). Therefore, the oncolytic capacity of MVM, H-1, and other parvoviruses against glioblastoma may be largely related to the failure of PKR activation. This conclusion is consistent with the widely studied permissiveness to parvovirus gene expression and toxicity of multiple human cells transformed by oncogenes and tumour suppressors genes (Mousset and Rommelaere 1982; Salome et al. 1990; Telerman et al. 1993), which disturb PKR-based antiviral innate immunity.

5. Parvovirus capsid assembly targets deregulated Raf signaling in glioblastoma

A virotherapy of glioma with potential clinical benefit should exploit synergy interactions between molecular targets upregulated in glioma cells, and viral factors involved in the replication or maturation of the therapeutic candidate. The genetic alterations undergoing malignant gliomas are multiple and complex, although some signaling pathways play major roles. Alterations in tyrosine kinase growth factor receptors (EGFR, PDGFR, MET and ERBB2), as those found in almost all World Health Organization (WHO) grade II, III and IV astrocytomas, result in constitutive downstream signaling of the RAS/RAF/MEK/ERK (MAPK) and PI3K/AKT pathways. The MAPK pathway is also important for glioma development as it is activated in most WHO grade I tumours. These epidemiological studies are consistent with experimental evidences in mouse models showing that the expression of activated KRAS, CRAF or BRAF in neural progenitor cells combined with either AKT activation, or Ink4aArf loss, leads to the development of high-grade gliomas in vivo (Robinson et al. 2010). In the MAPK signal cascade (see Figure 4), assembled membrane-associated complex formed by kinases and scaffold proteins transduces mitogenic and other stimuli from the cell surface to the nucleus (Marais and Marshall 1996).

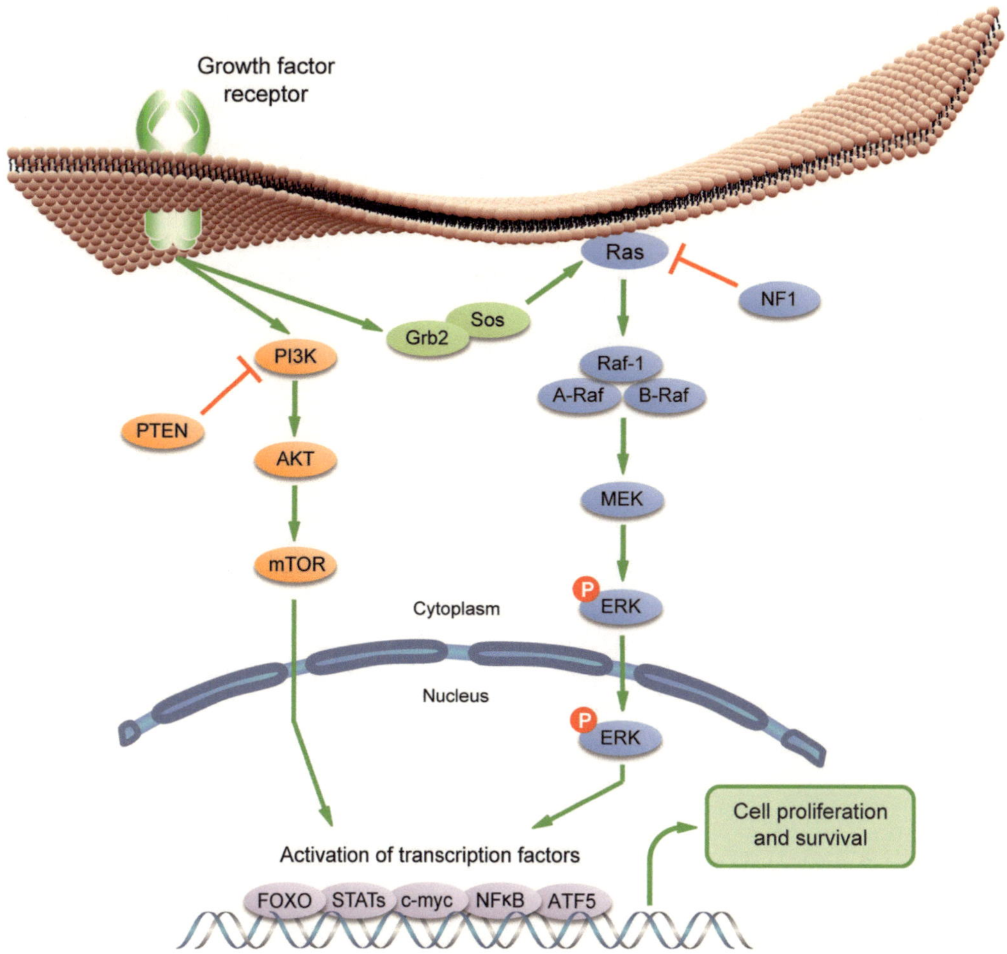

Fig. 4. Principal protein effectors of the signaling pathways altered in GBM. The two major pathways altered in GBM, the PI3K/AKT/mTOR and Ras/RAF/MEK/MAPK, may be activated from the membrane-coupled receptor. Arrows designate the activation cascades mainly due to phosphorylation. Two inhibitors, PTEN and NF1 (Van Meir et al. 2010), relevant for GBM development, are also outlined. Note the key role of RAF proteins complex as regulator of ERK nuclear translocation (references in the text).

The MEK1/2 proteins are the main downstream effectors of the activated RAF protein kinases, and subsequently they phosphorylate ERK, which dissociates from the complex and translocates into the nucleus (Khokhlatchev et al. 1998). Active ERK induces many transcription factors including ATF5, which expression inversely correlates with malignant glioma prognosis (Sheng et al. 2010). In glioma, the RAF kinase isoforms are constitutively activated, overexpressed, or mutated (Wellbrock et al. 2004; Lyustikman et al. 2008), and although most mutations map to BRAF (Davies et al. 2002), the activity of the complex may be regulated by CRAF, as it also acts as an effector of BRAF (Wan et al. 2004). Therefore, finding viral proteins that become specific substrate of the RAF kinases in infected cells may support anti-glioma therapeutic virotherapies.

The parvovirus capsid is composed of 60 protein subunits (named VP) folded in an eight-stranded antiparallel β-barrel motif (Tsao et al. 1991). From their synthesis in the cytoplasm, the VP proteins undergo a well-regulated assembly process that leads to the maturation of the infectious particle in the nucleus of permissive cells. In MVM, the VP1/VP2 capsid proteins are synthesized at an approximate 1/5 ratio, and rapidly assemble into two types of trimers in the cytoplasm at stoichiometric amounts (Riolobos et al. 2006). As outlined in Figure 5, in mammalian permissive cells these trimers are translocated into the nucleus driven by two nuclear-targeting sequences: (i) a non-conventional structured nuclear localization motif (NLM) evolutionary conserved in the parvovirus β-barrel (Lombardo et al. 2000); and (ii) a conventional nuclear localization sequence (NLS) found in the VP1 N-terminus (Lombardo et al. 2002; Vihinen-Ranta et al. 2002).

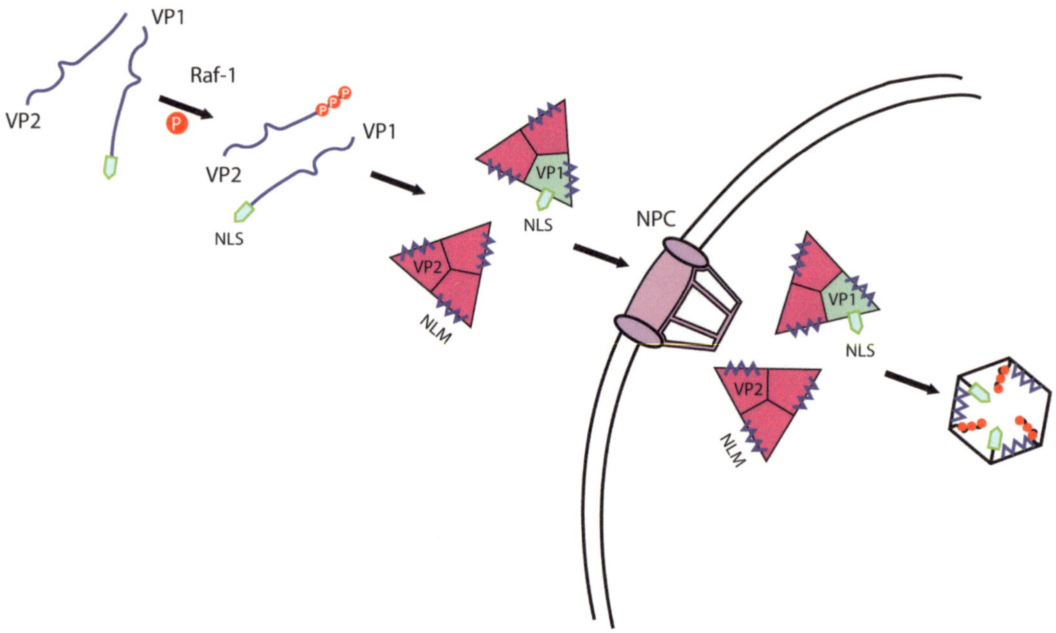

Fig. 5. Role of Raf-1 (C-Raf) in the nuclear transport of MVM capsid assembly intermediates. MVM capsid proteins (VP1 and VP2) assemble into two types of trimers at their 1/5 stoichiometry of synthesis. Trimers gain nuclear transport competence upon cytoplasmic Raf-1 phosphorylation (VP2 N-terminus is a major phosphorylated domain), and are driven into the nucleus by the NLM and NLS sequences exposed to the transport machinery. Inside the nucleus the fully assembled icosahedral capsid harbors the NLS and NLM facing to the particle inward. Abbreviations: NPC, nuclear pore complex; NLM, nuclear localization motif; NLS, nuclear localization sequence (based on Lombardo et al. 2000; Maroto et al. 2000; Riolobos et al. 2006; Riolobos et al. 2010).

The VP proteins of MVM undergo cytoplasmic phosphorylation by the Raf-1 kinase (Riolobos et al. 2010). Raf-1 (or C-RAF) (72-74 kDa) is a cytoplasmic major protein isoform of the conserved MAPK signaling module with intrinsic serine-threonine kinase activity. The phosphorylation of the VP capsid subunits by Raf-1 occurs at specific Ser/Thr sites *in vitro* yielding a characteristic 2-D phosphopeptides map found in the MVM infections (Maroto et al. 2000). The important role of Raf-1 phosphorylation in VP nuclear transport is best illustrated in heterologous cell systems devoid of Raf-1. For example, the expression of parvovirus VP proteins in insect cells resulted in non-phosphorylated VP trimers and aggregates (Riolobos et al. 2010) that, although at low efficiency, self-assembly into virus-like particles (VLPs) accumulating in the perinuclear region of the cytoplasm (Hernando et al. 2000; Yuan and Parrish 2001). However the co-expression of a constitutively active Raf-1 kinase in the insect cells, as the truncated mutant Raf-22W with transforming activity (Stanton et al. 1989), restored the phosphorylation and nuclear transport competence of the VP trimer (Riolobos et al. 2010).

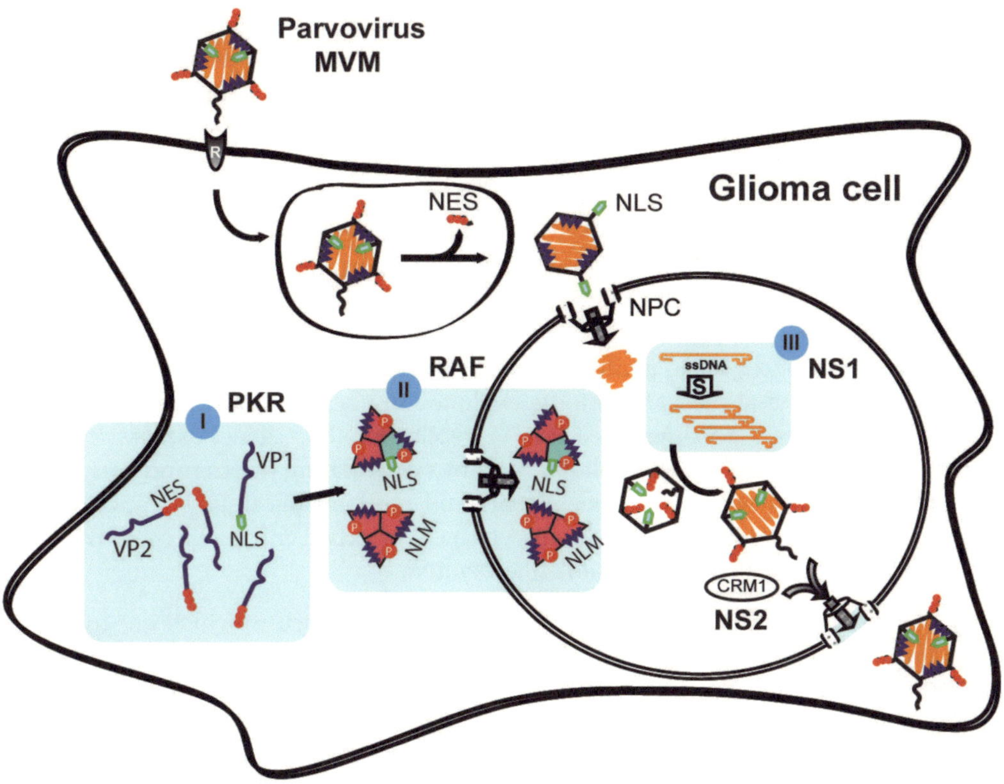

Fig. 6. Molecular overview of parvovirus MVM life cycle steps in glioma cells. **Virus Entry**: VP2 cleavage, Phospholipase activity and VP1 NLS externalization are required to deliver the genome across the NPC. **Capsid Assembly**: VP synthesis, phosphorylation and assembly into trimers lead to translocation into the nucleus by the NLM and NLS signals. **Maturation and Egress:** Viral DNA is amplified in the S phase and encapsidation presumably occurs in pre-assembled empty capsids. DNA-filled virions actively egress from the nucleus by the NES at VP2 n-terminus and CRM1-NS2-Nucleoporins mediation. For three processes (I, II, III), the cellular and viral factors found involved in the regulation of glioma-parvovirus interactions, are highlighted. NLS, nuclear localization sequence; NLM, nuclear localization motif; S, cell cycle dependent DNA synthesis; NES, nuclear export sequence; NPC, nuclear pore complex. CRM1, nuclear export factor (adapted with modifications from Maroto et al. 2004, and Valle et al. 2006).

The enhanced VP nuclear transport and MVM capsid assembly by oncogenic deregulated Raf-1 should facilitate parvovirus maturation in cancer cells. Indeed, in rat C6 and human U373MG glioblastoma cells infected with MVM, the characteristic pattern of VP phosphorylation by Raf-1 was conserved, correlating with a high activity of the MAPK signaling pathway (Riolobos et al. 2010). Moreover these glioblastomas were efficiently killed by MVM and the virus underwent productive maturation to high yields (Rubio et al. 2001). Given the difficulties encountered in searching effective chemotherapies against the Raf signaling cascade for cancer treatment (Madhunapantula and Robertson 2008; Newton 2010), the above mentioned findings may support MVM and related parvoviruses as replicative inhibitors specifically targeting glioblastomas with deregulated Raf signaling.

6. Conclusions

We have summarized in this chapter some molecular mechanisms involved in glioma-MVM interactions. Figure 6 illustrates some major events of MVM life cycle, highlighting those three steps at which the interaction of this parvovirus with glioma cells was found to be modulated. Final comments related to these findings are in brief : (i) Identifying the relevance of PKR translational control for MVM cytotoxic infection in U373MG glioblastoma, connects the parvoviral oncolysis with a common mechanism exhibited by other oncolytic viruses to preferentially infect tumour cells with deregulated IFN and other innate antiviral responses; (ii) Raf-1 requirement for MVM nuclear capsid assembly not only assignes parvoviral oncolysis to an important kinase upregulated in human cancer, but also underlies a novel general mechanism to be exploited in oncolytic virotherapy; (iii) the lack of correlation between NS1-mediated MVM replication and gene expression may be important to better understand the cellular machinery regulating theses processes in normal vs. tumour cells. It is likely that other signals and mechanisms tightly regulated during MVM life cycle steps (see Figure 6) be also found perturbed in cancer cells, what could provide additional targets for anti-glioma intervention.

Finally, the dependence of parvovirus infection on cellular factors which are functionally dysregulated in a cancer-specific manner may bring two important benefits: (i) the use of parvoviruses as markers of host-cell perturbations (e.g. signaling) coupled to transformation, and (ii) it may allow to apply these simple viruses as specific therapeutic agents against precise types of glioblastomas showing permissive genetic profiles, toward a personalized parvoviral anti-cancer virotherapy.

7. Acknowledgments

The experimental contributions of the following past members of the laboratory is gratefully acknowledged: S. Guerra, E. Hernando, E. Lombardo, A. López-Bueno, B. Maroto, J. C. Ramirez, L. Riolobos, M.- P. Rubio, N. Valle, and I. Ventoso. We are indebted to Michael Kann (Bourdeaux) for collaborative support on nuclear transport studies, and to Peter Tattersall (Yale, CT) and Jean Rommelaere (DKFZ, Heidelberg) for generous thoughtful advices along the years.

This work was supported by grants from the Spanish Ministerio de Ciencia e Innovación (SAF2008-03238) and Comunidad de Madrid (S-SAL/0185/2006) to the laboratory of J.M.A.

The Centro de Biología Molecular "Severo Ochoa" (CSIC-UAM) is in part supported by an institutional grant from Fundación Ramón Areces.

8. References

Balachandran, S. and Barber, G.N. 2000. Vesicular stomatitis virus (VSV) therapy of tumors. IUBMB Life 50(2): 135-138.

Balachandran, S. and Barber, G.N. 2004. Defective translational control facilitates vesicular stomatitis virus oncolysis. Cancer cell 5(1): 51-65.

Bashir, T., Horlein, R., Rommelaere, J., and Willwand, K. 2000. Cyclin A activates the DNA polymerase delta -dependent elongation machinery in vitro: A parvovirus DNA replication model. Proc Natl Acad Sci U S A 97(10): 5522-5527.

Beretta, L., Gabbay, M., Berger, R., Hanash, S.M., and Sonenberg, N. 1996. Expression of the protein kinase PKR in modulated by IRF-1 and is reduced in 5q- associated leukemias. Oncogene 12(7): 1593-1596.

Berns, N. and Parrish, C.R. 2007. in Parvoviridae. Lippincott Willians and Wilkins, Philadelphia, PA.

Bushell, M. and Sarnow, P. 2002. Hijacking the translation apparatus by RNA viruses. J Cell Biol 158(3): 395-399.

Cascallo, M., Capella, G., Mazo, A., and Alemany, R. 2003. Ras-dependent oncolysis with an adenovirus VAI mutant. Cancer research 63(17): 5544-5550.

Chapman, S.M. and Agbandje-McKenna, M. 2006. Atomic structure of viral particles. in Parvoviruses (ed. J.R. Kerr, S.F. Cotmore, M.E. Bloom, R.M. Linden, and C.R. Parrish), pp. 107-123. Hodder A., London, UK.

Christensen, J., Cotmore, S.F., and Tattersall, P. 1997. Parvovirus initiation factor PIF: a novel human DNA-binding factor which coordinately recognizes two ACGT motifs. J Virol 71(8): 5733-5741.

Christensen, J., Cotmore, S.F., and Tattersall, P. 2001. Minute virus of mice initiator protein NS1 and a host KDWK family transcription factor must form a precise ternary complex with origin DNA for nicking to occur. J Virol 75(15): 7009-7017.

Clarke, J., Butowski, N., and Chang, S. 2010. Recent advances in therapy for glioblastoma. Arch Neurol 67(3): 279-283.

Clemens, K.E. and Pintel, D.J. 1988. The two transcription units of the autonomous parvovirus minute virus of mice are transcribed in a temporal order. J Virol 62(4): 1448-1451.

Cornelis, J.J., Becquart, P., Duponchel, N., Salome, N., Avalosse, B.L., Namba, M., and Rommelaere, J. 1988. Transformation of human fibroblasts by ionizing radiation, a chemical carcinogen, or simian virus 40 correlates with an increase in susceptibility to the autonomous parvoviruses H-1 virus and minute virus of mice. J Virol 62(5): 1679-1686.

Cotmore, S.F. and Tattersall, P. 1987. The autonomously replicating parvoviruses of vertebrates. Adv Virus Res 33: 91-174.

Cotmore, S.F. and Tattersall, P. 1995. DNA replication in the autonomous parvovirus. Semin Virol 6(11): 271-281.

Cotmore, S.F. and Tattersall, P. 2007. Parvoviral host range and cell entry mechanisms. Adv Virus Res 70: 183-232.

Davies, H., Bignell, G.R., Cox, C., Stephens, P., Edkins, S., Clegg, S., Teague, J., Woffendin, H., Garnett, M.J., Bottomley, W., Davis, N., Dicks, E., Ewing, R., Floyd, Y., Gray, K., Hall, S., Hawes, R., Hughes, J., Kosmidou, V., Menzies, A., Mould, C., Parker, A., Stevens, C., Watt, S., Hooper, S., Wilson, R., Jayatilake, H., Gusterson, B.A., Cooper, C., Shipley, J., Hargrave, D., Pritchard-Jones, K., Maitland, N., Chenevix-Trench, G., Riggins, G.J., Bigner, D.D., Palmieri, G., Cossu, A., Flanagan, A., Nicholson, A., Ho, J.W., Leung, S.Y., Yuen, S.T., Weber, B.L., Seigler, H.F., Darrow, T.L., Paterson, H., Marais, R., Marshall, C.J., Wooster, R., Stratton, M.R., and Futreal, P.A. 2002. Mutations of the BRAF gene in human cancer. Nature 417(6892): 949-954.

Dever, T.E. 2002. Gene-specific regulation by general translation factors. Cell 108(4): 545-556.

Dey, M., Cao, C., Dar, A.C., Tamura, T., Ozato, K., Sicheri, F., and Dever, T.E. 2005. Mechanistic link between PKR dimerization, autophosphorylation, and eIF2alpha substrate recognition. Cell 122(6): 901-913.

Di Piazza, M., Mader, C., Geletneky, K., Herrero, Y.C.M., Weber, E., Schlehofer, J., Deleu, L., and Rommelaere, J. 2007. Cytosolic activation of cathepsins mediates parvovirus H-1-induced killing of cisplatin and TRAIL-resistant glioma cells. J Virol 81(8): 4186-4198.

Dupressoir, T., Vanacker, J.M., Cornelis, J.J., Duponchel, N., and Rommelaere, J. 1989. Inhibition by parvovirus H-1 of the formation of tumors in nude mice and colonies in vitro by transformed human mammary epithelial cells. Cancer research 49(12): 3203-3208.

Eager, R.M. and Nemunaitis, J. 2011. Clinical development directions in oncolytic viral therapy. Cancer Gene Ther 18(5): 305-317.

Elde, N.C., Child, S.J., Geballe, A.P., and Malik, H.S. 2009. Protein kinase R reveals an evolutionary model for defeating viral mimicry. Nature 457(7228): 485-489.

Farassati, F., Yang, A.D., and Lee, P.W. 2001. Oncogenes in Ras signalling pathway dictate host-cell permissiveness to herpes simplex virus 1. Nat Cell Biol 3(8): 745-750.

Friedrich, I., Eizenbach, M., Sajman, J., Ben-Bassat, H., and Levitzki, A. 2005. A cellular screening assay to test the ability of PKR to induce cell death in mammalian cells. Mol Ther 12(5): 969-975.

Gale, M., Jr., Blakely, C.M., Kwieciszewski, B., Tan, S.L., Dossett, M., Tang, N.M., Korth, M.J., Polyak, S.J., Gretch, D.R., and Katze, M.G. 1998. Control of PKR protein kinase by hepatitis C virus nonstructural 5A protein: molecular mechanisms of kinase regulation. Molecular and cellular biology 18(9): 5208-5218.

Geletneky, K., Hartkopf, A.D., Krempien, R., Rommelaere, J., and Schlehofer, J.R. 2010a. Improved killing of human high-grade glioma cells by combining ionizing radiation with oncolytic parvovirus H-1 infection. J Biomed Biotechnol 2010: 350748.

Geletneky, K., Kiprianova, I., Ayache, A., Koch, R., Herrero, Y.C.M., Deleu, L., Sommer, C., Thomas, N., Rommelaere, J., and Schlehofer, J.R. 2010b. Regression of advanced rat and human gliomas by local or systemic treatment with oncolytic parvovirus H-1 in rat models. Neuro Oncol. 12: 804-814.

Haseley, A., Alvarez-Breckenridge, C., Chaudhury, A.R., and Kaur, B. 2009. Advances in oncolytic virus therapy for glioma. *Recent Pat CNS Drug Discov* 4(1): 1-13.

He, B., Gross, M., and Roizman, B. 1997. The gamma(1)34.5 protein of herpes simplex virus 1 complexes with protein phosphatase 1alpha to dephosphorylate the alpha subunit of the eukaryotic translation initiation factor 2 and preclude the shutoff of protein synthesis by double-stranded RNA-activated protein kinase. Proc Natl Acad Sci U S A 94(3): 843-848.

Hernando, E., Llamas-Saiz, A.L., Foces-Foces, C., McKenna, R., Portman, I., Agbandje-McKenna, M., and Almendral, J.M. 2000. Biochemical and physical characterization of parvovirus minute virus of mice virus-like particles. Virology 267(2): 299-309.

Herrero, Y.C.M., Cornelis, J.J., Herold-Mende, C., Rommelaere, J., Schlehofer, J.R., and Geletneky, K. 2004. Parvovirus H-1 infection of human glioma cells leads to complete viral replication and efficient cell killing. International journal of cancer 109(1): 76-84.

Khokhlatchev, A.V., Canagarajah, B., Wilsbacher, J., Robinson, M., Atkinson, M., Goldsmith, E., and Cobb, M.H. 1998. Phosphorylation of the MAP kinase ERK2 promotes its homodimerization and nuclear translocation. Cell 93(4): 605-615.

Kiprianova, I., Thomas, N., Ayache, A., Fischer, M., Leuchs, B., Klein, M., Rommelaere, J., and Schlehofer, J.R. 2011. Regression of glioma in rat models by intranasal application of parvovirus H-1. Clin Cancer Res. 17: 5333-5342.

Kitajewski, J., Schneider, R.J., Safer, B., Munemitsu, S.M., Samuel, C.E., Thimmappaya, B., and Shenk, T. 1986. Adenovirus VAI RNA antagonizes the antiviral action of interferon by preventing activation of the interferon-induced eIF-2 alpha kinase. Cell 45(2): 195-200.

Kroeger, K.M., Muhammad, A.K., Baker, G.J., Assi, H., Wibowo, M.K., Xiong, W., Yagiz, K., Candolfi, M., Lowenstein, P.R., and Castro, M.G. 2010. Gene therapy and virotherapy: novel therapeutic approaches for brain tumors. *Discov Med* 10(53): 293-304.

Lombardo, E., Ramirez, J.C., Agbandje-McKenna, M., and Almendral, J.M. 2000. A beta-stranded motif drives capsid protein oligomers of the parvovirus minute virus of mice into the nucleus for viral assembly. J Virol 74(8): 3804-3814.

Lombardo, E., Ramirez, J.C., Garcia, J., and Almendral, J.M. 2002. Complementary roles of multiple nuclear targeting signals in the capsid proteins of the parvovirus minute virus of mice during assembly and onset of infection. J Virol 76(14): 7049-7059.

Lu, Y., Wambach, M., Katze, M.G., and Krug, R.M. 1995. Binding of the influenza virus NS1 protein to double-stranded RNA inhibits the activation of the protein kinase that phosphorylates the elF-2 translation initiation factor. Virology 214(1): 222-228.

Lyustikman, Y., Momota, H., Pao, W., and Holland, E.C. 2008. Constitutive activation of Raf-1 induces glioma formation in mice. Neoplasia (New York, NY 10(5): 501-510.

Madhunapantula, S.V. and Robertson, G.P. 2008. Is B-Raf a good therapeutic target for melanoma and other malignancies? Cancer research 68(1): 5-8.

Mangiola, A., Anile, C., Pompucci, A., Capone, G., Rigante, L., and De Bonis, P. 2010. Glioblastoma therapy: going beyond Hercules Columns. Expert Rev Neurother 10(4): 507-514.

Marais, R. and Marshall, C.J. 1996. Control of the ERK MAP kinase cascade by Ras and Raf. Cancer Surv 27: 101-125.

Markert, J.M., Medlock, M.D., Rabkin, S.D., Gillespie, G.Y., Todo, T., Hunter, W.D., Palmer, C.A., Feigenbaum, F., Tornatore, C., Tufaro, F., and Martuza, R.L. 2000. Conditionally replicating herpes simplex virus mutant, G207 for the treatment of malignant glioma: results of a phase I trial. Gene Ther 7(10): 867-874.

Maroto, B., Ramirez, J.C., and Almendral, J.M. 2000. Phosphorylation status of the parvovirus minute virus of mice particle: mapping and biological relevance of the major phosphorylation sites. J Virol 74(23): 10892-10902.

Maroto, B., Valle, N., Saffrich, R., and Almendral, J.M. 2004. Nuclear export of the nonenveloped parvovirus virion is directed by an unordered protein signal exposed on the capsid surface. J Virol 78(19): 10685-10694.

Mousset, S. and Rommelaere, J. 1982. Minute virus of mice inhibits cell transformation by simian virus 40. Nature 300(5892): 537-539.

Mousset, S. and Rommelaere, J. 1982. Minute virus of mice inhibits cell transformation by simian virus 40. Nature 300(5892): 537-539.

Mundschau, L.J. and Faller, D.V. 1992. Oncogenic ras induces an inhibitor of double-stranded RNA-dependent eukaryotic initiation factor 2 alpha-kinase activation. The Journal of biological chemistry 267(32): 23092-23098.

Nayak, R. and Pintel, D.J. 2007a. Adeno-associated viruses can induce phosphorylation of eIF2alpha via PKR activation, which can be overcome by helper adenovirus type 5 virus-associated RNA. J Virol 81(21): 11908-11916.

Nayak, R. and Pintel, D.J. 2007b. Positive and negative effects of adenovirus type 5 helper functions on adeno-associated virus type 5 (AAV5) protein accumulation govern AAV5 virus production. J Virol 81(5): 2205-2212.

Newton, H.B. 2010. Overview of the Molecular Genetics and Molecular Chemotherapy of GBM. in Glioblastoma Molecular Mechanisms of Pathogenesis and Current Therapeutic Strategies (ed. S.K. Ray).

Nuesch, J.P., Cotmore, S.F., and Tattersall, P. 1995. Sequence motifs in the replicator protein of parvovirus MVM essential for nicking and covalent attachment to the viral origin: identification of the linking tyrosine. Virology 209(1): 122-135.

Parato, K.A., Senger, D., Forsyth, P.A., and Bell, J.C. 2005. Recent progress in the battle between oncolytic viruses and tumours. Nature reviews 5(12): 965-976.

Riolobos, L., Reguera, J., Mateu, M.G., and Almendral, J.M. 2006. Nuclear transport of trimeric assembly intermediates exerts a morphogenetic control on the icosahedral parvovirus capsid. J Mol Biol 357(3): 1026-1038.

Riolobos, L., Valle, N., Hernando, E., Maroto, B., Kann, M., and Almendral, J.M. 2010. Viral oncolysis that targets Raf-1 signaling control of nuclear transport. J Virol 84(4): 2090-2099.

Robinson, J.P., VanBrocklin, M.W., Guilbeault, A.R., Signorelli, D.L., Brandner, S., and Holmen, S.L. 2010. Activated BRAF induces gliomas in mice when combined with Ink4a/Arf loss or Akt activation. Oncogene 29(3): 335-344.

Rommelaere, J., Geletneky, K., Angelova, A.L., Daeffler, L., Dinsart, C., Kiprianova, I., Schlehofer, J.R., and Raykov, Z. 2010. Oncolytic parvoviruses as cancer therapeutics. Cytokine Growth Factor Rev 21(2-3): 185-195.

Rubio, M.P., Guerra, S., and Almendral, J.M. 2001. Genome replication and postencapsidation functions mapping to the nonstructural gene restrict the host range of a murine parvovirus in human cells. J Virol 75(23): 11573-11582.

Salome, N., van Hille, B., Duponchel, N., Meneguzzi, G., Cuzin, F., Rommelaere, J., and Cornelis, J.J. 1990. Sensitization of transformed rat cells to parvovirus MVMp is restricted to specific oncogenes. Oncogene 5(1): 123-130.

Schneider, R.J. and Mohr, I. 2003. Translation initiation and viral tricks. Trends Biochem Sci 28(3): 130-136.

Shah, A.C., Parker, J.N., Gillespie, G.Y., Lakeman, F.D., Meleth, S., Markert, J.M., and Cassady, K.A. 2007. Enhanced antiglioma activity of chimeric HCMV/HSV-1 oncolytic viruses. Gene Ther 14(13): 1045-1054.

Sheng, Z., Li, L., Zhu, L.J., Smith, T.W., Demers, A., Ross, A.H., Moser, R.P., and Green, M.R. 2010. A genome-wide RNA interference screen reveals an essential CREB3L2-ATF5-MCL1 survival pathway in malignant glioma with therapeutic implications. Nat Med 16(6): 671-677.

Shir, A. and Levitzki, A. 2002. Inhibition of glioma growth by tumor-specific activation of double-stranded RNA-dependent protein kinase PKR. Nat Biotechnol 20(9): 895-900.

Stanton, V.P., Jr., Nichols, D.W., Laudano, A.P., and Cooper, G.M. 1989. Definition of the human raf amino-terminal regulatory region by deletion mutagenesis. Molecular and cellular biology 9(2): 639-647.

Strong, J.E., Coffey, M.C., Tang, D., Sabinin, P., and Lee, P.W. 1998. The molecular basis of viral oncolysis: usurpation of the Ras signaling pathway by reovirus. EMBO J 17(12): 3351-3362.

Telerman, A., Tuynder, M., Dupressoir, T., Robaye, B., Sigaux, F., Shaulian, E., Oren, M., Rommelaere, J., and Amson, R. 1993. A model for tumor suppression using H-1 parvovirus. Proc Natl Acad Sci U S A 90(18): 8702-8706.

Tijssen, P., Agbandje-McKenna, M., Almendral, J.M., Bergoin, M., Flegel, T.W., Hedman, K., Kleinschmidt, J., Li, Y., Pintel, D.J., and Tattersall, P. 2011. ICTV Ninth Report in press.

Toolan, H. and Ledinko, N. 1965. Growth and cytopathogenicity of H-viruses in human and simian cell cultures. Nature 208(5012): 812-813.

Tsao, J., Chapman, M.S., Agbandje, M., Keller, W., Smith, K., Wu, H., Luo, M., Smith, T.J., Rossmann, M.G., Compans, R.W., and et al. 1991. The three-dimensional structure of canine parvovirus and its functional implications. Science (New York, NY 251(5000): 1456-1464.

Valle, N., Riolobos, L., and Almendral, J.M. 2006. Synthesis, post-translational modification and trafficking of the parvovirus structural polypeptides. in Parvoviruses (ed. J.R. Kerr, S.F. Cotmore, M.E. Bloom, R.M. Linden, and C.R. Parrish). Hodder A., London, UK.

Van Meir, E.G., Hadjipanayis, C.G., Norden, A.D., Shu, H.K., Wen, P.Y., and Olson, J.J. 2010. Exciting new advances in neuro-oncology: the avenue to a cure for malignant glioma. CA Cancer J Clin 60(3): 166-193.

Ventoso, I., Berlanga, J.J., and Almendral, J.M. 2010. Translation control by protein kinase R restricts minute virus of mice infection: role in parvovirus oncolysis. J Virol 84(10): 5043-5051.

Vihinen-Ranta, M., Wang, D., Weichert, W.S., and Parrish, C.R. 2002. The VP1 N-terminal sequence of canine parvovirus affects nuclear transport of capsids and efficient cell infection. J Virol 76(4): 1884-1891.

Wan, P.T., Garnett, M.J., Roe, S.M., Lee, S., Niculescu-Duvaz, D., Good, V.M., Jones, C.M., Marshall, C.J., Springer, C.J., Barford, D., and Marais, R. 2004. Mechanism of activation of the RAF-ERK signaling pathway by oncogenic mutations of B-RAF. Cell 116(6): 855-867.

Wellbrock, C., Karasarides, M., and Marais, R. 2004. The RAF proteins take centre stage. Nat Rev Mol Cell Biol 5(11): 875-885.

Wen, P.Y. and Kesari, S. 2008. Malignant gliomas in adults. N Engl J Med 359(5): 492-507.

Wollmann, G., Tattersall, P., and van den Pol, A.N. 2005. Targeting human glioblastoma cells: comparison of nine viruses with oncolytic potential. J Virol 79(10): 6005-6022.

Yoon, C.H., Lee, E.S., Lim, D.S., and Bae, Y.S. 2009. PKR, a p53 target gene, plays a crucial role in the tumor-suppressor function of p53. Proc Natl Acad Sci U S A 106(19): 7852-7857.

Yuan, W. and Parrish, C.R. 2001. Canine parvovirus capsid assembly and differences in mammalian and insect cells. Virology 279(2): 546-557.

9

The Potential and Challenges of siRNA-Based Targeted Therapy for Treatment of Patients with Glioblastoma

M. Verreault[1,3,*], S. Yip[3,4], B. Toyota[5] and M.B. Bally[1,2,3]
[1]*Experimental Therapeutics, British Columbia Cancer Agency, Vancouver, BC*
[2]*Faculty of Pharmaceutical Sciences, University of British Columbia, Vancouver,*
[3]*Department of Pathology and Laboratory Medicine,*
University of British Columbia, Vancouver,
[4]*Department of Pathology and Laboratory Medicine,*
British Columbia Cancer Agency, Vancouver,
[5]*Division of Neurosurgery, British Columbia Cancer Agency, Vancouver, BC*
Canada

1. Introduction

Brain tumor is the second leading cause of cancer-related death in children under age of 20. An estimated total of 62,930 new cases of primary brain tumors in United States (CBTRUS, 2010) and 2,600 in Canada (CCS, 2010) were expected to be diagnosed in 2010 in adults and children. This includes both malignant (23,720 in US) and non-malignant (39,210 in US) brain tumors (CBTRUS, 2010). The most common (80%) form of malignant primary brain tumor originates from the neuroglial cells and is referred to as glioma (CBTRUS, 2010). Tumors originating from the astrocytes constitute 76% of cases of gliomas, and glioblastoma (GBM) is the most common malignant form of glioma (53.8%) (CBTRUS, 2010). Despite aggressive therapeutic interventions, 90% of patients are expected to succumb to the disease within five years after diagnosis (Stupp et al., 2005). Research is desperately needed to improve our understanding of the disease and to define strategies that will increase the efficacy of our treatment options.

2. Clinical and molecular features of GBM

GBM is a highly malignant type of primary brain cancer which mainly affects patients in their fifties and older. It is classified as a grade IV tumor using the World Health Organization (WHO) grading system and is associated with a median survival of approximately 12-15 months compared to 48 months for diffuse astrocytoma (WHO grade II), its lower grade counterpart (Louis et al., 2007). Secondary GBMs progress after a period of growth from low-grade gliomas (LGGs), while *de novo* GBMs arise rapidly into the most

* Corresponding Author

malignant form without the typical period of indolent growth associated with secondary GBMs. The latter preferentially affects older patients and is frequently associated with amplification of the epidermal growth factor receptor (*EGFR)* locus and inactivation of the phosphatase and tensin homolog *(PTEN)* tumor suppressor gene. Recent discovery of the recurrent R132H mutation in the isocitrate dehydrogenase 1 (*IDH1*) gene in a vast majority of secondary GBMs and a large percentage of LGGs further contributed to differentiate histologically similar GBM at the molecular level (Ichimura et al., 2009; Yan et al., 2009). In addition, the R132H *IDH1* genotype and the mutation of *TP53* are found to be frequently associated in secondary GBMs. Due to the aggressive biological phenotype of GBM, most patients present with acute headache, vomiting, occasional transient or partial blindness due to raised intracranial pressure, and local or general brain dysfunction, possibly leading to altered behavior or seizures (Brada et al., 2001; Chandana et al., 2008).

Current diagnosis and grading of gliomas are dependent on the histological analysis of biopsied or resected tumor tissue, together with immunohistochemistry and molecular testing on selected markers (Louis et al., 2007). Morphologic criteria are often arbitrary and based on the histological profile of tumor cells including 1) a high density of small and pleomorphic tumor cells that are characterized by large and elongated nuclei (Figure 1a), 2) the frequency of mitotic figures, 3) the presence of tumor necrosis that can be surrounded by dense accumulations of tumor cells (pseudopalisading necrosis, Figure 1b) and 4) the presence of microvascular proliferation (Figure 1c) (Gray, 2005; Prados M., 2002; Scherer, 1940). The presence of all these histological entities indicates an astrocytoma of WHO grade IV. Anaplastic astrocytoma, a WHO grade III tumor, does not have tumor necrosis or foci of microvascular proliferation. A feature that is common to all gliomas, regardless of grade and cell type, is the extent of local invasion and distant infiltration of the normal neuropil by the neoplastic cells. Histological correlations of this phenomenon were described by Scherer in 1940 (Scherer, 1940). Scherer described the aggregation and migration of glioma cells along normal blood vessels (perivascular satellitosis), neurons (perineuronal satellitosis), below the pial surface (subpial spread), and finally along large white matter tracts (intrafascicular growth). These "Scherer's secondary structures" are easily identified and constitute microscopic landmarks of glioma malignancy (Holland, 2000). However, accurate pathological classification of a tumor is often confounded by an undersampling bias, especially in cases of needle biopsies of large lesions. In addition, there is significant heterogeneity among gliomas at the genetic, epigenetic, and histological level (Walker C. et al., 2003).

There is little doubt that molecular heterogeneity contributes to the clonal evolution (Gerlinger & Swanton, 2010) within a tumor, which directly impacts clinical behavior such as treatment failure and disease recurrence (Yip et al., 2009). The example of the selection of GBM tumor cells carrying inactivating mutations in the mismatch repair gene mutS homolog 6 (*MSH6*) during treatment illustrates well this phenomenon and will be discussed further in section 5. Moreover, one microscopic field of GBM sample taken from the same patient can appear vastly different from another area. In addition, low and high-grade gliomas from different patients, with similar morphological appearance and of the same histological grade, can behave quite differently (Frazier et al., 2009; Krex et al., 2007; Yamanaka et al., 2006). Therefore, traditional histopathology alone is not sufficient to provide information with respect to prognostic and predictive substratification. Fortunately, molecular biomarkers are making inroads into the clinic diagnostic workup of brain tumors (Jansen et al., 2010; Yip et al., 2008).

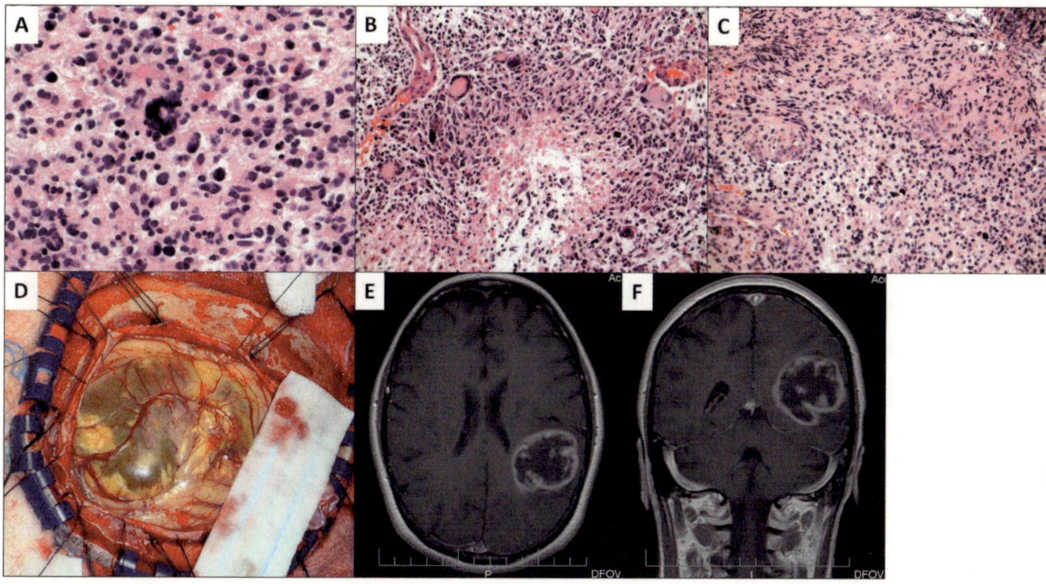

Fig. 1. Micro- and macroscopic view of a GBM tumor. a) Astrocytomas, both low and high grade, consist of neoplastic cells with elongated nuclei in association with variable amount of eosinophilic cytoplasm often extended into coarse processes. GBM often display an exaggerated degree of morphologic heterogeneity as seen in this figure, with tumor cells with bizarre and giant nuclei. b) Pseudopalisading necrosis is a cardinal feature of GBM and is characterized by an area of tissue necrosis surrounded immediately by a rim of viable tumor cells. The microenvironment in this region is often characterized by low oxygen tension (hence the necrosis) and activation of various hypoxia-mediated molecular pathways such as HIF-1α in the tumor cells (Kaur et al., 2005; Rong et al., 2006). c) Low magnification survey of a GBM showing multiple foci of microvascular proliferation (MVP) characterized by abnormal proliferation and hypertrophy of endothelial cells as a result of an overly pro-angiogenic environment. The presence of MVP automatically "upgrades" diagnosis from an astrocytoma to a WHO grade IV GBM. Foci of MVP are often found in areas with other malignant histological features including florid mitotic activity and tumor necrosis. d) Intraoperative picture of a GBM showing significant distortion of the gross morphology of the cerebral cortex resulting in expansion and discoloration of the gyri. e) and f) Magnetic resonance imaging (MRI) of a GBM using T1 sequence in conjunction with intravenous administration of gadolinium (GAD) dye. The tumor is represented in the axial (e) and coronal (f) planes, which is essential for localization of the lesion and surgical planning. The surfeit of tumor-associated and abnormally developed blood vessels (i.e. the MVP) with a defective blood-brain barrier (BBB) allows for penetration of GAD into the tissue, and accentuates areas of BBB breakdown. This so-called "contrast- enhancing" appearance is typical of high grade gliomas.

In addition to changes in nucleotide sequences within the genetic makeup of a cancer cell, the epigenome, defined by the profile of selective methylation of CpG-islands and complex covalent modifications of histone proteins, is equally important in defining malignant behavior (Ting et al., 2006). Epigenetic modifications result in transcriptional silencing or activation of affected gene or genes, and can have widespread consequences in the expression of genes important in survival, development, and growth regulation. Aberrant epigenetic changes in brain tumors are well documented (Fouse & Costello, 2009; Kim et al., 2006; Wu et al., 2010) and recently, The Cancer Genome Atlas (TCGA) consortium undertook a systematic large scale profiling of the GBM epigenomes (CGARN, 2008). The best-known brain tumor epigenetic biomarker is the hypermethylation of the O-6-methylguanine methyltransferase (*MGMT)* promoter. *MGMT* promoter hypermethylation correlates with an enhanced response to combined temozolomide (TMZ; Temodar®, Merck) chemotherapy and radiotherapy in patients with GBMs (Hegi et al., 2005), and predicts a better prognosis in elderly GBM patients (Gerstner et al., 2009). The discovery of the glioma-CpG Island Methylator Phenotype from epigenome-wide analysis of TCGA glioblastoma has also highlighted the potentials of the epigenome-wide approach (Noushmehr et al., 2010). The information obtained from genetic and epigenetic analyses of a tumor sample can be used to guide the decision of the treatment to offer the patient.

3. Standard of care and other therapeutic options

The current standard of care for GBM patients starts with maximal safe surgical resection. Patients might undergo repeated surgical resections to treat recurrent tumor growth (Wen & Kesari, 2008). As mentioned in the previous section, neoplastic cells from both low and high-grade glioma do share some common characteristics including the innate ability to infiltrate and invade surrounding normal brain tissue, which results in the distal spread of tumor cells at an early stage of the disease and the difficulty in clearly delineating the tumor margin. Surgical resection is followed by radiation therapy and concurrent TMZ, followed by adjuvant TMZ therapy (Clarke et al., 2010). TMZ is an alkylating agent, triggering cell death by the addition of DNA damaging alkyl groups on guanine bases (Newlands et al., 1997). The inclusion of TMZ in GBM standard of care improved the 2-year survival times from 10.4% to 26.5% (Stupp et al., 2005). However, the 5-year survival of GBM patients still remains less than 10% (CBTRUS, 2010; Stupp et al., 2009). As mentioned earlier, an important predictive factor in response to TMZ is the level of methylation of the *MGMT* promoter region found in the tumor. Promoter methylation of the *MGMT* gene prevents the expression of the MGMT enzyme capable of removing alkyl groups (Jacinto & Esteller, 2007). GBM tumors carrying a non-methylated promoter (40-55% of cases (Hegi et al., 2005; Sadones et al., 2009)) respond poorly to TMZ and there is currently no alternative treatment for these patients. At present, all patients with GBM are treated with TMZ with concurrent radiation therapy. Recurrent GBM tumors are often chemoresistant and exhibit accelerated growth rate (Cahill et al., 2007; Yip et al., 2009). Interestingly, a subset of patients with GBM who recurred after the initial treatment (surgery, radiation, TMZ) does respond to metronomic doses of TMZ. This treatment option consists of a dose-intensive daily intake of the drugs to maintain tumor suppression (Perry et al., 2010).

Before the introduction of TMZ as the standard of care for GBM patients, nitrosoureas were the foundation of GBM treatment for more than 30 years (Stupp et al., 2006). Among them, the alkylating agent carmustine (BiCNU®, Bristol-Myers Squibb) was used in conjunction with radiotherapy (Brandes et al., 2004a; Walker M. D. et al., 1978; Walker M. D. et al., 1980).

Severe pulmonary toxicity and limited efficacy of the drug due to insufficient drug delivery motivated the development of carmustine wafers (Gliadel®, Guilford Pharmaceuticals; Figure 2). Administration of carmustine using biodegradable polymer wafers provides a controlled release of the drug in the brain micro-environment while minimizing systemic toxicity (Lin & Kleinberg, 2008). However, recent trials showed that the system provides no additional benefit compared to TMZ (Adamson et al., 2009). A combination regimen consisting of the alkylating agents lomustine and procarbazine, and the microtubules destabilizer vincristine (PCV), has also been used extensively for the treatment of GBM (Kappelle et al., 2001). Yet, high incidence of hematological toxicities and inferior response rates in comparison to TMZ (Kappelle et al., 2001; Stupp et al., 2006) favored the establishment of TMZ as the current standard of care. The topoisomerase I inhibitor irinotecan (CPT-11; Camptosar®, Pharmacia & Upjohn) is a FDA-approved drug for colorectal cancer. Promising results for GBM patients in phase II trials were demonstrated with this compound, especially when used in combination with other agents such as TMZ or carmustine (Brandes et al., 2004b; Friedman et al., 2009; Turner et al., 2002; Vredenburgh et al., 2009), and it may soon be integrated among the Food and Drug Administration (FDA)-approved options for GBM patients. This compound is now recommended by the National Comprehensive Cancer Network for use in combination with bevacizumab (Avastin, Genentech/Roche) for GBM treatment (NCCN, 2011).

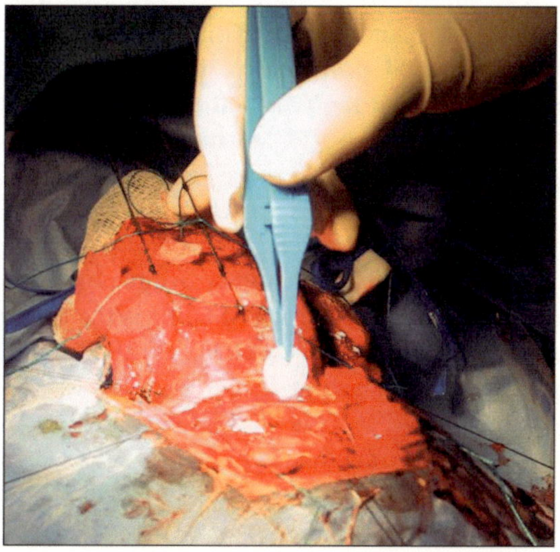

Fig. 2. Intraoperative picture of the placement of Gliadel® wafers into the resection cavity of a recurrent anaplastic oligoastrocytoma. The wafers, impregnated with the alkylating agent carmustine, deliver a locally concentrated dose of chemotherapeutic agent, reducing systemic toxicity.

More recently, targeted agents have been developed and showed some activity in GBM patients. Among them, a monoclonal antibody raised against the vascular endothelial growth factor (VEGF), bevacizumab, was recently approved by the FDA for the treatment of recurrent GBM, as several clinical trials demonstrated its efficacy as a single agent to prolong the progression-free survival of patients (Friedman et al., 2009; Kreisl et al., 2009).

However, results have been disappointing in terms of improvements in median survival, and a clinical trial is currently ongoing and was designed to investigate the value of combining bevacizumab with TMZ (Chinot et al., 2011). It is hoped that bevacizumab therapy can induce a normalization of the tumor vasculature (see section 10) and thus improve the homogenous delivery of the cytotoxic agent TMZ. The EGFR inhibitors gefitinib (Iressa®, AstraZeneca Canada Inc.) and erlotinib (Tarceva®, Roche) have also shown some efficacy in the treatment of malignant glioma (Raizer et al., 2010; Rich et al., 2004), but response rates have been variable and unpredictable (Stupp et al., 2006). Imatinib mesylate (Gleevec®, Novartis) was developed to specifically inhibit Bcr-Abl signal transduction in chronic myeloid leukemia, and was later shown to also inhibit c-Kit and platelet-derived growth factor receptor (PDGFR) activity. The latter finding supported clinical testing of imatinib for GBM treatment, and similarly to the EGFR inhibitors, response rates were variable but promising (Razis et al., 2009; Wen et al., 2006). Other targeted therapy compounds currently evaluated for use in GBM treatment are described in section 5.

4. Challenges

One of the major challenges of GBM chemotherapy is the achievement of adequate drug concentration within the tumor itself, and this obstacle can largely be attributed to the presence of the BBB (Clarke et al., 2010). Unlike capillaries elsewhere in the body, endothelial cells of brain capillaries have tight junctions that are highly resistant to the passage of ions or small molecules and do not exhibit trans-endothelial transport (Fawcett, 1994). Moreover, the astrocytes and pericytes play an important role in regulating this barrier through molecular cross-talk involving adhesion and tight-junction molecules, the integrins and other extra-cellular matrix (ECM) molecules (reviewed in (Wolburg et al., 2009)). The BBB in GBM tumors exhibits more frequent fenestrations, a loss of tight intercellular junctions and less developed astrocytic pericapillary sheath, all factors contributing to increasing its permeability (Engerhard et al., 1999) (Figure 3). However, this compromised BBB still acts as an obstacle for many drugs (Pardridge, 2007). Therefore, the main limitation for drug choice in the treatment of GBM is the capacity of the compound to penetrate the BBB. Two main mechanisms by which a synthetic drug molecule can cross the BBB are: 1) by transmembrane diffusion or 2) through transporters (Banks, 2009). Most drugs used for management of GBM (e.g. TMZ, carmustine) are small and lipophilic molecules that cross the BBB by transmembrane diffusion. This mechanism is a non-saturable process that depends on molecular diffusion through cell membranes. Factors influencing this process include a good balance between liposolubility (penetration through cell membrane) and hydrosolubility (to improve drug circulation and presentation to the BBB) which are influenced by chemical structure, size and charge (Banks, 2009). The capacity to escape the ATP-Binding Cassette (ABC) transporters, such as the P-glycoprotein (Begley, 2004a) responsible for brain-to-blood efflux, is also important. Saturable transport systems (i.e. ligand transporters) can be used to improve the pharmacokinetic profile of a substance and to target uptake into specific regions of the central nervous system (CNS) (Banks, 2009). Analogs of transporter ligands have been developed for various CNS pathologies (Begley, 2004b). Alternatively, influx transporters can be targeted in a "Trojan-horse" like strategy (i.e. molecules that do not cross the BBB are coupled to ligand molecules that do) but unfortunately, these chemical modifications often result in a decrease in ligand uptake or routing of the hybrid compound to lysosome compartments for degradation (Banks, 2009).

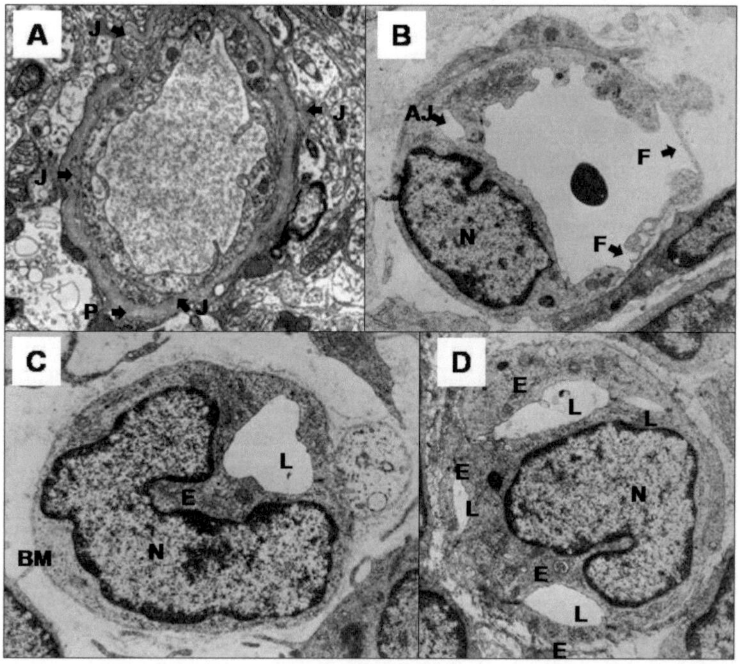

Fig. 3. Electron micrograph showing the structure of brain capillaries from normal and tumor tissue. a) This normal brain capillary is made of two endothelial cells bound together with tight junctions (J) and forming a thin and regular layer around the lumen. Processes of pericytes (P) can be seen embedded in the basement membrane. b, c, d) Capillaries from astrocytoma tumors are lined by immature endothelial cells (E) of irregular thickness and with hyperplastic nuclei (N), discontinuous basement membrane (BM) and a decreased presence of pericytes or astrocytic processes. Abnormal intercellular junctions (AJ), fenestrations (F) and irregular slit-like lumen (L) can be seen in these micrographs. Adapted from (Deane & Lantos, 1981; Rojiani & Dorovini-Zis, 1996).

5. The targets and therapeutic effects

In the case where therapeutic agents capable of crossing the BBB, such as TMZ or irinotecan, are available and do exhibit considerable anticancer activity, the most significant problem for GBM cancer patients is repopulation of malignant cells following treatment, causing inevitable relapse (CBTRUS, 2010; Stupp et al., 2005). For example, recent identification of the somatic inactivation of the mismatch repair gene *MSH6* in a subgroup of recurrent GBM has highlighted the constant evolution of malignant glioma cells in the presence of selective pressure, in this case alkylator chemotherapy and concurrent radiotherapy. This initial discovery, achieved through whole kinome sequencing of two recurrent GBM, was bolstered by corroborative findings from the TCGA project studying a much larger number of GBM samples (CGARN, 2008; Hunter et al., 2006). Subsequent studies have also highlighted the importance of somatic *MSH6* integrity on the *in vivo* and *in vitro* growth of

GBM with direct impact on patient survival (Cahill et al., 2007; Yip et al., 2009). In fact, a careful evaluation of the TCGA data of the recurrent GBM cohort shows that a majority of the recurrent tumors with the *MSH6* hypermutation phenotype, a genetic signature of defects in the cellular mismatch repair (MMR) system, also have somatic mutations and epigenetic silencing affecting other members of the MMR family. This highlights a novel mechanism of tumor survival during alkylator therapy and is especially relevant in a cancer for which alkylators, such as TMZ, are used as the therapeutic mainstay. One possible explanation for this phenomenon is that a small number of GBM cells, prior to therapy, harbor mutations in the MMR genes and these cells are positively selected during therapy, leading to clonal expansion. Alternatively, and equally plausible, random mutations inactivating MMR genes during therapy could lead to outgrowth of a resistant clone of tumor cells which exhibits therapeutic resistance.

Although it is acknowledged that advances in GBM treatment will continue to rely on conventional treatment approaches (surgery, radiation and/or chemotherapy), the value of combining standard chemotherapy with targeted agents that increase tumor drug sensitivity is now being recognized (Krakstad & Chekenya, 2010). The goal of this effort is to target survival and/or proliferation-promoting proteins which are overexpressed, or have upregulated activity, in cancer cells. This approach has the additional benefit of overcoming resistance mechanisms due to the activation of single pathways (e.g. *MGMT*). Moreover, many trials have indicated that groups of cancer patients treated similarly on the basis of a histopathology classification (e.g. WHO II astrocytoma, WHO III anaplastic astrocytoma, and WHO IV glioblastoma) exhibit very different responses to the same treatment (Stupp et al., 2006), implying that various gene expression patterns underlying the disease phenotype may play a more important role in treatment outcomes. This observation highlights the necessity of developing tumor-targeted gene therapy treatments that would be personalized for the specific molecular lesions present in a patient's tumor.

Cancer is believed to be a genetic disease, arising as a result of genetic mutations that endow the cell with many specific functional capabilities (Vogelstein & Kinzler, 1993) such as cell proliferation, survival, invasion and metastasis (Hanahan & Weinberg, 2000). Recent advances in molecular genetics have enabled the development of methods to specifically target gene expression (small interfering RNA; siRNA or antisense oligonucleotides; ASO) or the activity of proteins (small molecule inhibitors; SMI). Our current understanding of cancer biology has made it clear that gene targeting therapies will provide an effective strategy to treat cancer. The next paragraphs will present an overview of the approaches used in targeted therapy for the treatment of malignant glioma. The targets and potential therapeutic effects will be discussed based on the six essential alterations in cell physiology that dictate malignant growth as described elsewhere (Hanahan & Weinberg, 2000,2011) and consist of the capacity for (I) sustaining proliferative signals and II) evading growth suppressors; (III) resisting cell death; (IV) inducing angiogenesis; (V) activating invasion and metastasis and (VI) enabling replicative immortality. Table 1 and 2 present a list of genes or associated protein targets that have been inhibited by means of non-viral gene silencing agents in orthotopic GBM pre-clinical or clinical studies (Table 1), or by SMI in GBM clinical trials phase II/III (Table 2). It is interesting to note that very few of these studies have assessed the efficacy of the targeted therapy agent in combination with standard chemotherapy or radiation.

Target	Experimental design	Agent	Benefit	Ref
Self-sufficiency in growth signals and insensitivity to growth suppressors				
EGFR	I.cr. U87 line in mice	shRNA in PEGylated immunolip. (h-Insuline R and m-Transferrin R) i.v.	Tumor growth inhibition and increased survival	(Zhang et al., 2004)
	I.cr U87 line in mice	ASO plasmid in PEGylated immunolip. (h-Insuline R and m-Transferrin R) i.v.	Tumor growth inhibition and increased survival	(Zhang et al., 2002)
PKC family	Phase II CTr	ASO i.v. (Aprinocarsen)	Minimal benefit	(Grossman et al., 2005)
UPA/UPAR	4910 line i.cr. in mice	shRNA i.p.	Tumor growth inhibition and increased survival	(Gondi et al., 2007)
Evasion of cell death				
Bcl-2	U251 line i.cr. in mice	siRNA cDNA i.p.	Enhanced efficacy of taxol on tumor growth inhibition	(George et al., 2008)
Survivin	U87 line i.cr. in mice	PEI-complexed siRNA i.t.	Increased survival	(Hendruschk et al., 2011)
Induction of angiogenesis				
Pleitrophin	U87 line i.cr. in mice	PEI-siRNA i.t.	Tumor growth inhibition	(Grzelinski et al., 2006)
Invasion and metastasis				
Cathepsin B	SNB19 line i.cr. in mice	shRNA i.t.	Tumor growth inhibition	(Gondi et al., 2004)
MMPs	SNB19 or U251 line i.cr. in mice	shRNA i.t.	Tumor growth inhibition and enhanced sensitivity to radiation	(Badiga et al., 2011; Lakka et al., 2005)
Tenascin-C	Phase I CTr	Long RNA molecule i.t.	Increased survival	(Wyszko et al., 2008; Zukiel et al., 2006)
Replicative immortality				
hTERT	SNB-19 and LN-18 lines i.cr. in mice	ASO in cat. lip.	Tumor growth inhibition. More active when combined with IFN-γ injections	(George et al., 2009)
	U373 line i.cr. in mice	ASO i.t.	Increased survival	(Mukai et al., 2000)
	U251MG i.cr. in rats	GRN183 ASO i.n.	Tumor growth inhibition and increased survival	(Hashizume et al., 2008)
Other function				
TGF-β	F98 line i.cr. in rats	Nanoparticle-complexed ASO i.p.	Increased survival when given with immunization	(Schneider et al., 2008)

Table 1. Protein targets that have been inhibited by means of non-viral gene silencing agents in orthotopic GBM pre-clinical studies or clinical trials (CTr) (definition of abbreviations is given at the beginning of this chapter)

Target	Experimental design	Agent	Benefit	Ref
Self-sufficiency in growth signals and insensitivity to growth suppressors				
EGFR	Phase II CTr	SMI Erlotinib (Tarceva®), Gefitinib (Iressa®) i.v.	Minimal as single-agent. Some efficacy with TMZ	(Franceschi et al., 2007; Prados M. D. et al., 2009; Raizer et al., 2010)
PKC family	Phase II/III CTr	SMI Enzastaurin	Minimal benefit	(Kreisl et al., 2010; Wick et al., 2010)
mTOR	Phase II CTr	SMI Temsirolimus i.v	Disease stabilization and increased survival	(Chang et al., 2005; Galanis et al., 2005)
Growth factors	Phase II CTr	SMI Suramin i.v	No benefit with radiotherapy	(Laterra et al., 2004)
Farnesyl-transferase	Phase II CTr	SMI Tipifarnib i.v	No benefit	(Cloughesy et al., 2006; Lustig et al., 2008)
HDAC	Phase II CTr	SMI Vorinostat i.v	Modest activity	(Galanis et al., 2009)
PDGF R	Phase II CTr	SMI Imatinib (Gleevec®) i.v	Variable response	(Razis et al., 2009; Wen et al., 2006)
Induction of angiogenesis				
VEGF	Phase II/III CTr	mAb Bevacizumab (Avastin) i.v.	Active, with and w/o irinotecan or TMZ and FDA-approved for recurrent disease	(Friedman et al., 2009; Kreisl et al., 2009; Lai et al., 2011)
Fibroblast growth factors	Phase II CTr	Thalidomide i.v.	Minimal benefit as a single agent, some benefit with carmustine or irinotecan	(Fadul et al., 2008; Fine et al., 2003; Marx et al., 2001)
Invasion and metastasis				
Integrins	Phase I/II CTr	SMI Cilengitide i.v.	Some activity with TMZ	(Stupp et al., 2010)

Table 2. Protein targets that have been inhibited by means of SMI or mAb in GBM clinical trials phase II/III (definition of abbreviations is given at the beginning of this chapter)

5.1 Self-sufficiency in growth signals and insensitivity to growth suppressors

Tumor cells generate many of their own growth signals, thereby reducing their dependence on stimulation from the normal tissue microenvironment (Hanahan & Weinberg, 2000,2011). Molecular strategies for achieving autonomy involve: I) alterations in extracellular growth signals, II) alterations in transducers of those signals, III) alterations in components enabling or preventing the cell to enter cell cycle (Hanahan & Weinberg, 2000). For example, protein overexpression of EGFR, involved in growth signal transduction, was reported in 60% of

GBM cases; EGFR gene amplification was reported in 40% of cases; EGFR truncated transcript encoding for a constitutive activity of the receptor was reported in 20% of cases and mutations of EGFR extracellular domain was reported in 15% of cases (Nicholas et al., 2006; Ohgaki et al., 2004). These mutations are quite often combined in the same tumor cell, leading to overactivation of EGFR pathways (Ekstrand et al., 1991; Idbaih et al., 2008). ASO- (Zhang et al., 2002) and RNA interference- (Zhang et al., 2004) mediated inhibition of EGFR has been shown to induce a strong reduction in tumor growth and increased the survival of orthotopic GBM tumor bearing mice. However, the inhibition of EGFR using SMI in clinical phase II trials was not representative of this success. As discussed earlier, erlotinib (Prados M. D. et al., 2009; Raizer et al., 2010) or gefitinib (Franceschi et al., 2007; Rich et al., 2004) SMI showed variable activity in GBM patients although better efficacy was seen when used in combination with TMZ. The constitutive activation of the PI3K/AKT pathway associated with the mutation of PTEN (60% of GBM cases) (Haas-Kogan et al., 1998; Knobbe et al., 2002) has also received considerable attention as it is generally associated with aggressive disease and poor prognosis (Ermoian et al., 2002; Rasheed et al., 1997; Schmidt et al., 1999). The mammalian target of rapamycin (mTOR) was identified as a major downstream effector in this pathway (Manning & Cantley, 2003). Phase II clinical trials using the mTOR SMI Temsirolimus (CCI-779) induced disease stabilization and an increase in survival in some GBM patients of phase II clinical trials (Chang et al., 2005; Galanis et al., 2005).

5.2 Evasion of cell death

The ability of tumor cell populations to expand in number is determined not only by the rate of cell proliferation but also by the rate of cell death. Acquired resistance toward programmed cell death, apoptosis, is a hallmark of most and perhaps all types of cancer (Hanahan & Weinberg, 2000,2011), causing the tumor to resist conditions that would normally kill cells. In this context, Bcl-2 targeted therapy has attracted the most attention with studies both in pre-clinical cancer models and patients (ASO Oblimersen, SMI AT-101). Although the potential of Bcl-2 targeting has not yet been demonstrated in GBM patients, one report showed that siRNA-mediated inhibition of Bcl-2 can increase the efficacy of taxol in a pre-clinical orthotopic model of GBM (George et al., 2008).

5.3 Induction of angiogenesis

Strong evidence indicates that the growth of GBM depends on angiogenesis (Jain et al., 2007; Norden et al., 2009). However, experimental models of GBM have shown that the resulting vessels are poorly organized and poorly functional, and it is believed that high levels of angiogenesis in GBM are associated with increased hypoxia and interstitial fluid pressure, which contribute to the disease malignancy and resistance to treatments (Blasberg et al., 1983; Groothuis et al., 1983). This aspect of GBM vasculature will be discussed further in section 10. Members of the VEGF family have emerged as prime mediators of angiogenesis in GBM (Jain et al., 2007). As already noted, several clinical trials have demonstrated the efficacy of bevacizumab, a monoclonal antibody (mAb) against VEGF as a single agent and in combination with TMZ or irinotecan to prolong the survival of patients (Friedman et al., 2009; Kreisl et al., 2009; Lai et al., 2011). Bevacizumab was recently approved by the FDA for the treatment of recurrent GBM and is showing promising efficacy in clinical trials for newly diagnosed GBM patients (Lai et al., 2008). Many other VEGF or VEGFR inhibitors are currently being tested in the clinic (Norden et al., 2009).

5.4 Invasion and metastasis

Proteins responsible for tissue invasion and metastatic behavior are often effectors allowing the cell to grow in the absence of ECM adhesion signals. The most obvious example is the integrins family, which is involved in ECM anchorage-independent growth of tumor cells, and provides the traction necessary for cell motility and invasion (reviewed in (Desgrosellier & Cheresh, 2010)). An integrin SMI, cilengitide, has shown some promising activity in GBM clinical trial phase I/II in combination with TMZ (Stupp et al., 2010), and is now moving to phase III (Carter, 2010). In addition, enzymes that are involved in the degradation of the ECM will allow cancer cells to invade surrounding brain tissue. Matrix-metalloproteinases (MMPs) were shown to play a central role in the proteolysis necessary for this process (Nakada et al., 2003). Intratumoral administration of a shRNA against MMP-9 inhibited tumor growth in an orthotopic GBM mouse model (Lakka et al., 2005). To date, no MMP inhibitors have made their way to a phase II clinical trial for GBM treatment. Moreover, the clinical evaluation of MMP inhibitors as single agents in cancers other than GBM has not been associated with significant anti-tumor responses (Brinker et al., 2008; Chu et al., 2007) and they will most likely show better efficacy in a combination setting.

5.5 Replicative immortality

Some studies suggest that at a given point during the course of tumor progression, evolving premalignant cell populations acquire the capacity to breach the mortality barrier (Hanahan & Weinberg, 2000); they become capable of unlimited replicative cycles. Overexpression of telomerase reverse transcriptase (hTERT), a unique ribonucleoprotein enzyme responsible for adding telomeric repeats onto 3' ends of chromosomes (Holt & Shay, 1999), could play an important role in the development of cellular immortality and oncogenesis. Telomerase activity has been detected in 89% of GBM cases and correlates with tumor grade (Le et al., 1998), whereas low expression of hTERT was shown to be associated with a better prognosis (Wager et al., 2008). Pre-clinical investigation of hTERT targeted therapy illustrates that downregulation of this gene results in tumor regression and increased survival in orthotopic GBM murine models (George et al., 2009; Mukai et al., 2000).

6. The potential of targeting multiple pathways

Hallmarks of cancer cell malignancy include upregulation or dysregulation of multiple pathways, with deregulations increasing in number as the cancer progresses. In contrast to this observation, the vast majority of clinical trials to date have focused on a single agent that targets a single molecular aberration. It is expected that a therapeutic modality targeting one of these dysregulated pathways will only result in modest benefits to patients in terms of disease-free survival time. Cellular proliferation, growth and death are regulated by an intricate network of cellular functions, and it is very likely that disturbances in the balance between these pathways will lead to the activation of compensating mechanisms in normal cells as well as cancer cells. While it is well understood that a combination of chemotherapeutic agents inclusive of drugs with differing mechanisms of action is generally more efficacious than single agent chemotherapy in the treatment of aggressive cancers, clinicians and scientists are now beginning to realize the benefits of combining agents targeting different biological pathways in order to effectively silence as many cancer phenotypes as possible.

The therapeutic value of targeting two different pathways is exemplified by some research data obtained by our laboratory (Verreault et al., 2011a). One of the most commonly reported molecular defects in GBM is the aberrant activation of the PI3K/AKT pathway, which is associated with increased proliferation rate, invasion, metastasis and poor prognosis (Ermoian et al., 2002; Haas-Kogan et al., 1998; Li X. Y. et al., 2010). Rictor, the rapamycin-insensitive companion of mTOR, is a protein member of the mTOR Complex 2 (mTORC2), and can activate AKT through direct phosphorylation at its serine 473 site (Sarbassov et al., 2004; Sarbassov et al., 2005; Sparks & Guertin, 2010). Elevated levels of Rictor were found in human GBM tumor tissue samples and cell lines when compared to normal brain tissue (Masri et al., 2007). Rictor and EGFR proteins were silenced alone and in combination by siRNA *in vitro* transfection in a panel of three human GBM lines (U251MG, U118MG and LN229). It was found that the co-silencing of Rictor and EGFR exerted effects on cell migration and sensitivity to chemotherapeutic drugs that were not observed by the single silencing of either target (Verreault et al., 2011a). The most striking evidence of the validity of this combined silencing came from the *in vivo* aspect of this study, which was done by intracranial inoculation in mice brains of U251MG cells expressing small hairpin RNA (shRNA) specific to each target. Silencing of EGFR or Rictor alone had no significant effect on tumor growth, but the dual silencing resulted in the eradication of the tumor (Verreault et al., 2011a). Also, tumor growth block in response to the combined suppression of EGFR and PI3K/AKT pathway was reported previously using the SMIs gefitinib and LY294002 in a GBM xenograft model (Fan et al., 2003), while monotherapy of each inhibitor had no impact on tumor burden. Taken together, these studies strongly support the value of inhibiting both EGFR and PI3K/mTORC2/Rictor/AKT pathways to achieve therapeutic effects that may not be observed by the single inhibition of either pathway, and provide compelling evidences of the potential of targeting multiple pro-oncogenic pathways in GBM.

7. Drug delivery to brain tumors

The idea of targeting gene expression at the level of transcription or translation has been mirrored by the emergence of gene therapy as a strategy to specifically silence the activity of any defective or overactive gene without the limiting step of SMI availability (Bumcrot et al., 2006). Since tumor cells have a different pattern of gene expression in comparison with normal cells, gene silencing can theoretically be used to specifically target tumor-associated genes or mutated genes without altering gene expression of normal cells (Helene, 1994). The most commonly used strategies employed to achieve gene silencing involve administration of ASOs or siRNAs that can inhibit the expression of specific proteins. However, the therapeutic value of this technology is proving difficult to establish, in part because of the lack of pharmaceutically viable products that can be administered orally, intravenously or intraperitoneally, and that can deliver the gene silencing agent to tumor cell populations in sufficient quantity to achieve target knockdown. Despite the fact that we are still learning to navigate the technology of RNAi in order to achieve optimal benefits with minimal side-effects, the high specificity and potency of siRNAs, together with the unlimited possibility of designs for siRNAs against any genes, make this technology an attractive option for targeted therapy. Once a viable option for safe and effective delivery to the tumor is defined, RNAi will be regarded as the most powerful tool for designing personalized treatment strategies. Some of the strategies that have been developed and explored pre-clinically for gene silencing agent delivery to brain tumors are discussed below, with references to successful achievements in the clinic for chemotherapeutic agent delivery.

7.1 Bypassing the blood-brain barrier

As discussed earlier, the BBB constitutes one of the main barriers to the development of new therapeutics for GBM treatment. Hence, a great deal of research has been focused on defining strategies aimed at bypassing the BBB and increasing delivery of therapeutics. One of these strategies consists of a direct intratumoral (i.t.) injection, and has been successfully used in pre-clinical brain tumor models for delivery of gene silencing agents (George et al., 2009; Gondi et al., 2004; Lakka et al., 2005; Thakker et al., 2005), and in the clinic for chemotherapeutic agents (Boiardi et al., 2005; Patchell et al., 2002). The only clinical trial testing the efficacy of RNAi in GBM was done by local delivery of a 146 nucleotides long RNA molecule (ATN-RNA) targeting Tenascin-C mRNA (Wyszko et al., 2008; Zukiel et al., 2006). Although its role in GBM pathology is still unclear, the expression of the ECM glycoprotein Tenascin-C was found to correlate with tumor grade (Pas et al., 2006). Treatment with ATN-RNA was associated with increased survival in GBM patients and these results constitute the first demonstration of a potential clinical application for RNAi in the treatment of GBM. Convention-enhanced delivery (CED) is another technique tested in the clinic for local delivery, and consists of placing catheters into the surgical cavity after the resection procedure and to deliver antineoplastic agents through the catheters using positive pressure (0.5 to 15.0μl/min). This technique was shown to increase the anti-tumor efficacy of paclitaxel (Lidar et al., 2004) and of the recombinant protein Cintredekin besudotox (Kunwar et al., 2007) in GBM patients. CED was also used to deliver siRNAs to the CNS of non-human primates, and resulted in a durable and specific silencing of the selected target (Querbes et al., 2009). Carmustine wafers (Gliadel) are currently used in the clinic and represent a good example of local delivery (Figure 2). In this system, carmustine is incorporated in a hydrophobic matrix made of a polyanhydride polymer that protects the agent from hydrolysis (Brem et al., 1994; Grossman et al., 1992). After tumor resection, the wafer discs are implanted at the surface of the resection cavity and the drug is slowly released for a period of three weeks (Brem et al., 1991). Although wafers have shown some promising efficacy when combined with TMZ (Gururangan et al., 2001), it is not indicated for patients with infiltrative or multifocal tumors. It is believed that local administration does not allow access to infiltrative cancer cells that are a predominant hallmark of GBM, and this is especially true for macro-molecules such as ASOs or siRNAs.

In order to overcome the limitations of direct i.t. administration of agents, other routes of administration have been explored, including systemic administration (intraperitoneal (i.p.) and intravenous (i.v.)), some of which integrating the use of delivery systems (Table 1). Challenges and opportunities for these strategies will be discussed in the following section. Interestingly, the intranasal (i.n.) route of delivery was recently shown to promote a rapid and efficient delivery of molecules that do not cross the BBB to the brain (Thorne et al.,

1995). The i.n. technique allows for a noninvasive bypass of the BBB via the nasal mucosa, through the olfactory and trigeminal nerves, directly to the brain and cerebrospinal fluid (Thorne et al., 2004). The ASO GRN163 specific to hTERT was successfully delivered to pre-clinical orthotopic tumors using this technique (Hashizume et al., 2008). The i.n. technique was also used in a phase I/II clinical trial to administer perillyl alcohol, a Ras inhibitor, and results suggested some antitumor activity without any toxicity in GBM patients (da Fonseca et al., 2008). These studies, together with other pre-clinical reports (Sakane et al., 1999; Thorne et al., 2004; Wang D. et al., 2006; Wang F. et al., 2003), suggest that the i.n. route of administration may be of great therapeutic value for treatment of brain tumors and could be part of the solution to the issue of polynucleotide therapeutics delivery. It should be noted, however, that material delivery in tissues other than the brain (liver, kidney, heart, muscles) was also detected following i.n. administration (Thorne et al., 2004), suggesting the need for combining this administration route with delivery systems that would improve specificity to the tumor. The currently accepted mechanisms of transport following intranasal administration are the intraneuronal transport following endocytosis or an extracellular diffusion along the nerves (Thorne et al., 1995). Thus it is clear that the size limitation imposed by these routes may restrict the possible delivery systems that could be used.

7.2 Limitation to systemic administration

Strategies used to administer agents through systemic administration include simple infusion as well as more sophisticated delivery systems designed to promote intracellular delivery. In this context, the success of gene silencing therapy for cancer depends in large part on stable and tumor-specific delivery, which can be achieved only if therapeutic molecules can survive as active agents as they cross various biological barriers. These barriers are i) degradation in the blood or uptake by the liver, ii) passage from the circulation across the BBB and into the extravascular space within the tumor, ii) passage into cytoplasm of target cells, iv) release from the carrier and/or the endosomes if associated with a carrier system or internalized via endocytosis, v) escape from nucleases in tumor cell's cytoplasm and vi) binding to target mRNA. As described earlier, the BBB consists of endothelial cells, pericytes, astrocytes endfeet and neuronal cells that are organized in such way to confer a unique selective permeability to the CNS vascular network (Rubin & Staddon, 1999), restricting the passive transport of most therapeutic molecules (Pardridge, 2007). Some success in delivering molecules across the BBB has been made with long circulating carrier systems (see section 8) that can take advantage of the fact that tumor-associated BBB consists of poorly formed vascular endothelium that is more permeable to circulating macromolecules than the normal BBB (Patel et al., 2009). Strategies to open the BBB have also been explored and include osmotic disruption (Bellavance et al., 2008), the use of vasomodulators to increase permeability (Ningaraj et al., 2003), or the use of potassium channel agonists to increase the formation of transport vesicles (Ningaraj, 2006).

Although it has been shown that siRNAs are more stable in cells than a single-stranded antisense molecule (Bertrand et al., 2002), naked RNA sequences injected *in vivo* are rapidly eliminated and have a short duration of effect (Khan et al., 2004). Pre-clinical studies suggest that this can be overcome by use of multiple i.v. or i.p. injections of naked siRNAs (Filleur et al., 2003), and can lead to successful downregulation of the target in intracranial tumor (George et al., 2008). However, other studies reported very little accumulation of siRNA in the brain following i.v. administration, and preferential accumulation was observed in the liver and the kidneys (Braasch et al., 2004; De Paula et al., 2007; Santel et al., 2006). Other reports show that a high-pressure delivery technique could increase delivery of siRNAs given i.v. (Lewis et al., 2002; McCaffrey et al., 2002; Song et al., 2003) or i.p (Heidel et al., 2004), but no evidence of delivery to the brain was shown (Lewis et al., 2002). Moreover, this technique is not relevant to human therapies as it involves high pressure and massive volume delivery schemes to generate transiently high local intravascular pressure (Lieberman et al., 2003; Shuey et al., 2002). It is now widely recognized that if siRNAs are to be used in the clinic for GBM patients, they will have to be formulated with a delivery system strategy in order to increase the agent's half-life and tumor specific delivery.

8. Lipid nanoparticle delivery systems

Studies over the last few decades have established that liposomal nanoparticle (LNP) formulations of selected antineoplastic agents can be more effective than a drug administered in its free form, due to their capacity to increase drug circulation time. Further, increased tumor delivery is observed due to the increased permeability of blood vessels in the tumor environment, a process referred to as the "enhanced permeability and retention effect" (EPR) (Maeda et al., 2009). Conventional LNPs, which consist of bilayer lipid vesicles, are prepared with phospholipids (e.g. phosphatidylcholine or phosphatidylglycerol) (Storm & Crommelin, 1998). The incorporation of cholesterol in these formulations influences the mechanical strength and permeability of LNP membranes (Ohvo-Rekila et al., 2002). Stealth LNP can also be made by coating the LNP surface with the hydrophilic polymer polyethylene glycol (PEG), which provides a barrier against interactions with molecular and cellular components in the plasma compartment (Storm & Crommelin, 1998) and can engender remarkable increases in plasma longevity of the carrier (Park et al., 2004). The FDA-approved and commercially available doxorubicin LNP formulation (Caelyx®, Schering-Plough or Doxil®, Centocor Ortho Biotech Inc) is an example of a PEG-coated formulation (Barenholz, 2007).

Liposomal formulations have shown some success in the delivery of drugs to brain tumors. Caelyx® was reported to be less toxic in the clinic than the unencapsulated form (Judson et al., 2001; O'Brien et al., 2004; Porter & Rifkin, 2007); when used to treat malignant glioma, stabilization of the disease (reduction of tumor volume of < 50% or a < 25% increase in tumor volume for more than 8 weeks) was observed (Fabel et al., 2001; Hau et al., 2004). An orthotopic GBM pre-clinical study showed anti-vascular activity of doxorubicin when encapsulated in LNPs, and these effects were not observed with the free form of the drug or in normal brain tissue (Zhou et al., 2002). Other pre-clinical studies showed that liposomal formulations of irinotecan are more efficacious than the unencapsulated form in brain tumors (Krauze et al., 2007; Noble et al., 2006; Verreault et al., 2011b) and in colorectal and adenocarcinoma tumors (Hattori et al., 2009; Messerer et al., 2004; Ramsay et al., 2008). More specifically, our laboratory has established that Irinophore C™ (IrC™), a LPN formulation of irinotecan, exhibits improved anti-cancer efficacy compared to the free drug in a GBM orthotopic model (Verreault et al., 2011b). We demonstrated that the presence in the brain of irinotecan and its active metabolite SN-38 is extended following administration of IrC™ compared to irinotecan. At equivalent doses (50 mg/kg), the average survival of GBM-tumor bearing animals was improved of 17% compared to the free drug-treated group (49.1% compared to untreated animals). Further, a repeated dose tolerability study showed that IrC™ is much better tolerated than the free drug. This increase in tolerability permitted the administration of 100mg/kg IrC™ doses, which provided an increase in average survival of 83% compared to the untreated group. These studies demonstrate the potential of LNP delivery systems to improve chemotherapeutic drug delivery to brain tumors and consequently, to increase drug therapeutic effects. Interestingly, very little effort has been made in the development of SMI that could be administered in LNPs. It appears that if the expertise and knowledge that was gained over the last decades in the field of lipid-based delivery systems was directed towards improving SMI delivery to brain tumors, potential therapeutic success could have already been achieved.

In developing lipid-based delivery systems for gene silencing agents, the goal is to design a system that simultaneously achieves high efficiency (defined by delivery and release of the agent to the disease site), prolonged effects and low toxicity (Lundstrom & Boulikas, 2003). Small cationic LNPs can interact with negatively charged DNA or RNA, leading to the formation of complexes with a prolonged half-life in the circulation (Cattel et al., 2004) and capable of promoting cellular internalization (Storm & Crommelin, 1998). A report showed that hTERT-targeted ASO delivery using cationic LNPs resulted in increased survival of intracranial tumor bearing mice (Mukai et al., 2000). Numerous other studies have been done using i.v. or i.p. injections of siRNAs (Aigner, 2008; Sioud & Sorensen, 2003; Sorensen D. R. et al., 2003) or ASOs (Shoji & Nakashima, 2004) complexed with cationic LNPs in cancer models other than brain tumor. These techniques led to good silencing efficiency with no significant signs of toxicity. It is important to mention that some studies have demonstrated immune system activation induced by common cationic lipids following systemic administration (Freimark et al., 1998; Li S. et al., 1999; Scheule et al., 1997). Furthermore, another limitation to the therapeutic use of positively charged complexes is that they are cleared rapidly following intravenous administration (Nishikawa et al., 1998) as they bind to proteins in the plasma and form aggregates which are eliminated by non-target cells (Ogris et al., 1999). Since neutralized complexes have proven to be less efficient, cationic complexes possessing hydrophilic steric barriers, achieved through the use of surface-grafted polymers like PEG, have been pursued to address the problem of plasma protein binding and rapid elimination (Allen et al., 2002). PEG-immunoliposomes (made by adding antibodies at the surface of LNPs, see section 9) are able to efficiently deliver ASO (Zhang et al., 2002) and siRNAs (Zhang et al., 2004) to orthotopic brain tumors following systemic administration. Stable nucleic-acid-lipid particles (SNALP) consist of lipid bilayer particles prepared with a mixture of cationic and fusogenic lipids, and have been shown to exhibit the stability, small size, low surface charge and low toxicity required for *in vivo* administration (Morrissey et al., 2005), and to promote efficient siRNA cellular uptake (Heyes et al., 2005). The lipid particles are coated with PEG molecules which dissociates from the SNALP rapidly after administration, thus transforming the carrier into a transfection-competent entity (Ambegia et al., 2005). SNALP-formulated siRNA have shown improved circulation time and increased downregulation efficacy in mice and nonhuman primates liver (Judge et al., 2009; Morrissey et al., 2005; Zimmermann et al., 2006), and recent modifications to the lipid composition have engendered a substantial 10-fold improvement in activity *in vivo* (Semple et al., 2010). Alternatives to cationic lipids complexed with therapeutic polynucleotides are also being explored to overcome the limitations observed with current formulations. In particular, reductions in *in vivo* toxicity and targeting efficiency for a certain cell population are a main focus. These options are discussed further in a previously published review (Verreault et al., 2006).

9. Targeted delivery

The concept of targeted delivery has been suggested by many to be the solution to the obstacle of siRNA delivery to brain tumors (Lichota et al., 2009; Prakash et al., 2010). An efficient targeted delivery strategy should promote specific crossing of the therapeutic material across tumor-associated BBB, passage through cancer cell membranes, and prevention of accumulation in healthy tissue. Antibody-coupled liposomes (immunoliposomes) combine the capacity of LNPs to increase nucleic acid half-life in the blood compartment with specific targeting to tumor sites. One of the first attempts to deliver material to the brain using immunoliposomes was done by coupling the monoclonal antibody OX26 specific against the transferrin receptor (Huwyler et al., 1996) to PEGylated liposomes made with DSPE lipids. The transferrin receptor is present at the surface of normal brain capillary endothelial cells and is upregulated in brain tumor tissue (Recht et al., 1990). Following i.v. injection of OX26 coupled-DSPE-PEG immunoliposomes encapsulating the chemotherapeutic agent daunomycin, an average of 0.03% of the injected dose of daunomycin was measured in the brain of rats after 60 min, while only 0.008% of injected daunomycin dose was measured following administration of free daunomycin or non-OX26-conjugated daunomycin DSPE-PEG carrier (Huwyler et al., 1996). The use of mouse transferrin receptor-targeted immunoliposomes has also shown success in the delivery of bigger molecules such as DNA plasmids (Shi et al., 2001) or siRNAs (Pirollo et al., 2006) to brain tumors.

It can be speculated that many other types of antibodies specific against GBM cells or micro-environment antigens could also be used to produce immunoliposomes that would increase delivery of nucleic acid sequences to the tumor tissue. For example, the arginine-glycine-aspartic acid (RGD) motif of fibronectin has been used to target delivery of siRNAs in a s.c. model of neuroblastoma (Schiffelers et al., 2004). RGD binds to integrins that are expressed on activated endothelial cells found in tumor vasculature of many advanced cancers including GBM (Gladson & Cheresh, 1991). *In vivo* studies demonstrated the accumulation of CY5.5-RGD in cells and vessels of orthotopic GBM tumors following i.v. injection (Hsu et al., 2006), supporting its potential use for siRNA targeted delivery to GBM tumors. Tumor-associated endothelial cells in GBM have higher levels of VEGFR2 than normal endothelial cells (Charalambous et al., 2006). Targeted delivery specific to the VEGFR2 receptor could also be used to specifically deliver material across the brain tumor-associated BBB. CD44 is a surface receptor overexpressed in GBM tumor cells (Axelsen et al., 2007) and is another example of GBM-specific marker that could be used for immunoliposome targeting. Further, antigens found at the surface of brain tumor initiating cells (BTIC) (e.g. CD133) (Altaner, 2008; Guo et al., 2006) could potentially allow for specific delivery of silencing agents against defective genes in these cells. BTIC are a sub-population of cells that have the ability to reconstitute the overall tumor cell population and are typically more resistant to chemotherapy and radiation than the rest of the tumor cell population (Hadjipanayis & Van Meir, 2009). It is now believed that treatment resistance and eventual relapse result in part from a failure to eliminate BTICs (Xie & Chin, 2008). It is important to note that CD133 is also expressed in normal stem cells (Tarnok et al., 2009) and use of this antigen for targeted delivery could negatively impact healthy CD133+ cells. Therefore, it appears necessary to combine several targeted delivery strategies to achieve both efficacy and specificity. For example, use of immunoliposomes specific to human insulin receptor and mouse transferrin receptor was more effective at delivering nucleic acid molecules to brain tumors cells than a carrier specific to mouse transferrin receptor only in a human xenograft murine model (Zhang et al., 2003). This dual receptor targeting strategy was used to deliver ASOs or shRNA plasmids to orthotopic brain tumors (Zhang et al., 2004; Zhang et al., 2002) and resulted in 88-100% increase in animals' lifespan when compared to untreated animals. Thus, a treatment aimed at targeting BTIC could include a proportion of transferrin and insulin targeting immunoliposomes that would also incorporate antibodies against the CD133 marker. Such system could increase the likelihood that all targeted CD133+ cells are part of the tumor tissue. The complex and heterogeneous nature of brain tumors seems to require multivalency of delivery systems in order to achieve highly specific and efficient siRNA delivery. Targeted delivery systems will also have to be versatile, allowing the encapsulation of diverse combinations of siRNA (e.g. against EGFR and Rictor) selected based on the patient's tumor genetic profile.

Interestingly, the capacity of exogenous neural stem cells (NSC) administered directly into the brain parenchyma, the cerebral ventricles or even in the systemic circulation to migrate great distances into sites of intracranial pathology has triggered the interest of using these cells as anti-cancer therapeutics vehicles (reviewed in (Yip et al., 2006)). Indeed, exogenous NSCs were shown to be able to accumulate around brain tumors and to track tumor cells migrating into the surrounding tissue (Aboody et al., 2000). This unique tropism of NSCs for gliomas has motivated the development "genetically-armed" NSC to target cancer cells through the delivery of a variety of therapeutic gene products. NSCs have been produced to express cytokines to enhance the immune response against the tumor (Benedetti et al., 2000; Ehtesham et al., 2002b), the proapoptotic protein TRAIL (Ehtesham et al., 2002a) or the pro-drug converting enzyme cytosine deaminase (Aboody et al., 2000). Given the potential of NSCs to deliver therapeutic agents in a specific and sustained manner to brain tumors, it will be interesting to evaluate whether shRNA-expressing NSCs could be used to secrete and deliver siRNAs in the vicinity of tumors and invading tumor cells. These therapeutic NSCs can also be designed to express bioluminescence or red fluorescence (Shah et al., 2005; Yip & Shah, 2008). Hence, it is hoped that therapeutic NSCs could be used as biological, motile and dynamic diagnostic tools as well as specific delivery systems for therapeutic agents in gliomas, especially for infiltrating tumor cells in the close vicinity to normal CNS structures and therefore not remediable by traditional therapy (Shah et al., 2005; Yip & Shah, 2008). However, it is not sure whether therapeutic NSCs have the ability to transgress the abnormal tumor-associated vasculature, and research into the underlying molecular mechanism and clinical utility of these cells is active and ongoing.

10. Opportunity for improving tumor drug delivery by vascular normalization

Pre-clinical models showed that GBM tumors are poorly perfused (Blasberg et al., 1983; Groothuis et al., 1983) due to factors such as reduced blood flow rates, elevated hematocrit and interstitial fluid pressure, and an increase in geometric resistance (Baish et al., 1996; Vajkoczy & Menger, 2000; Vajkoczy et al., 1998; Yuan et al., 1994). The microvasculature of GBM was characterized as tortuous and fenestrated vessels with diameters that are larger than normal (Vajkoczy & Menger, 2004) and discontinuous basement membrane which rarely encloses pericytes (Deane & Lantos, 1981). The poorly organized architecture of GBM vessels, illustrated in figure 3, impedes vascular function and reduces drug delivery to the tumor tissue. In glioma (Kamoun et al., 2009; Sorensen A. G. et al., 2009; Winkler et al., 2004), tumor vascular normalization has been described as the specific activity of an agent (e.g. antiangiogenic therapy) against proliferating vasculature, which results in the growth inhibition of new vessels, the pruning of immature and inefficient tumor vessels, and the normalization of surviving vasculature by increasing the fraction of pericyte-covered vessels, restoring the abnormally thick and irregular basement membrane and reducing the high vascular permeability of these vessels (Baffert et al., 2006; Jain, 2001). The normalization of tumor vessels appears to be transient in nature, but was suggested to create a window where blood flow is improved, leading to an opportunity to improve delivery of other drugs (Jain, 2005). In GBM patients, a "vascular normalization index", defined by changes in vascular permeability (K_{trans} values), microvessel volume and circulating collagen IV, was found to be closely associated with overall survival and progression-free survival in response to Cediranib, a pan-VEGFR inhibitor (Sorensen A. G. et al., 2009). Pre-clinically, the delivery of TMZ in an intracranial model of glioma was increased after treatment with the angiogenesis inhibitor SU5416. It was suggested that SU5416 restored capillary architecture and decreased interstitial fluid pressure (Ma et al., 2003), allowing for an increase in TMZ delivery to the tumor tissue. Our laboratory has recently reported that IrC™ therapy (once weekly for three weeks) can lead to normalization of GBM blood vessel structure and function (Verreault et al., 2011c). IrC™ treatment restored the basement membrane architecture of the tumor vasculature, reduced blood vessel diameters and reduced vessel permeability to the fluorescent dye Hoechst 33342, suggesting a restoration of the vessel architecture and function to a more normal state (Verreault et al., 2011c). Treatment also increased the quantity of vessel in the center of tumors, suggesting a more homogeneous distribution of blood across the entire tumor (Verreault et al., 2011c). Further, IrC™ significantly reduced K_{trans} values calculated from Dynamic Contrast Enhanced Magnetic Resonance Imaging (DCE-MRI) studies (Verreault et al., 2011c), which was also suggestive of a decrease in vessel permeability (O'Connor et al., 2007). Taken together, these observations strongly suggested an improvement in vascular function: the tumor blood vessels in tumors from animals treated with IrC™ were behaving more like vessels in the normal brain. Thus, IrC™ exerts a dual mechanism of action in GBM tumors. As described in section 8, the therapeutic activity of irinotecan is improved by the extended exposure of tumor cells to the drug provided by the drug carrier (Verreault et al., 2011b). Moreover, the effects of the formulation on the tumor micro-environment may increase the delivery and efficacy of a second agent (Verreault et al., 2011c). This dual mechanism may provide an opportunity for designing a therapy which would encompass the cytotoxic activity of an optimized chemotherapeutic agent together with the increase in tumor delivery of an antibody-coupled carrier encapsulating siRNAs specific to pro-malignancy genes. It can be expected that such therapy could lead to significant therapeutic benefits for GBM patients. Studies designed to evaluate the capacity of IrC™ therapy to increase delivery and efficacy of TMZ in GBM are currently ongoing.

11. Conclusion

It is widely recognized that there is a tremendous potential in the use of targeted therapy agents to treat GBM and, importantly, to become the therapeutic modality of choice when developing target-specific personalized treatment options. The following three main areas of investigation could lead to improved treatment outcome in GBM: (i) Use of targeted agents in combination with conventional treatment options: the capacity of SMIs or siRNAs to enhance the activity of chemotherapeutic agents or radiation should be tested in established

GBM orthotopic models and in clinical studies. (ii) Use of targeted agents customized therapy: the anti-tumor efficacy of SMIs or siRNAs should be tested using GBM tumors arising from orthotopic inoculation of tumor cells isolated from patient tumor biopsies for which a list of genetic defects (e.g. EGFR amplification, PTEN mutation) is available. (iii) Use of delivery systems to circumvent the obstacles of delivery to brain tumors and improve efficacy of targeted agents and chemotherapeutics: antibody-coupled carriers could be designed to improve delivery to the tumor, and the ligand specificity of such a carrier could be made based on immunohistopathology analysis of each individual tumor.

Chapter summary

- The most significant problem for GBM cancer patients is repopulation of malignant cells following treatment, causing inevitable relapse. This is thought to be the result of genetic mutations that endow the cell with many specific functional capabilities such as cell proliferation, survival, invasion and metastasis. Although it is acknowledged that advances in GBM treatment will continue to rely on conventional treatment approaches (surgery, radiation and/or chemotherapy), the value of combining standard chemotherapy with targeted agents that increase tumor drug sensitivity is now being recognized.
- Several targeted therapy approaches are currently being evaluated in GBM pre-clinical and clinical studies using SMI, ASOs and RNAi-based compounds (siRNA or shRNA), and the targets include proteins involved in sustaining proliferative signals, evading growth suppressors, resisting cell death, inducing angiogenesis, activating invasion and metastasis and enabling replicative immortality.
- The potential benefits of combining agents targeting different biological pathways in order to effectively silence as many cancer phenotypes as possible is also being recognized.
- Another major challenge of GBM treatment is the achievement of adequate concentration of the therapeutic agent within the tumor itself, and this obstacle can largely be attributed to the presence of the BBB. Strategies that are currently being tested to overcome this obstacle include the bypass of the BBB using alternative delivery routes (i.t., CED, i.n., "genetically-armed" NSCs) or the use of delivery systems (LNPs, immunoliposomes) which have been shown to promote a more efficient and specific delivery of therapeutics to brain tumors following intravenous administration.
- The poorly organized architecture of GBM vessels is thought to impede vascular function and to reduce drug delivery to the tumor tissue, and the normalization of GBM vasculature has been approached in an attempt to improve drug delivery to brain tumors.

It has become clear that delivery systems, whether they are lipid-based, polymer-based or antibody-conjugated, can have a significant benefit in enhancing stability of drugs, facilitating delivery to tumor sites and perhaps delivery to the intracellular compartments containing the molecular targets. Moreover, the reduced toxicity profile associated with many liposomal drug formulations compared to the free form of the drug (Mayer et al., 1995; O'Brien et al., 2004) could be used to administer higher doses that would lead to increased drug delivery to brain tumors. To date, the full potential of this technology has not been explored in GBM and may constitute a significant opportunity for delivery of targeted therapeutic approaches that encompass the use of multiple therapeutics all designed to inhibit phenotypes of GBM that contribute to its aggressive behavior.

It is now obvious that conventional treatment approaches for patients affected by GBM must change if improved treatment outcomes are going to be achieved. One important avenue would be to determine how many treatment agents must be included in order to achieve GBM cure. While most combination clinical trials will typically test 2 or 3 agents, it may be necessary to consider using 5 or even 10 different compounds that will block or eradicate all tumorigenic phenotypes of a cancer. Obviously, the design complexity of these trials may be a limiting factor. However, pre-clinical approaches where animals are inoculated orthotopically with tumor cells from patient samples could allow for testing several combination therapy options in a model that is more representative of the clinical reality than conventional models using commercially available cell lines. Moreover, non-invasive imaging using cancer cell lines expressing fluorescent proteins (e.g. mKate2 or mCherry proteins (Verreault et al., 2011d)) or bioluminescence (Maes et al., 2009) will facilitate the use of such models by providing immediate information on treatment response. It can be expected that the future of GBM treatment will incorporate information acquired from pre-clinical models obtained from orthotopic inoculation of patients' tumor samples to guide treatment decisions for these particular patients. We can be hopeful that the personalization of therapy options will improve treatment outcomes for individuals diagnosed with this devastating cancer.

12. References

Aboody, K.S., Brown, A., Rainov, N.G. et al. (2000). Neural stem cells display extensive tropism for pathology in adult brain: evidence from intracranial gliomas. *Proceedings of the National Academy of Sciences of the United States of America*, Vol. 97, No. 23, pp. (12846-51), ISBN: 0027-8424.

Adamson, C., Kanu, O.O., Mehta, A.I. et al. (2009). Glioblastoma multiforme: a review of where we have been and where we are going. *Expert Opin Investig Drugs*, Vol. 18, No. 8, pp. (1061-83), ISBN: 1744-7658.

Aigner, A. (2008). Cellular delivery in vivo of siRNA-based therapeutics. *Curr Pharm Des*, Vol. 14, No. 34, pp. (3603-19), ISBN: 1873-4286.

Allen, C., Dos Santos, N., Gallagher, R. et al. (2002). Controlling the physical behavior and biological performance of liposome formulations through use of surface grafted poly(ethylene glycol). *Biosci Rep*, Vol. 22, No. 2, pp. (225-50), ISBN: 0144-8463.

Altaner, C. (2008). Glioblastoma and stem cells. *Neoplasma*, Vol. 55, No. 5, pp. (369-74), ISBN: 0028-2685.

Ambegia, E., Ansell, S., Cullis, P., Heyes, J., Palmer, L. & MacLachlan, I. (2005). Stabilized plasmid-lipid particles containing PEG-diacylglycerols exhibit extended circulation lifetimes and tumor selective gene expression. *Biochimica et biophysica acta*, Vol. 1669, No. 2, pp. (155-63), ISBN: 0006-3002.

Axelsen, J.B., Lotem, J., Sachs, L. & Domany, E. (2007). Genes overexpressed in different human solid cancers exhibit different tissue-specific expression profiles. *Proc Natl Acad Sci USA*, Vol. 104, No. 32, pp. (13122-13127), ISBN: 0027-8424.

Badiga, A.V., Chetty, C., Kesanakurti, D. et al. (2011). MMP-2 siRNA inhibits radiation-enhanced invasiveness in glioma cells. *PloS one*, Vol. 6, No. 6, pp. (e20614), ISBN: 1932-6203.

Baffert, F., Le, T., Sennino, B. et al. (2006). Cellular changes in normal blood capillaries undergoing regression after inhibition of VEGF signaling. *Am J Physiol Heart Circ Physiol*, Vol. 290, No. 2, pp. (H547-59), ISBN: 0363-6135.

Baish, J.W., Gazit, Y., Berk, D.A., Nozue, M., Baxter, L.T. & Jain, R.K. (1996). Role of tumor vascular architecture in nutrient and drug delivery: an invasion percolation-based network model. *Microvasc Res*, Vol. 51, No. 3, pp. (327-46), ISBN: 0026-2862.

Banks, W.A. (2009). Characteristics of compounds that cross the blood-brain barrier. *BMC Neurol*, Vol. 9 Suppl 1, No. pp. (S3), ISBN: 1471-2377.

Barenholz, Y. (2007). Amphipathic weak base loading into preformed liposomes having a transmembrane ammonium ion gradient: from the bench to approved Doxil. *Liposome Technology: Entrapment of drugs and other materials into liposomes*, Vol. 2, No. 3rd edition, pp. (1-25), ISBN: 978-0-8493-8828-6.

Begley, D.J. (2004a). ABC transporters and the blood-brain barrier. *Curr Pharm Des*, Vol. 10, No. 12, pp. (1295-312), ISBN: 1381-6128.

Begley, D.J. (2004b). Delivery of therapeutic agents to the central nervous system: the problems and the possibilities. *Pharmacol Ther*, Vol. 104, No. 1, pp. (29-45), ISBN: 0163-7258.

Bellavance, M.A., Blanchette, M. & Fortin, D. (2008). Recent advances in blood-brain barrier disruption as a CNS delivery strategy. *AAPS J*, Vol. 10, No. 1, pp. (166-77), ISBN: 1550-7416.

Benedetti, S., Pirola, B., Pollo, B. et al. (2000). Gene therapy of experimental brain tumors using neural progenitor cells. *Nature medicine*, Vol. 6, No. 4, pp. (447-50), ISBN: 1078-8956.

Bertrand, J.R., Pottier, M., Vekris, A., Opolon, P., Maksimenko, A. & Malvy, C. (2002). Comparison of antisense oligonucleotides and siRNAs in cell culture and in vivo. *Biochem Biophys Res Commun*, Vol. 296, No. 4, pp. (1000-4), ISBN: 0006-291X.

Blasberg, R.G., Kobayashi, T., Horowitz, M. et al. (1983). Regional blood flow in ethylnitrosourea-induced brain tumors. *Ann Neurol*, Vol. 14, No. 2, pp. (189-201), ISBN: 0364-5134.

Boiardi, A., Bartolomei, M., Silvani, A. et al. (2005). Intratumoral delivery of mitoxantrone in association with 90-Y radioimmunotherapy (RIT) in recurrent glioblastoma. *J Neurooncol*, Vol. 72, No. 2, pp. (125-31), ISBN: 0167-594X.

Braasch, D.A., Paroo, Z., Constantinescu, A. et al. (2004). Biodistribution of phosphodiester and phosphorothioate siRNA. *Bioorg Med Chem Lett*, Vol. 14, No. 5, pp. (1139-43), ISBN: 0960-894X.

Brada, M., Collins, V.P., Dorward, N.L. & Thomas, D.G.T. (2001). Tumours of the brain and spinal cord in adults. *Oxford Textbook of Oncology* Vol. 2, No. 2nd edition, pp. (2707-2753), ISBN: 0-19-262926-3.

Brandes, A.A., Tosoni, A., Amista, P. et al. (2004a). How effective is BCNU in recurrent glioblastoma in the modern era? A phase II trial. *Neurology*, Vol. 63, No. 7, pp. (1281-4), ISBN: 1526-632X.

Brandes, A.A., Tosoni, A., Basso, U. et al. (2004b). Second-line chemotherapy with irinotecan plus carmustine in glioblastoma recurrent or progressive after first-line temozolomide chemotherapy: a phase II study of the Gruppo Italiano Cooperativo di Neuro-Oncologia (GICNO). *J Clin Oncol*, Vol. 22, No. 23, pp. (4779-4786), ISBN: 0732-183X.

Brem, H., Mahaley, M.S., Jr., Vick, N.A. et al. (1991). Interstitial chemotherapy with drug polymer implants for the treatment of recurrent gliomas. *J Neurosurg*, Vol. 74, No. 3, pp. (441-6), ISBN: 0022-3085.

Brem, H., Tamargo, R.J., Olivi, A. et al. (1994). Biodegradable polymers for controlled delivery of chemotherapy with and without radiation therapy in the monkey brain. *J Neurosurg*, Vol. 80, No. 2, pp. (283-90), ISBN: 0022-3085.

Brinker, B.T., Krown, S.E., Lee, J.Y. et al. (2008). Phase 1/2 trial of BMS-275291 in patients with human immunodeficiency virus-related Kaposi sarcoma: a multicenter trial of the AIDS Malignancy Consortium. *Cancer*, Vol. 112, No. 5, pp. (1083-8), ISBN: 0008-543X.

Bumcrot, D., Manoharan, M., Koteliansky, V. & Sah, D.W. (2006). RNAi therapeutics: a potential new class of pharmaceutical drugs. *Nat Chem Biol*, Vol. 2, No. 12, pp. (711-9), ISBN: 1552-4450.

Cahill, D.P., Levine, K.K., Betensky, R.A. et al. (2007). Loss of the mismatch repair protein MSH6 in human glioblastomas is associated with tumor progression during temozolomide treatment. *Clinical cancer research : an official journal of the American Association for Cancer Research*, Vol. 13, No. 7, pp. (2038-45), ISBN: 1078-0432.

Carter, A. (2010). Integrins as target: first phase III trial launches, but questions remain. *J Natl Cancer Inst*, Vol. 102, No. 10, pp. (675-7), ISBN: 1460-2105.

Cattel, L., Ceruti, M. & Dosio, F. (2004). From conventional to stealth liposomes: a new Frontier in cancer chemotherapy. *J Chemother*, Vol. 16 Suppl 4, No. pp. (94-7), ISBN: 1120-009X.

CBTRUS. (2010). Statistical Report: Primary Brain and Central Nervous System Tumors Diagnosed in the United States in 2004-2006. *In: Central Brain Tumor Registry of the United States, Hinsdale, IL.*, Vol. Accessed in February 2011, No. pp. (Available from: www.cbtrus.org), ISBN:

CCS. (2010). Statistics for brain cancer. *In: Canadian Cancer Society*, Vol. Accessed in February 2011, No. pp. (Available from: www.cancer.ca), ISBN:

CGARN. (2008). Comprehensive genomic characterization defines human glioblastoma genes and core pathways. *Nature*, Vol. 455, No. 7216, pp. (1061-8), ISBN: 1476-4687.

Chandana, S.R., Movva, S., Arora, M. & Singh, T. (2008). Primary brain tumors in adults. *Am Fam Physician*, Vol. 77, No. 10, pp. (1423-30), ISBN: 0002-838X.

Chang, S.M., Wen, P., Cloughesy, T. et al. (2005). Phase II study of CCI-779 in patients with recurrent glioblastoma multiforme. *Invest New Drugs*, Vol. 23, No. 4, pp. (357-61), ISBN: 0167-6997.

Charalambous, C., Chen, T.C. & Hofman, F.M. (2006). Characteristics of tumor-associated endothelial cells derived from glioblastoma multiforme. *Neurosurg Focus*, Vol. 20, No. 4, pp. (E22), ISBN: 1092-0684.

Chinot, O.L., de La Motte Rouge, T., Moore, N. et al. (2011). AVAglio: Phase 3 trial of bevacizumab plus temozolomide and radiotherapy in newly diagnosed glioblastoma multiforme. *Advances in therapy*, Vol. 28, No. 4, pp. (334-40), ISBN: 1865-8652.

Chu, Q.S., Forouzesh, B., Syed, S. et al. (2007). A phase II and pharmacological study of the matrix metalloproteinase inhibitor (MMPI) COL-3 in patients with advanced soft tissue sarcomas. *Invest New Drugs*, Vol. 25, No. 4, pp. (359-67), ISBN: 0167-6997.

Clarke, J., Butowski, N. & Chang, S. (2010). Recent advances in therapy for glioblastoma. *Arch Neurol*, Vol. 67, No. 3, pp. (279-283), ISBN: 1538-3687.

Cloughesy, T.F., Wen, P.Y., Robins, H.I. et al. (2006). Phase II trial of tipifarnib in patients with recurrent malignant glioma either receiving or not receiving enzyme-inducing antiepileptic drugs: a North American Brain Tumor Consortium Study. *J Clin Oncol*, Vol. 24, No. 22, pp. (3651-6), ISBN: 1527-7755.

da Fonseca, C.O., Linden, R., Futuro, D., Gattass, C.R. & Quirico-Santos, T. (2008). Ras pathway activation in gliomas: a strategic target for intranasal administration of perillyl alcohol. *Arch Immunol Ther Exp (Warsz)*, Vol. 56, No. 4, pp. (267-76), ISBN: 0004-069X.

De Paula, D., Bentley, M.V. & Mahato, R.I. (2007). Hydrophobization and bioconjugation for enhanced siRNA delivery and targeting. *RNA*, Vol. 13, No. 4, pp. (431-56), ISBN: 1355-8382.

Deane, B.R. & Lantos, P.L. (1981). The vasculature of experimental brain tumours. Part 1. A sequential light and electron microscope study of angiogenesis. *J Neurol Sci*, Vol. 49, No. 1, pp. (55-66), ISBN: 0022-510X.

Desgrosellier, J.S. & Cheresh, D.A. (2010). Integrins in cancer: biological implications and therapeutic opportunities. *Nat Rev Cancer*, Vol. 10, No. 1, pp. (9-22), ISBN: 1474-1768.

Ehtesham, M., Kabos, P., Gutierrez, M.A. et al. (2002a). Induction of glioblastoma apoptosis using neural stem cell-mediated delivery of tumor necrosis factor-related apoptosis-inducing ligand. *Cancer research*, Vol. 62, No. 24, pp. (7170-4), ISBN: 0008-5472.

Ehtesham, M., Kabos, P., Kabosova, A., Neuman, T., Black, K.L. & Yu, J.S. (2002b). The use of interleukin 12-secreting neural stem cells for the treatment of intracranial glioma. *Cancer research*, Vol. 62, No. 20, pp. (5657-63), ISBN: 0008-5472.

Ekstrand, A.J., James, C.D., Cavenee, W.K., Seliger, B., Pettersson, R.F. & Collins, V.P. (1991). Genes for epidermal growth factor receptor, transforming growth factor alpha, and epidermal growth factor and their expression in human gliomas in vivo. *Cancer Res*, Vol. 51, No. 8, pp. (2164-72), ISBN: 0008-5472.

Engerhard, H.H., Groothuis, D.G. & Coons, S.W. (1999). Chapter 11: The Blood-Brain barrier: Structure, Function, and Response to Neoplasia & Chapter 20: Anatomy and Growth Patterns of Diffuse Gliomas. *The Gliomas*, Vol. 1, No. 1, pp. (115-121), ISBN: 0721648258.

Ermoian, R.P., Furniss, C.S., Lamborn, K.R. et al. (2002). Dysregulation of PTEN and protein kinase B is associated with glioma histology and patient survival. *Clin Cancer Res*, Vol. 8, No. 5, pp. (1100-6), ISBN: 1078-0432.

Fabel, K., Dietrich, J., Hau, P. et al. (2001). Long-term stabilization in patients with malignant glioma after treatment with liposomal doxorubicin. *Cancer*, Vol. 92, No. 7, pp. (1936-42), ISBN: 0008-543X.

Fadul, C.E., Kingman, L.S., Meyer, L.P. et al. (2008). A phase II study of thalidomide and irinotecan for treatment of glioblastoma multiforme. *J Neurooncol*, Vol. 90, No. 2, pp. (229-35), ISBN: 0167-594X.

Fan, Q.W., Specht, K.M., Zhang, C., Goldenberg, D.D., Shokat, K.M. & Weiss, W.A. (2003). Combinatorial efficacy achieved through two-point blockade within a signaling pathway-a chemical genetic approach. *Cancer Res*, Vol. 63, No. 24, pp. (8930-8), ISBN: 0008-5472.

Fawcett, D.W. (1994). Section 11: The nervous tissue. *A textbook of histology*, Vol. 1, No. 12th edition, pp. (336-339), ISBN: 0412046911

Filleur, S., Courtin, A., Ait-Si-Ali, S. et al. (2003). SiRNA-mediated inhibition of vascular endothelial growth factor severely limits tumor resistance to antiangiogenic thrombospondin-1 and slows tumor vascularization and growth. *Cancer Res*, Vol. 63, No. 14, pp. (3919-22), ISBN: 0008-5472.

Fine, H.A., Wen, P.Y., Maher, E.A. et al. (2003). Phase II trial of thalidomide and carmustine for patients with recurrent high-grade gliomas. *J Clin Oncol*, Vol. 21, No. 12, pp. (2299-304), ISBN: 0732-183X.

Fouse, S.D. & Costello, J.F. (2009). Epigenetics of neurological cancers. *Future oncology*, Vol. 5, No. 10, pp. (1615-29), ISBN: 1744-8301.

Franceschi, E., Cavallo, G., Lonardi, S. et al. (2007). Gefitinib in patients with progressive high-grade gliomas: a multicentre phase II study by Gruppo Italiano Cooperativo di Neuro-Oncologia (GICNO). *Br J Cancer*, Vol. 96, No. 7, pp. (1047-51), ISBN: 0007-0920.

Frazier, J.L., Johnson, M.W., Burger, P.C., Weingart, J.D. & Quinones-Hinojosa, A. (2009). Rapid malignant transformation of low-grade astrocytomas: report of 2 cases and review of the literature. *Surgical neurology*, Vol. Aug 6, No. pp. ISBN: 1879-3339.

Freimark, B.D., Blezinger, H.P., Florack, V.J. et al. (1998). Cationic lipids enhance cytokine and cell influx levels in the lung following administration of plasmid: cationic lipid complexes. *J Immunol*, Vol. 160, No. 9, pp. (4580-6), ISBN: 0022-1767.

Friedman, H.S., Prados, M.D., Wen, P.Y. et al. (2009). Bevacizumab alone and in combination with irinotecan in recurrent glioblastoma. *J Clin Oncol*, Vol. 27, No. 28, pp. (4733-40), ISBN: 1527-7755.

Galanis, E., Buckner, J.C., Maurer, M.J. et al. (2005). Phase II trial of temsirolimus (CCI-779) in recurrent glioblastoma multiforme: a North Central Cancer Treatment Group Study. *J Clin Oncol*, Vol. 23, No. 23, pp. (5294-304), ISBN: 0732-183X.

Galanis, E., Jaeckle, K.A., Maurer, M.J. et al. (2009). Phase II trial of vorinostat in recurrent glioblastoma multiforme: a north central cancer treatment group study. *J Clin Oncol*, Vol. 27, No. 12, pp. (2052-8), ISBN: 1527-7755.

George, J., Banik, N.L. & Ray, S.K. (2008). Combination of taxol and Bcl-2 siRNA induces apoptosis in human glioblastoma cells and inhibits invasion, angiogenesis, and tumor growth. *J Cell Mol Med*, Vol. No. pp. ISBN: 1582-4934.

George, J., Banik, N.L. & Ray, S.K. (2009). Combination of hTERT knockdown and IFN-gamma treatment inhibited angiogenesis and tumor progression in glioblastoma. *Clin Cancer Res*, Vol. 15, No. 23, pp. (7186-95), ISBN: 1078-0432.

Gerlinger, M. & Swanton, C. (2010). How Darwinian models inform therapeutic failure initiated by clonal heterogeneity in cancer medicine. *British journal of cancer*, Vol. 103, No. 8, pp. (1139-43), ISBN: 1532-1827.

Gerstner, E.R., Yip, S., Wang, D.L., Louis, D.N., Iafrate, A.J. & Batchelor, T.T. (2009). Mgmt methylation is a prognostic biomarker in elderly patients with newly diagnosed glioblastoma. *Neurology*, Vol. 73, No. 18, pp. (1509-10), ISBN: 1526-632X.

Gladson, C.L. & Cheresh, D.A. (1991). Glioblastoma expression of vitronectin and the alpha v beta 3 integrin. Adhesion mechanism for transformed glial cells. *J Clin Invest*, Vol. 88, No. 6, pp. (1924-32), ISBN: 0021-9738.

Gondi, C.S., Lakka, S.S., Dinh, D.H., Olivero, W.C., Gujrati, M. & Rao, J.S. (2004). RNAi-mediated inhibition of cathepsin B and uPAR leads to decreased cell invasion, angiogenesis and tumor growth in gliomas. *Oncogene*, Vol. 23, No. 52, pp. (8486-96), ISBN: 0950-9232.

Gondi, C.S., Lakka, S.S., Dinh, D.H., Olivero, W.C., Gujrati, M. & Rao, J.S. (2007). Intraperitoneal injection of a hairpin RNA-expressing plasmid targeting urokinase-type plasminogen activator (uPA) receptor and uPA retards angiogenesis and inhibits intracranial tumor growth in nude mice. *Clin Cancer Res*, Vol. 13, No. 14, pp. (4051-60), ISBN: 1078-0432.

Gray, H. (2005). Chapter 22: Cerebral Hemisphere & Chapter 23: Basal Ganglia. *Gray's Anatomy: The anatomical basis of Clinical Practice* Vol. 1, No. 39th edition, pp. (387-430), ISBN: 0443071683.

Groothuis, D.R., Pasternak, J.F., Fischer, J.M., Blasberg, R.G., Bigner, D.D. & Vick, N.A. (1983). Regional measurements of blood flow in experimental RG-2 rat gliomas. *Cancer Res*, Vol. 43, No. 7, pp. (3362-7), ISBN: 0008-5472.

Grossman, S.A., Alavi, J.B., Supko, J.G. et al. (2005). Efficacy and toxicity of the antisense oligonucleotide aprinocarsen directed against protein kinase C-alpha delivered as a 21-day continuous intravenous infusion in patients with recurrent high-grade astrocytomas. *Neuro Oncol*, Vol. 7, No. 1, pp. (32-40), ISBN: 1522-8517.

Grossman, S.A., Reinhard, C., Colvin, O.M. et al. (1992). The intracerebral distribution of BCNU delivered by surgically implanted biodegradable polymers. *J Neurosurg*, Vol. 76, No. 4, pp. (640-7), ISBN: 0022-3085.

Grzelinski, M., Urban-Klein, B., Martens, T. et al. (2006). RNA interference-mediated gene silencing of pleiotrophin through polyethylenimine-complexed small interfering RNAs in vivo exerts antitumoral effects in glioblastoma xenografts. *Hum Gene Ther*, Vol. 17, No. 7, pp. (751-66), ISBN: 1043-0342.

Guo, W., Lasky, J.L., 3rd & Wu, H. (2006). Cancer stem cells. *Pediatr Res*, Vol. 59, No. 4 Pt 2, pp. (59R-64R), ISBN: 0031-3998.

Gururangan, S., Cokgor, L., Rich, J.N. et al. (2001). Phase I study of Gliadel wafers plus temozolomide in adults with recurrent supratentorial high-grade gliomas. *Neuro Oncol*, Vol. 3, No. 4, pp. (246-50), ISBN: 1522-8517.

Haas-Kogan, D., Shalev, N., Wong, M., Mills, G., Yount, G. & Stokoe, D. (1998). Protein kinase B (PKB/Akt) activity is elevated in glioblastoma cells due to mutation of the tumor suppressor PTEN/MMAC. *Curr Biol*, Vol. 8, No. 21, pp. (1195-8), ISBN: 0960-9822.

Hadjipanayis, C.G. & Van Meir, E.G. (2009). Tumor initiating cells in malignant gliomas: biology and implications for therapy. *J Mol Med*, Vol. 87, No. 4, pp. (363-74), ISBN: 1432-1440.

Hanahan, D. & Weinberg, R.A. (2000). The hallmarks of cancer. *Cell*, Vol. 100, No. 1, pp. (57-70), ISBN: 0092-8674.

Hanahan, D. & Weinberg, R.A. (2011). Hallmarks of cancer: the next generation. *Cell*, Vol. 144, No. 5, pp. (646-74), ISBN: 1097-4172.

Hashizume, R., Ozawa, T., Gryaznov, S.M. et al. (2008). New therapeutic approach for brain tumors: Intranasal delivery of telomerase inhibitor GRN163. *Neuro Oncol*, Vol. 10, No. 2, pp. (112-20), ISBN: 1522-8517.

Hattori, Y., Shi, L., Ding, W. et al. (2009). Novel irinotecan-loaded liposome using phytic acid with high therapeutic efficacy for colon tumors. *J Control Release*, Vol. 136, No. 1, pp. (30-7), ISBN: 1873-4995.

Hau, P., Fabel, K., Baumgart, U. et al. (2004). Pegylated liposomal doxorubicin-efficacy in patients with recurrent high-grade glioma. *Cancer*, Vol. 100, No. 6, pp. (1199-207), ISBN: 0008-543X.

Hegi, M.E., Diserens, A.C., Gorlia, T. et al. (2005). MGMT gene silencing and benefit from temozolomide in glioblastoma. *N Engl J Med*, Vol. 352, No. 10, pp. (997-1003), ISBN: 1533-4406.

Heidel, J.D., Hu, S., Liu, X.F., Triche, T.J. & Davis, M.E. (2004). Lack of interferon response in animals to naked siRNAs. *Nat Biotechnol*, Vol. 22, No. 12, pp. (1579-82), ISBN: 1087-0156.

Helene, C. (1994). Control of oncogene expression by antisense nucleic acids. *Eur J Cancer*, Vol. 30A, No. 11, pp. (1721-6), ISBN: 0959-8049.

Hendruschk, S., Wiedemuth, R., Aigner, A. et al. (2011). RNA interference targeting survivin exerts antitumoral effects in vitro and in established glioma xenografts in vivo. *Neuro-oncology*, Vol. No. pp. ISBN: 1523-5866.

Heyes, J., Palmer, L., Bremner, K. & MacLachlan, I. (2005). Cationic lipid saturation influences intracellular delivery of encapsulated nucleic acids. *Journal of controlled release*, Vol. 107, No. 2, pp. (276-87), ISBN: 0168-3659.

Holland, E.C. (2000). Glioblastoma multiforme: the terminator. *Proceedings of the National Academy of Sciences of the United States of America*, Vol. 97, No. 12, pp. (6242-4), ISBN: 0027-8424.

Holt, S.E. & Shay, J.W. (1999). Role of telomerase in cellular proliferation and cancer. *J Cell Physiol*, Vol. 180, No. 1, pp. (10-8), ISBN: 0021-9541.

Hsu, A.R., Hou, L.C., Veeravagu, A. et al. (2006). In vivo near-infrared fluorescence imaging of integrin alphavbeta3 in an orthotopic glioblastoma model. *Mol Imaging Biol*, Vol. 8, No. 6, pp. (315-23), ISBN: 1536-1632.

Hunter, C., Smith, R., Cahill, D.P. et al. (2006). A hypermutation phenotype and somatic MSH6 mutations in recurrent human malignant gliomas after alkylator chemotherapy. *Cancer research*, Vol. 66, No. 8, pp. (3987-91), ISBN: 0008-5472.

Huwyler, J., Wu, D. & Pardridge, W.M. (1996). Brain drug delivery of small molecules using immunoliposomes. *Proc Natl Acad Sci U S A*, Vol. 93, No. 24, pp. (14164-9), ISBN: 0027-8424.

Ichimura, K., Pearson, D.M., Kocialkowski, S. et al. (2009). IDH1 mutations are present in the majority of common adult gliomas but rare in primary glioblastomas. *Neuro-oncology*, Vol. 11, No. 4, pp. (341-7), ISBN: 1522-8517.

Idbaih, A., Ducray, F., Sierra Del Rio, M., Hoang-Xuan, K. & Delattre, J.Y. (2008). Therapeutic application of noncytotoxic molecular targeted therapy in gliomas: growth factor receptors and angiogenesis inhibitors. *Oncologist*, Vol. 13, No. 9, pp. (978-92), ISBN: 1549-490X.

Jacinto, F.V. & Esteller, M. (2007). MGMT hypermethylation: a prognostic foe, a predictive friend. *DNA Repair (Amst)*, Vol. 6, No. 8, pp. (1155-60), ISBN: 1568-7864.

Jain, R.K. (2001). Normalizing tumor vasculature with anti-angiogenic therapy: a new paradigm for combination therapy. *Nat Med*, Vol. 7, No. 9, pp. (987-9), ISBN: 1078-8956.

Jain, R.K. (2005). Normalization of tumor vasculature: an emerging concept in antiangiogenic therapy. *Science*, Vol. 307, No. 5706, pp. (58-62), ISBN: 1095-9203.

Jain, R.K., di Tomaso, E., Duda, D.G., Loeffler, J.S., Sorensen, A.G. & Batchelor, T.T. (2007). Angiogenesis in brain tumours. *Nat Rev Neurosci*, Vol. 8, No. 8, pp. (610-22), ISBN: 1471-003X.

Jansen, M., Yip, S. & Louis, D.N. (2010). Molecular pathology in adult gliomas: diagnostic, prognostic, and predictive markers. *Lancet neurology*, Vol. 9, No. 7, pp. (717-26), ISBN: 1474-4465.

Judge, A.D., Robbins, M., Tavakoli, I. et al. (2009). Confirming the RNAi-mediated mechanism of action of siRNA-based cancer therapeutics in mice. *The Journal of clinical investigation*, Vol. 119, No. 3, pp. (661-73), ISBN: 1558-8238.

Judson, I., Radford, J.A., Harris, M. et al. (2001). Randomised phase II trial of pegylated liposomal doxorubicin (DOXIL/CAELYX) versus doxorubicin in the treatment of advanced or metastatic soft tissue sarcoma: a study by the EORTC Soft Tissue and Bone Sarcoma Group. *Eur J Cancer*, Vol. 37, No. 7, pp. (870-7), ISBN: 0959-8049.

Kamoun, W.S., Ley, C.D., Farrar, C.T. et al. (2009). Edema control by cediranib, a vascular endothelial growth factor receptor-targeted kinase inhibitor, prolongs survival despite persistent brain tumor growth in mice. *J Clin Oncol*, Vol. 27, No. 15, pp. (2542-52), ISBN: 1527-7755.

Kappelle, A.C., Postma, T.J., Taphoorn, M.J. et al. (2001). PCV chemotherapy for recurrent glioblastoma multiforme. *Neurology*, Vol. 56, No. 1, pp. (118-20), ISBN: 0028-3878.

Kaur, B., Khwaja, F.W., Severson, E.A., Matheny, S.L., Brat, D.J. & Van Meir, E.G. (2005). Hypoxia and the hypoxia-inducible-factor pathway in glioma growth and angiogenesis. *Neuro-oncology*, Vol. 7, No. 2, pp. (134-53), ISBN: 1522-8517.

Khan, A., Benboubetra, M., Sayyed, P.Z. et al. (2004). Sustained polymeric delivery of gene silencing antisense ODNs, siRNA, DNAzymes and ribozymes: in vitro and in vivo studies. *J Drug Target*, Vol. 12, No. 6, pp. (393-404), ISBN: 1061-186X.

Kim, T.Y., Zhong, S., Fields, C.R., Kim, J.H. & Robertson, K.D. (2006). Epigenomic profiling reveals novel and frequent targets of aberrant DNA methylation-mediated silencing in malignant glioma. *Cancer research*, Vol. 66, No. 15, pp. (7490-501), ISBN: 0008-5472.

Knobbe, C.B., Merlo, A. & Reifenberger, G. (2002). Pten signaling in gliomas. *Neuro Oncol*, Vol. 4, No. 3, pp. (196-211), ISBN: 1522-8517.

Krakstad, C. & Chekenya, M. (2010). Survival signalling and apoptosis resistance in glioblastomas: opportunities for targeted therapeutics. *Mol Cancer*, Vol. 9, No. pp. (135), ISBN: 1476-4598.

Krauze, M.T., Noble, C.O., Kawaguchi, T. et al. (2007). Convection-enhanced delivery of nanoliposomal CPT-11 (irinotecan) and PEGylated liposomal doxorubicin (Doxil) in rodent intracranial brain tumor xenografts. *Neuro Oncol*, Vol. 9, No. 4, pp. (393-403), ISBN: 1522-8517.

Kreisl, T.N., Kim, L., Moore, K. et al. (2009). Phase II trial of single-agent bevacizumab followed by bevacizumab plus irinotecan at tumor progression in recurrent glioblastoma. *J Clin Oncol*, Vol. 27, No. 5, pp. (740-5), ISBN: 1527-7755.

Kreisl, T.N., Kotliarova, S., Butman, J.A. et al. (2010). A phase I/II trial of enzastaurin in patients with recurrent high-grade gliomas. *Neuro Oncol*, Vol. 12, No. 2, pp. (181-9), ISBN: 1523-5866.

Krex, D., Klink, B., Hartmann, C. et al. (2007). Long-term survival with glioblastoma multiforme. *Brain : a journal of neurology*, Vol. 130, No. 10, pp. (2596-606), ISBN: 1460-2156.

Kunwar, S., Prados, M.D., Chang, S.M. et al. (2007). Direct intracerebral delivery of cintredekin besudotox (IL13-PE38QQR) in recurrent malignant glioma: a report by the Cintredekin Besudotox Intraparenchymal Study Group. *J Clin Oncol*, Vol. 25, No. 7, pp. (837-44), ISBN: 1527-7755.

Lai, A., Filka, E., McGibbon, B. et al. (2008). Phase II pilot study of bevacizumab in combination with temozolomide and regional radiation therapy for up-front treatment of patients with newly diagnosed glioblastoma multiforme: interim analysis of safety and tolerability. *Int J Radiat Oncol Biol Phys*, Vol. 71, No. 5, pp. (1372-80), ISBN: 0360-3016.

Lai, A., Tran, A., Nghiemphu, P.L. et al. (2011). Phase II study of bevacizumab plus temozolomide during and after radiation therapy for patients with newly diagnosed glioblastoma multiforme. *J Clin Oncol*, Vol. 29, No. 2, pp. (142-8), ISBN: 1527-7755.

Lakka, S.S., Gondi, C.S., Dinh, D.H. et al. (2005). Specific interference of urokinase-type plasminogen activator receptor and matrix metalloproteinase-9 gene expression induced by double-stranded RNA results in decreased invasion, tumor growth, and angiogenesis in gliomas. *J Biol Chem*, Vol. 280, No. 23, pp. (21882-92), ISBN: 0021-9258.

Laterra, J.J., Grossman, S.A., Carson, K.A., Lesser, G.J., Hochberg, F.H. & Gilbert, M.R. (2004). Suramin and radiotherapy in newly diagnosed glioblastoma: phase 2 NABTT CNS Consortium study. *Neuro Oncol*, Vol. 6, No. 1, pp. (15-20), ISBN: 1522-8517.

Le, S., Zhu, J.J., Anthony, D.C., Greider, C.W. & Black, P.M. (1998). Telomerase activity in human gliomas. *Neurosurgery*, Vol. 42, No. 5, pp. (1120-5), ISBN: 0148-396X.

Lewis, D.L., Hagstrom, J.E., Loomis, A.G., Wolff, J.A. & Herweijer, H. (2002). Efficient delivery of siRNA for inhibition of gene expression in postnatal mice. *Nat Genet*, Vol. 32, No. 1, pp. (107-8), ISBN: 1061-4036.

Li, S., Wu, S.P., Whitmore, M. et al. (1999). Effect of immune response on gene transfer to the lung via systemic administration of cationic lipidic vectors. *Am J Physiol*, Vol. 276, No. 5 Pt 1, pp. (L796-804), ISBN: 0002-9513.

Li, X.Y., Zhang, L.Q., Zhang, X.G. et al. (2010). Association between AKT/mTOR signalling pathway and malignancy grade of human gliomas. *J Neurooncol*, Vol. No. pp. (Epub), ISBN: 1573-7373.

Lichota, J., Skjorringe, T., Thomsen, L.B. & Moos, T. (2009). Macromolecular drug transport into the brain using targeted therapy. *J Neurochem*, Vol. 113, No. 1, pp. (1-13), ISBN: 1471-4159.

Lidar, Z., Mardor, Y., Jonas, T. et al. (2004). Convection-enhanced delivery of paclitaxel for the treatment of recurrent malignant glioma: a phase I/II clinical study. *J Neurosurg*, Vol. 100, No. 3, pp. (472-9), ISBN: 0022-3085.

Lieberman, J., Song, E., Lee, S.K. & Shankar, P. (2003). Interfering with disease: opportunities and roadblocks to harnessing RNA interference. *Trends Mol Med*, Vol. 9, No. 9, pp. (397-403), ISBN: 1471-4914.

Lin, S.H. & Kleinberg, L.R. (2008). Carmustine wafers: localized delivery of chemotherapeutic agents in CNS malignancies. *Expert Rev Anticancer Ther*, Vol. 8, No. 3, pp. (343-59), ISBN: 1744-8328.

Louis, D.N., Ohgaki, H., Wiestler, O.D. et al. (2007). The 2007 WHO classification of tumours of the central nervous system. *Acta neuropathologica*, Vol. 114, No. 2, pp. (97-109), ISBN: 0001-6322.

Lundstrom, K. & Boulikas, T. (2003). Viral and non-viral vectors in gene therapy: technology development and clinical trials. *Technol Cancer Res Treat*, Vol. 2, No. 5, pp. (471-86), ISBN: 1533-0346.

Lustig, R., Mikkelsen, T., Lesser, G. et al. (2008). Phase II preradiation R115777 (tipifarnib) in newly diagnosed GBM with residual enhancing disease. *Neuro Oncol*, Vol. 10, No. 6, pp. (1004-9), ISBN: 1522-8517.

Ma, J., Li, S., Reed, K., Guo, P. & Gallo, J.M. (2003). Pharmacodynamic-mediated effects of the angiogenesis inhibitor SU5416 on the tumor disposition of temozolomide in subcutaneous and intracerebral glioma xenograft models. *J Pharmacol Exp Ther*, Vol. 305, No. 3, pp. (833-9), ISBN: 0022-3565.

Maeda, H., Bharate, G.Y. & Daruwalla, J. (2009). Polymeric drugs for efficient tumor-targeted drug delivery based on EPR-effect. *Eur J Pharm Biopharm*, Vol. 71, No. 3, pp. (409-19), ISBN: 1873-3441.

Maes, W., Deroose, C., Reumers, V. et al. (2009). In vivo bioluminescence imaging in an experimental mouse model for dendritic cell based immunotherapy against malignant glioma. *J Neurooncol*, Vol. 91, No. 2, pp. (127-39), ISBN: 0167-594X.

Manning, B.D. & Cantley, L.C. (2003). United at last: the tuberous sclerosis complex gene products connect the phosphoinositide 3-kinase/Akt pathway to mammalian target of rapamycin (mTOR) signalling. *Biochem Soc Trans*, Vol. 31, No. Pt 3, pp. (573-8), ISBN: 0300-5127.

Marx, G.M., Pavlakis, N., McCowatt, S. et al. (2001). Phase II study of thalidomide in the treatment of recurrent glioblastoma multiforme. *J Neurooncol*, Vol. 54, No. 1, pp. (31-8), ISBN: 0167-594X.

Masri, J., Bernath, A., Martin, J. et al. (2007). mTORC2 activity is elevated in gliomas and promotes growth and cell motility via overexpression of rictor. *Cancer Res*, Vol. 67, No. 24, pp. (11712-20), ISBN: 1538-7445.

Mayer, L.D., Masin, D., Nayar, R., Boman, N.L. & Bally, M.B. (1995). Pharmacology of liposomal vincristine in mice bearing L1210 ascitic and B16/BL6 solid tumours. *Br J Cancer*, Vol. 71, No. 3, pp. (482-8), ISBN: 0007-0920.

McCaffrey, A.P., Meuse, L., Pham, T.T., Conklin, D.S., Hannon, G.J. & Kay, M.A. (2002). RNA interference in adult mice. *Nature*, Vol. 418, No. 6893, pp. (38-9), ISBN: 0028-0836.

Messerer, C.L., Ramsay, E.C., Waterhouse, D. et al. (2004). Liposomal irinotecan: formulation development and therapeutic assessment in murine xenograft models of colorectal cancer. *Clin Cancer Res*, Vol. 10, No. 19, pp. (6638-49), ISBN: 1078-0432.

Morrissey, D.V., Lockridge, J.A., Shaw, L. et al. (2005). Potent and persistent in vivo anti-HBV activity of chemically modified siRNAs. *Nature biotechnology*, Vol. 23, No. 8, pp. (1002-7), ISBN: 1087-0156.

Mukai, S., Kondo, Y., Koga, S., Komata, T., Barna, B.P. & Kondo, S. (2000). 2-5A antisense telomerase RNA therapy for intracranial malignant gliomas. *Cancer Res*, Vol. 60, No. 16, pp. (4461-7), ISBN: 0008-5472.

Nakada, M., Okada, Y. & Yamashita, J. (2003). The role of matrix metalloproteinases in glioma invasion. *Front Biosci*, Vol. 8, No. 1, pp. (e261-9), ISBN: 1093-4715.

NCCN. (2011). National Comprehensive Cancer Network Clinical Practice Guidelines in Oncology. *In: Anaplastic Glioma/Glioblastoma*, Vol. Accessed in February 2011, No. pp. (Available from: www.nccn.org), ISBN:

Newlands, E.S., Stevens, M.F., Wedge, S.R., Wheelhouse, R.T. & Brock, C. (1997). Temozolomide: a review of its discovery, chemical properties, pre-clinical development and clinical trials. *Cancer Treat Rev*, Vol. 23, No. 1, pp. (35-61), ISBN: 0305-7372.

Nicholas, M.K., Lukas, R.V., Jafri, N.F., Faoro, L. & Salgia, R. (2006). Epidermal growth factor receptor - mediated signal transduction in the development and therapy of gliomas. *Clin Cancer Res*, Vol. 12, No. 24, pp. (7261-70), ISBN: 1078-0432.

Ningaraj, N.S. (2006). Drug delivery to brain tumours: challenges and progress. *Expert Opin Drug Deliv*, Vol. 3, No. 4, pp. (499-509), ISBN: 1742-5247.

Ningaraj, N.S., Rao, M. & Black, K.L. (2003). Calcium-dependent potassium channels as a target protein for modulation of the blood-brain tumor barrier. *Drug News Perspect*, Vol. 16, No. 5, pp. (291-8), ISBN: 0214-0934.

Nishikawa, M., Takemura, S., Takakura, Y. & Hashida, M. (1998). Targeted delivery of plasmid DNA to hepatocytes in vivo: optimization of the pharmacokinetics of plasmid DNA/galactosylated poly(L-lysine) complexes by controlling their physicochemical properties. *J Pharmacol Exp Ther*, Vol. 287, No. 1, pp. (408-15), ISBN: 0022-3565.

Noble, C.O., Krauze, M.T., Drummond, D.C. et al. (2006). Novel nanoliposomal CPT-11 infused by convection-enhanced delivery in intracranial tumors: pharmacology and efficacy. *Cancer Res*, Vol. 66, No. 5, pp. (2801-6), ISBN: 0008-5472.

Norden, A.D., Drappatz, J. & Wen, P.Y. (2009). Antiangiogenic therapies for high-grade glioma. *Nat Rev Neurol*, Vol. 5, No. 11, pp. (610-20), ISBN: 1759-4766.

Noushmehr, H., Weisenberger, D.J., Diefes, K. et al. (2010). Identification of a CpG island methylator phenotype that defines a distinct subgroup of glioma. *Cancer Cell*, Vol. 17, No. 5, pp. (510-22), ISBN: 1878-3686.

O'Brien, M.E., Wigler, N., Inbar, M. et al. (2004). Reduced cardiotoxicity and comparable efficacy in a phase III trial of pegylated liposomal doxorubicin HCl (CAELYX/Doxil) versus conventional doxorubicin for first-line treatment of metastatic breast cancer. *Ann Oncol*, Vol. 15, No. 3, pp. (440-9), ISBN: 0923-7534.

O'Connor, J.P., Jackson, A., Parker, G.J. & Jayson, G.C. (2007). DCE-MRI biomarkers in the clinical evaluation of antiangiogenic and vascular disrupting agents. *Br J Cancer*, Vol. 96, No. 2, pp. (189-95), ISBN: 0007-0920.

Ogris, M., Brunner, S., Schuller, S., Kircheis, R. & Wagner, E. (1999). PEGylated DNA/transferrin-PEI complexes: reduced interaction with blood components, extended circulation in blood and potential for systemic gene delivery. *Gene Ther*, Vol. 6, No. 4, pp. (595-605), ISBN: 0969-7128.

Ohgaki, H., Dessen, P., Jourde, B. et al. (2004). Genetic pathways to glioblastoma: a population-based study. *Cancer Res*, Vol. 64, No. 19, pp. (6892-9), ISBN: 0008-5472.

Ohvo-Rekila, H., Ramstedt, B., Leppimaki, P. & Slotte, J.P. (2002). Cholesterol interactions with phospholipids in membranes. *Prog Lipid Res*, Vol. 41, No. 1, pp. (66-97), ISBN: 0163-7827.

Pardridge, W.M. (2007). Blood-brain barrier delivery. *Drug Discov Today*, Vol. 12, No. 1-2, pp. (54-61), ISBN: 1359-6446.

Park, J.W., Benz, C.C. & Martin, F.J. (2004). Future directions of liposome- and immunoliposome-based cancer therapeutics. *Semin Oncol*, Vol. 31, No. 6 Suppl 13, pp. (196-205), ISBN: 0093-7754.

Pas, J., Wyszko, E., Rolle, K. et al. (2006). Analysis of structure and function of tenascin-C. *Int J Biochem Cell Biol*, Vol. 38, No. 9, pp. (1594-602), ISBN: 1357-2725.

Patchell, R.A., Regine, W.F., Ashton, P. et al. (2002). A phase I trial of continuously infused intratumoral bleomycin for the treatment of recurrent glioblastoma multiforme. *J Neurooncol*, Vol. 60, No. 1, pp. (37-42), ISBN: 0167-594X.

Patel, M.M., Goyal, B.R., Bhadada, S.V., Bhatt, J.S. & Amin, A.F. (2009). Getting into the brain: approaches to enhance brain drug delivery. *CNS Drugs*, Vol. 23, No. 1, pp. (35-58), ISBN: 1172-7047.

Perry, J.R., Belanger, K., Mason, W.P. et al. (2010). Phase II trial of continuous dose-intense temozolomide in recurrent malignant glioma: RESCUE study. *Journal of clinical oncology : official journal of the American Society of Clinical Oncology*, Vol. 28, No. 12, pp. (2051-7), ISBN: 1527-7755.

Pirollo, K.F., Zon, G., Rait, A. et al. (2006). Tumor-targeting nanoimmunoliposome complex for short interfering RNA delivery. *Hum Gene Ther*, Vol. 17, No. 1, pp. (117-24), ISBN: 1043-0342.

Porter, C.A. & Rifkin, R.M. (2007). Clinical benefits and economic analysis of pegylated liposomal doxorubicin/vincristine/dexamethasone versus doxorubicin/vincristine/dexamethasone in patients with newly diagnosed multiple myeloma. *Clin Lymphoma Myeloma*, Vol. 7 No. Suppl 4, pp. (S150-5), ISBN: 1557-9190.

Prados, M. (2002). Histology of Primary Tumors of the Central Nervous System. *American Cancer Society Atlas of Clinical Oncology: Brain Cancer*, Vol. 1, No. 1, pp. (29-103), ISBN: 1550090984

Prados, M.D., Chang, S.M., Butowski, N. et al. (2009). Phase II study of erlotinib plus temozolomide during and after radiation therapy in patients with newly diagnosed glioblastoma multiforme or gliosarcoma. *J Clin Oncol*, Vol. 27, No. 4, pp. (579-84), ISBN: 1527-7755.

Prakash, S., Malhotra, M. & Rengaswamy, V. (2010). Nonviral siRNA delivery for gene silencing in neurodegenerative diseases. *Methods Mol Biol*, Vol. 623, No. pp. (211-29), ISBN: 1940-6029.

Querbes, W., Ge, P., Zhang, W. et al. (2009). Direct CNS delivery of siRNA mediates robust silencing in oligodendrocytes. *Oligonucleotides*, Vol. 19, No. 1, pp. (23-29), ISBN: 1557-8526.

Raizer, J.J., Abrey, L.E., Lassman, A.B. et al. (2010). A phase II trial of erlotinib in patients with recurrent malignant gliomas and nonprogressive glioblastoma multiforme postradiation therapy. *Neuro Oncol*, Vol. 12, No. 1, pp. (95-103), ISBN: 1523-5866.

Ramsay, E., Alnajim, J., Anantha, M. et al. (2008). A novel liposomal irinotecan formulation with significant anti-tumour activity: use of the divalent cation ionophore A23187 and copper-containing liposomes to improve drug retention. *Eur J Pharm Biopharm*, Vol. 68, No. 3, pp. (607-17), ISBN: 0939-6411.

Rasheed, B.K., Stenzel, T.T., McLendon, R.E. et al. (1997). PTEN gene mutations are seen in high-grade but not in low-grade gliomas. *Cancer Res*, Vol. 57, No. 19, pp. (4187-90), ISBN: 0008-5472.

Razis, E., Selviaridis, P., Labropoulos, S. et al. (2009). Phase II study of neoadjuvant imatinib in glioblastoma: evaluation of clinical and molecular effects of the treatment. *Clin Cancer Res*, Vol. 15, No. 19, pp. (6258-66), ISBN: 1078-0432.

Recht, L., Torres, C.O., Smith, T.W., Raso, V. & Griffin, T.W. (1990). Transferrin receptor in normal and neoplastic brain tissue: implications for brain-tumor immunotherapy. *J Neurosurg*, Vol. 72, No. 6, pp. (941-5), ISBN: 0022-3085.

Rich, J.N., Reardon, D.A., Peery, T. et al. (2004). Phase II trial of gefitinib in recurrent glioblastoma. *J Clin Oncol*, Vol. 22, No. 1, pp. (133-42), ISBN: 0732-183X.

Rojiani, A.M. & Dorovini-Zis, K. (1996). Glomeruloid vascular structures in glioblastoma multiforme: an immunohistochemical and ultrastructural study. *J Neurosurg*, Vol. 85, No. 6, pp. (1078-84), ISBN: 0022-3085.

Rong, Y., Durden, D.L., Van Meir, E.G. & Brat, D.J. (2006). 'Pseudopalisading' necrosis in glioblastoma: a familiar morphologic feature that links vascular pathology, hypoxia, and angiogenesis. *Journal of neuropathology and experimental neurology*, Vol. 65, No. 6, pp. (529-39), ISBN: 0022-3069.

Rubin, L.L. & Staddon, J.M. (1999). The cell biology of the blood-brain barrier. *Annu Rev Neurosci*, Vol. 22, No. pp. (11-28), ISBN: 0147-006X.

Sadones, J., Michotte, A., Veld, P. et al. (2009). MGMT promoter hypermethylation correlates with a survival benefit from temozolomide in patients with recurrent anaplastic astrocytoma but not glioblastoma. *Eur J Cancer*, Vol. 45, No. 1, pp. (146-53), ISBN: 1879-0852.

Sakane, T., Yamashita, S., Yata, N. & Sezaki, H. (1999). Transnasal delivery of 5-fluorouracil to the brain in the rat. *J Drug Target*, Vol. 7, No. 3, pp. (233-40), ISBN: 1061-186X.

Santel, A., Aleku, M., Keil, O. et al. (2006). A novel siRNA-lipoplex technology for RNA interference in the mouse vascular endothelium. *Gene Ther*, Vol. 13, No. 16, pp. (1222-34), ISBN: 0969-7128.

Sarbassov, D.D., Ali, S.M., Kim, D.H. et al. (2004). Rictor, a novel binding partner of mTOR, defines a rapamycin-insensitive and raptor-independent pathway that regulates the cytoskeleton. *Curr Biol*, Vol. 14, No. 14, pp. (1296-302), ISBN: 0960-9822.

Sarbassov, D.D., Guertin, D.A., Ali, S.M. & Sabatini, D.M. (2005). Phosphorylation and regulation of Akt/PKB by the rictor-mTOR complex. *Science*, Vol. 307, No. 5712, pp. (1098-101), ISBN: 1095-9203.

Scherer, H.J. (1940). The forms of growth in gliomas and their practical significance. *Brain*, Vol. 1, No. 63, pp. (1-35), ISBN: NA.

Scheule, R.K., St George, J.A., Bagley, R.G. et al. (1997). Basis of pulmonary toxicity associated with cationic lipid-mediated gene transfer to the mammalian lung. *Hum Gene Ther*, Vol. 8, No. 6, pp. (689-707), ISBN: 1043-0342.

Schiffelers, R.M., Ansari, A., Xu, J. et al. (2004). Cancer siRNA therapy by tumor selective delivery with ligand-targeted sterically stabilized nanoparticle. *Nucleic Acids Res*, Vol. 32, No. 19, pp. (e149), ISBN: 1362-4962.

Schmidt, E.E., Ichimura, K., Goike, H.M., Moshref, A., Liu, L. & Collins, V.P. (1999). Mutational profile of the PTEN gene in primary human astrocytic tumors and cultivated xenografts. *J Neuropathol Exp Neurol*, Vol. 58, No. 11, pp. (1170-83), ISBN: 0022-3069.

Schneider, T., Becker, A., Ringe, K., Reinhold, A., Firsching, R. & Sabel, B.A. (2008). Brain tumor therapy by combined vaccination and antisense oligonucleotide delivery with nanoparticles. *Journal of neuroimmunology*, Vol. 195, No. 1-2, pp. (21-7), ISBN: 0165-5728.

Semple, S.C., Akinc, A., Chen, J. et al. (2010). Rational design of cationic lipids for siRNA delivery. *Nature biotechnology*, Vol. 28, No. 2, pp. (172-6), ISBN: 1546-1696.

Shah, K., Bureau, E., Kim, D.E. et al. (2005). Glioma therapy and real-time imaging of neural precursor cell migration and tumor regression. *Annals of neurology*, Vol. 57, No. 1, pp. (34-41), ISBN: 0364-5134.

Shi, N., Zhang, Y., Zhu, C., Boado, R.J. & Pardridge, W.M. (2001). Brain-specific expression of an exogenous gene after i.v. administration. *Proc Natl Acad Sci U S A*, Vol. 98, No. 22, pp. (12754-9), ISBN: 0027-8424.

Shoji, Y. & Nakashima, H. (2004). Current status of delivery systems to improve target efficacy of oligonucleotides. *Curr Pharm Des*, Vol. 10, No. 7, pp. (785-96), ISBN: 1381-6128.

Shuey, D.J., McCallus, D.E. & Giordano, T. (2002). RNAi: gene-silencing in therapeutic intervention. *Drug Discov Today*, Vol. 7, No. 20, pp. (1040-6), ISBN: 1359-6446.

Sioud, M. & Sorensen, D.R. (2003). Cationic liposome-mediated delivery of siRNAs in adult mice. *Biochem Biophys Res Commun*, Vol. 312, No. 4, pp. (1220-5), ISBN: 0006-291X.

Song, E., Lee, S.K., Wang, J. et al. (2003). RNA interference targeting Fas protects mice from fulminant hepatitis. *Nat Med*, Vol. 9, No. 3, pp. (347-51), ISBN: 1078-8956.

Sorensen, A.G., Batchelor, T.T., Zhang, W.T. et al. (2009). A "vascular normalization index" as potential mechanistic biomarker to predict survival after a single dose of cediranib in recurrent glioblastoma patients. *Cancer Res*, Vol. 69, No. 13, pp. (5296-300), ISBN: 1538-7445.

Sorensen, D.R., Leirdal, M. & Sioud, M. (2003). Gene silencing by systemic delivery of synthetic siRNAs in adult mice. *J Mol Biol*, Vol. 327, No. 4, pp. (761-6), ISBN: 0022-2836.

Sparks, C.A. & Guertin, D.A. (2010). Targeting mTOR: prospects for mTOR complex 2 inhibitors in cancer therapy. *Oncogene*, Vol. 29, No. 26, pp. (3733-44), ISBN: 1476-5594.

Storm, G. & Crommelin, D.J.A. (1998). Liposomes: quo vadis? *Pharmaceutical Science & Technology Today*, Vol. 1, No. 1, pp. (19-31), ISBN: 1461-5347.

Stupp, R., Hegi, M.E., Mason, W.P. et al. (2009). Effects of radiotherapy with concomitant and adjuvant temozolomide versus radiotherapy alone on survival in glioblastoma in a randomised phase III study: 5-year analysis of the EORTC-NCIC trial. *Lancet Oncol*, Vol. 10, No. 5, pp. (459-66), ISBN: 1474-5488.

Stupp, R., Hegi, M.E., Neyns, B. et al. (2010). Phase I/IIa study of cilengitide and temozolomide with concomitant radiotherapy followed by cilengitide and temozolomide maintenance therapy in patients with newly diagnosed glioblastoma. *J Clin Oncol*, Vol. 28, No. 16, pp. (2712-8), ISBN: 1527-7755.

Stupp, R., Hegi, M.E., van den Bent, M.J. et al. (2006). Changing paradigms--an update on the multidisciplinary management of malignant glioma. *Oncologist*, Vol. 11, No. 2, pp. (165-80), ISBN: 1083-7159.

Stupp, R., Mason, W.P., van den Bent, M.J. et al. (2005). Radiotherapy plus concomitant and adjuvant temozolomide for glioblastoma. *N Engl J Med*, Vol. 352, No. 10, pp. (987-96), ISBN: 1533-4406.

Tarnok, A., Ulrich, H. & Bocsi, J. (2009). Phenotypes of stem cells from diverse origin. *Cytometry A*, Vol. 77, No. 1, pp. (6-10), ISBN: 1552-4930.

Thakker, D.R., Natt, F., Husken, D. et al. (2005). siRNA-mediated knockdown of the serotonin transporter in the adult mouse brain. *Mol Psychiatry*, Vol. 10, No. 8, pp. (782-9, 714), ISBN: 1359-4184.

Thorne, R.G., Emory, C.R., Ala, T.A. & Frey, W.H., 2nd. (1995). Quantitative analysis of the olfactory pathway for drug delivery to the brain. *Brain Res*, Vol. 692, No. 1-2, pp. (278-82), ISBN: 0006-8993.

Thorne, R.G., Pronk, G.J., Padmanabhan, V. & Frey, W.H., 2nd. (2004). Delivery of insulin-like growth factor-I to the rat brain and spinal cord along olfactory and trigeminal pathways following intranasal administration. *Neuroscience*, Vol. 127, No. 2, pp. (481-96), ISBN: 0306-4522.

Ting, A.H., McGarvey, K.M. & Baylin, S.B. (2006). The cancer epigenome--components and functional correlates. *Genes & development*, Vol. 20, No. 23, pp. (3215-31), ISBN: 0890-9369.

Turner, C.D., Gururangan, S., Eastwood, J. et al. (2002). Phase II study of irinotecan (CPT-11) in children with high-risk malignant brain tumors: the Duke experience. *Neuro Oncol*, Vol. 4, No. 2, pp. (102-108), ISBN: 1522-8517.

Vajkoczy, P. & Menger, M.D. (2000). Vascular microenvironment in gliomas. *J Neurooncol*, Vol. 50, No. 1-2, pp. (99-108), ISBN: 0167-594X.

Vajkoczy, P. & Menger, M.D. (2004). Vascular microenvironment in gliomas. *Cancer Treat Res*, Vol. 117, No. pp. (249-62), ISBN: 0927-3042.

Vajkoczy, P., Schilling, L., Ullrich, A., Schmiedek, P. & Menger, M.D. (1998). Characterization of angiogenesis and microcirculation of high-grade glioma: an intravital multifluorescence microscopic approach in the athymic nude mouse. *J Cereb Blood Flow Metab*, Vol. 18, No. 5, pp. (510-20), ISBN: 0271-678X.

Verreault, M., Stegeman, A., Warburton, C., Strutt, D., Masin, D. & Bally, M. (2011a). Combined RNAi mediated suppression of Rictor and EGFR inhibits tumor growth in an orthotopic glioblastoma tumor model. *In revision for Plos One*.

Verreault, M., Strutt, D., Masin, D. et al. (2011b). Irinophore C™, a lipid-based nanoparticulate formulation of irinotecan, is more effective than free irinotecan when used to treat an orthotopic glioblastoma model. *J Control Release*, Oct 5, [Epub ahead of print]

Verreault, M., Strutt, D., Masin, D. et al. (2011c). Vascular normalization in orthotopic glioblastoma following intravenous treatment with lipid-based nanoparticulate formulations of irinotecan (Irinophore CTM), doxorubicin (Caelyx®) or vincristine. *BMC Cancer*, Vol. Apr 8, No. 11, pp. (124).

Verreault, M., Strutt, D., Masin, D., Fink, D., Gill, R. & Bally, M. (2011d). Development of glioblastoma cell lines expressing red fluorescence for non-invasive live imaging of intracranial tumors *Anticancer Research*, Vol. 31, No. 6, pp. (2161-71).

Verreault, M., Webb, M.S., Ramsay, E.C. & Bally, M.B. (2006). Gene silencing in the development of personalized cancer treatment: the targets, the agents and the delivery systems. *Curr Gene Ther*, Vol. 6, No. 4, pp. (505-33), ISBN: 1566-5232.

Vogelstein, B. & Kinzler, K.W. (1993). The multistep nature of cancer. *Trends Genet*, Vol. 9, No. 4, pp. (138-41), ISBN: 0168-9525.

Vredenburgh, J.J., Desjardins, A., Reardon, D.A. & Friedman, H.S. (2009). Experience with irinotecan for the treatment of malignant glioma. *Neuro Oncol*, Vol. 11, No. 1, pp. (80-91), ISBN: 1522-8517.

Wager, M., Menei, P., Guilhot, J. et al. (2008). Prognostic molecular markers with no impact on decision-making: the paradox of gliomas based on a prospective study. *Br J Cancer*, Vol. 98, No. 11, pp. (1830-8), ISBN: 1532-1827.

Walker, C., du Plessis, D.G., Joyce, K.A. et al. (2003). Phenotype versus genotype in gliomas displaying inter- or intratumoral histological heterogeneity. *Clinical cancer research : an official journal of the American Association for Cancer Research*, Vol. 9, No. 13, pp. (4841-51), ISBN: 1078-0432.

Walker, M.D., Alexander, E., Jr., Hunt, W.E. et al. (1978). Evaluation of BCNU and/or radiotherapy in the treatment of anaplastic gliomas. A cooperative clinical trial. *J Neurosurg*, Vol. 49, No. 3, pp. (333-43), ISBN: 0022-3085.

Walker, M.D., Green, S.B., Byar, D.P. et al. (1980). Randomized comparisons of radiotherapy and nitrosoureas for the treatment of malignant glioma after surgery. *N Engl J Med*, Vol. 303, No. 23, pp. (1323-9), ISBN: 0028-4793.

Wang, D., Gao, Y. & Yun, L. (2006). Study on brain targeting of raltitrexed following intranasal administration in rats. *Cancer Chemother Pharmacol*, Vol. 57, No. 1, pp. (97-104), ISBN: 0344-5704.

Wang, F., Jiang, X. & Lu, W. (2003). Profiles of methotrexate in blood and CSF following intranasal and intravenous administration to rats. *Int J Pharm*, Vol. 263, No. 1-2, pp. (1-7), ISBN: 0378-5173.

Wen, P.Y. & Kesari, S. (2008). Malignant gliomas in adults. *The New England journal of medicine*, Vol. 359, No. 5, pp. (492-507), ISBN: 1533-4406.

Wen, P.Y., Yung, W.K., Lamborn, K.R. et al. (2006). Phase I/II study of imatinib mesylate for recurrent malignant gliomas: North American Brain Tumor Consortium Study 99-08. *Clin Cancer Res*, Vol. 12, No. 16, pp. (4899-907), ISBN: 1078-0432.

Wick, W., Puduvalli, V.K., Chamberlain, M.C. et al. (2010). Phase III study of enzastaurin compared with lomustine in the treatment of recurrent intracranial glioblastoma. *J Clin Oncol*, Vol. 28, No. 7, pp. (1168-74), ISBN: 1527-7755.

Winkler, F., Kozin, S.V., Tong, R.T. et al. (2004). Kinetics of vascular normalization by VEGFR2 blockade governs brain tumor response to radiation: role of oxygenation, angiopoietin-1, and matrix metalloproteinases. *Cancer Cell*, Vol. 6, No. 6, pp. (553-63), ISBN: 1535-6108.

Wolburg, H., Noell, S., Mack, A., Wolburg-Buchholz, K. & Fallier-Becker, P. (2009). Brain endothelial cells and the glio-vascular complex. *Cell Tissue Res*, Vol. 335, No. 1, pp. (75-96), ISBN: 1432-0878.

Wu, X., Rauch, T.A., Zhong, X. et al. (2010). CpG island hypermethylation in human astrocytomas. *Cancer research*, Vol. 70, No. 7, pp. (2718-27), ISBN: 1538-7445.

Wyszko, E., Rolle, K., Nowak, S. et al. (2008). A multivariate analysis of patients with brain tumors treated with ATN-RNA. *Acta Pol Pharm*, Vol. 65, No. 6, pp. (677-84), ISBN: 0001-6837.

Xie, Z. & Chin, L.S. (2008). Molecular and cell biology of brain tumor stem cells: lessons from neural progenitor/stem cells. *Neurosurg Focus*, Vol. 24, No. 3-4, pp. (E25), ISBN: 1092-0684.

Yamanaka, R., Arao, T., Yajima, N. et al. (2006). Identification of expressed genes characterizing long-term survival in malignant glioma patients. *Oncogene*, Vol. 25, No. 44, pp. (5994-6002), ISBN: 0950-9232.

Yan, H., Parsons, D.W., Jin, G. et al. (2009). IDH1 and IDH2 mutations in gliomas. *The New England journal of medicine*, Vol. 360, No. 8, pp. (765-73), ISBN: 1533-4406.

Yip, S., Iafrate, A.J. & Louis, D.N. (2008). Molecular diagnostic testing in malignant gliomas: a practical update on predictive markers. *Journal of neuropathology and experimental neurology*, Vol. 67, No. 1, pp. (1-15), ISBN: 0022-3069.

Yip, S., Miao, J., Cahill, D.P. et al. (2009). MSH6 mutations arise in glioblastomas during temozolomide therapy and mediate temozolomide resistance. *Clinical cancer research : an official journal of the American Association for Cancer Research*, Vol. 15, No. 14, pp. (4622-9), ISBN: 1078-0432.

Yip, S., Sabetrasekh, R., Sidman, R.L. & Snyder, E.Y. (2006). Neural stem cells as novel cancer therapeutic vehicles. *European journal of cancer*, Vol. 42, No. 9, pp. (1298-308), ISBN: 0959-8049.

Yip, S. & Shah, K. (2008). Stem-cell based therapies for brain tumors. *Current opinion in molecular therapeutics*, Vol. 10, No. 4, pp. (334-42), ISBN: 1464-8431.

Yuan, F., Salehi, H.A., Boucher, Y., Vasthare, U.S., Tuma, R.F. & Jain, R.K. (1994). Vascular permeability and microcirculation of gliomas and mammary carcinomas transplanted in rat and mouse cranial windows. *Cancer Res*, Vol. 54, No. 17, pp. (4564-8), ISBN: 0008-5472.

Zhang, Y., Boado, R.J. & Pardridge, W.M. (2003). Marked enhancement in gene expression by targeting the human insulin receptor. *J Gene Med*, Vol. 5, No. 2, pp. (157-63), ISBN: 1099-498X.

Zhang, Y., Zhang, Y.F., Bryant, J., Charles, A., Boado, R.J. & Pardridge, W.M. (2004). Intravenous RNA interference gene therapy targeting the human epidermal growth factor receptor prolongs survival in intracranial brain cancer. *Clin Cancer Res*, Vol. 10, No. 11, pp. (3667-77), ISBN: 1078-0432.

Zhang, Y., Zhu, C. & Pardridge, W.M. (2002). Antisense gene therapy of brain cancer with an artificial virus gene delivery system. *Mol Ther*, Vol. 6, No. 1, pp. (67-72), ISBN: 1525-0016.

Zhou, R., Mazurchuk, R. & Straubinger, R.M. (2002). Antivasculature effects of doxorubicin-containing liposomes in an intracranial rat brain tumor model. *Cancer Res*, Vol. 62, No. 9, pp. (2561-6), ISBN: 0008-5472.

Zimmermann, T.S., Lee, A.C., Akinc, A. et al. (2006). RNAi-mediated gene silencing in non-human primates. *Nature*, Vol. 441, No. 7089, pp. (111-4), ISBN: 1476-4687.

Zukiel, R., Nowak, S., Wyszko, E. et al. (2006). Suppression of human brain tumor with interference RNA specific for tenascin-C. *Cancer Biol Ther*, Vol. 5, No. 8, pp. (1002-7), ISBN: 1538-4047.

10

Hypoxia Responsive Vectors Targeting Astrocytes in Glioma

Manas R. Biswal[1], Howard M. Prentice[2] and Janet C. Blanks[1,2*]
[1]*Center for Complex Systems and Brain Sciences, Charles E. Schmidt College of Science,*
[2]*Charles E. Schmidt College of Medicine,*
Florida Atlantic University, Boca Raton, Fl
USA

1. Introduction

Gliomas are the most common brain tumor in the central nervous system (CNS). The majority of malignant gliomas arise from neoplastic transformation of resident astrocytes. Gliomas are very aggressive tumors since they are characterized by widespread invasion of brain tissue. The exact pathogenesis and underlying mechanisms for glioma cell infiltration are currently unclear. Cell-cell interaction and tissue microenvironment play an important role in tumor progression leading to modification and infiltration of surrounding tissue. The hypoxic microenvironment contributes to abnormal neovascularization of the glioma.

Uncontrolled cellular proliferation, abnormal angiogenesis and invasion of surrounding tissue make these tumors difficult to treat. Poor prognosis and ineffective treatments for glioma point to the necessity of developing new therapeutic strategies. The use of gene therapy to deliver a therapeutic gene may successfully overcome the failure of conventional therapies. Although non-cell specific and unregulated promoters have been used to target gliomas, it is possible that unregulated vectors elicit damage in cells that do not require the therapeutic protein. Thus it may be of value to design a regulated, tissue-specific vector to express a therapeutic protein in a specific cell type and to regulate it according to the local tissue environment.

The hypoxic microenvironment is known to play a major role in several conditions including cerebral ischemia, retinal angiogenesis, gliomas, and other cancers. Hypoxia inducible factor 1 alpha (HIF-1α), the most common transcription factor induced during hypoxia, binds to a hypoxia regulated enhancer (HRE) region of oxygen sensitive genes leading to their transcription. By taking advantage of hypoxia for regulating foreign gene expression, a hypoxia regulated vector could be exploited to modify the cells that reside within the target tissue. Use of a cell-specific promoter would be an added advantage to restrict gene expression only in certain cells.

Our recently developed vector platform works in a manner such that in an hypoxic environment, HIF-1α will bind to the HRE region and express the foreign protein in a cell-

* Corresponding Author

specific manner. These vectors were designed to prevent neovascularization in the eye. Using a hypoxia regulated, retinal pigment epithelial cell (RPE)-specific promoter, a vector was developed which leads to expression of a therapeutic gene only in RPE cells. By driving expression of the human endostatin gene, this vector prevented neovascularization in the laser induced mouse model of choroidal neovascularization. Another gene therapy vector was constructed using the human GFAP promoter along with several hypoxia regulated enhancer and silencer elements. Both of these vectors have been tested in different cell lines to show specificity and hypoxic-inducibility. The regulated promoter is active only during the conditions of hypoxia, and shows significantly enhanced induction of reporter genes, especially in primary rat astrocytes in culture.

Our hypoxia-regulated, astrocyte-specific vector has the capacity to restrict its expression to astrocytes and can be expressed only in the hypoxic microenvironment thus remaining inactive both under hypoxic and normoxic conditions in other cells. This vector has a unique potential for treating pathology in which astrocytes and an hypoxic environment play a major role in disease progression. Our goal is to use our regulated astrocyte-specific promoter in vectors designed to target gliomas in which both astrocytes and a hypoxic microenvironment are involved. Potential therapeutic proteins can be added to the downstream region of the promoter to prevent abnormal angiogenesis, induce apoptosis in tumor cells and/or prevent invasion and infiltration of the glioma. The following points will be discussed in section 2 through 6.

a. Importance of gene therapy to target gliomas utilizing the hypoxic micro-environment.
b. Design and testing of hypoxia-regulated astrocyte- specific promoter.
c. Vector choice and route of delivery.
d. Therapeutic window for treatment of gliomas.
e. Future directions and limitations of proposed treatment.

2. Importance of gene therapy to target gliomas utilizing the hypoxic micro-environment

Gliomas are tumors of the CNS which arise from glial cells. They are divided into several types depending on clinical features and histopathology. According to the WHO classification, gliomas can be classified into fours grades depending upon their malignancies: Grade 1 covers benign tumors (e.g. pilocytic astrocytoma), and group II to IV are malignant neoplasias which differ in aggressiveness. The most aggressive glioblastoma belongs to group IV. Histopathologically, gliomas are divided into astrocytomas, oligodendrocytomas and glioblastomas depending upon the type of macroglial cell. The most common form of gliomas in humans is the astrocytoma, and the most aggressive form of astrocytomas is glioblastoma multiforme (GBM.)

Gliomas are characterized by their active propagation through nervous tissue. There is a limitation of space for glioma growth in the CNS due to existence of firm boundaries (skull for the brain and vertebra for the spinal cord). In order to grow, gliomas must clear space by actively eliminating the surrounding healthy cells and actively propagate neoplasmic cells in the brain parenchyma. Malignant gliomas produce space for expansion by secreting increased amounts of excitatory neurotransmitters which kill neighboring neurons. First, they express metalloproteinases which assist in breaking down the extracellular matrix and producing migrating channels. Second, glioma cells are able to undergo substantial shrinkage, which helps them attain an elongated shape and thus penetrate into narrow interstitial compartments.

Poor prognosis, short survival time and poor response to chemotherapeutic drug intervention make glioma a devastating disease. The reason for the poor efficacy of these agents includes the selectivity of the blood brain barrier, the heterogeneity and low immunogenicity of gliomas and appropriate selection of chemotherapy-resistant clones. New therapeutic strategies are therefore needed to treat this devastating tumor. Since multiple genes determine the severity of glioma progression and invasion, theoretically the design of a therapeutic strategy could be targeted utilizing the tumor microenvironment. A major set of therapeutic targets could involve changes in the molecular pathways associated with the hypoxic environment.

2.1 Molecular basis of glioma

Molecular and genetic approaches have provided dramatic insights into glioma biology. As part of the intensive effort to determine the process of glioma formation, several molecular defects have been implicated in gliomas. These genes affect encoded proteins involved in several critical biologic processes, including signal transduction, cell growth, cell cycle control or proliferation, apoptosis and differentiation.

An hypoxic microenvironment is a frequent characteristic of GBM since these tumors exhibit abnormal neovascularization, irregular blood flow, and a high rate of oxygen consumption by the rapidly proliferating malignant cells. Regions of low oxygen concentration are a characteristic feature of growing tumors and are frequently found around necrotic areas. Hypoxic microenvironments are powerful stimuli for the expression of genes involved in tumor cell proliferation, angiogenesis and immuno-suppression. Tumor hypoxia activates a complex set of cellular responses which are differentially regulated by two members of hypoxia-inducible transcription factors family; hypoxia inducible factors 1 and 2 (HIF-1 and HIF-2). It has been shown that HIFs control tumor stem cell phenotype and the acquisition or maintenance of stem cell properties (Seidel et al., 2010).

2.2 Significance of hypoxia in glioma

Histological studies suggest that gliomas are abnormally vascularized due to highly proliferating tumor cells which exhibit slow or inefficient blood flow. Evans et al have shown that the physiological oxygen concentration varies between 2.5% to 12.5% in healthy brain tissue. The majority of GBMs examined showed mild to moderate/severe hypoxia with oxygen concentration ranging between 0.5% to 2.5% to (pO2 = 20-40mm Hg) for mild hypoxia and 0.5%-0.1 % (pO2 0.75mm to 4 mm Hg) for moderate/severe hypoxia (Evans et al., 2004a, Evans et al., 2004b, Evans et al., 2008). Although some researchers do not include moderate hypoxia as major factor in the pathogensis of glioma, an oxygen tension of 0.5% to 2.5% would likely be appropriate to model the hypoxic environment since HIF-1 elevation occurs in GBM patients (Kaynar et al., 2008).

There are several cellular responses to hypoxia and all are controlled by the expression of different transcription factors which are called hypoxia inducible factors (HIF-1-3α). These transcription factors produce dimerization with HIF-1β which is expressed constitutively followed by translocation to the nucleus. Under normal conditions, HIF1 α is expressed ubiquitously at low levels in all organs. The HIF-1α subunit has an oxygen-dependent degradation domain which leads to rapid ubiquination and degradation by the proteasome **(Figure 1)**. During hypoxia, the hydroxylation of HIF-1α is inhibited, leading to accumulation of HIF-1α protein. The accumulated HIF-1 binds to hypoxia responsive regions (HREs) of several genes inducing their transcription. Many of these genes play a critical role in important aspects of cancer biology: angiogenesis, cell survival, chemotherapy, radiation-resistance, genomic instability, invasion and metastasis, and glucose metabolism (Bar et al., 2010).

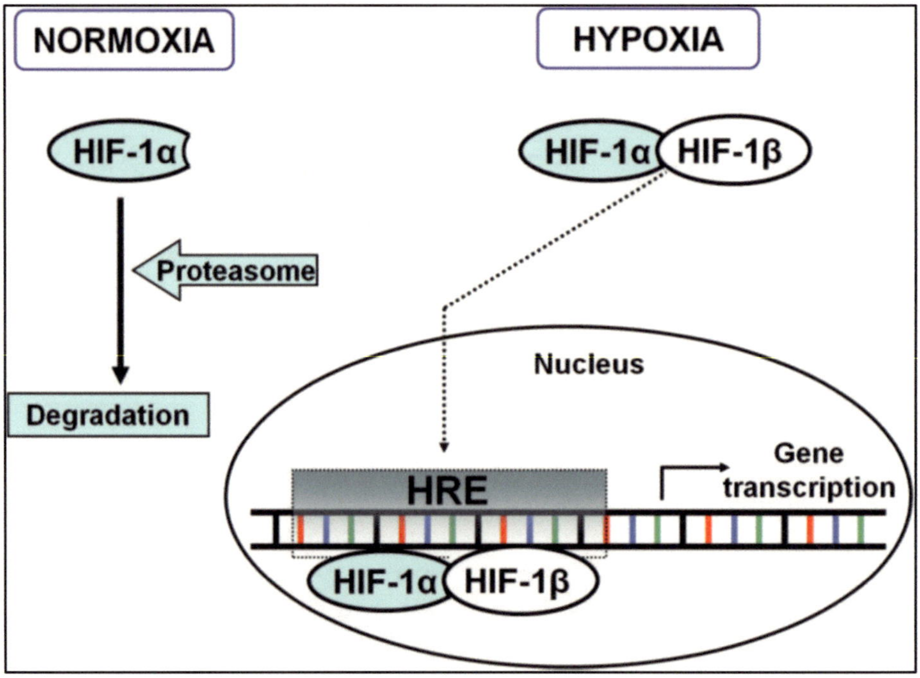

Fig. 1. Hypoxia induces the expression of hypoxia inducible factors (HIF-1) which are composed of two subunits HIF-1α and HIF-1β. During normoxia HIF-1α is degraded by the proteasomal ubiquitination. In absence of oxygen HIF-1α is stabilized by binding with HIF-1β to form HIF-1. The HIF-1 translocates into the nucleus and binds to sequence of hypoxia responsiveelement (HRE) of several genes to induce the gene transcription.

2.3 Hypoxia promotes angiogenesis, glioma cell migration and immunosuppression

Hypoxia induced HIFs act as a proangiogenic switch to drive angiogenesis in gliomas. HIF is expressed inside tumor cells and astrocytes in response to changes in oxygen availability of the surrounding tissue. HIF-1 stimulates the expression of the potent angiogenic factor, vascular endothelial growth factor (VEGF). VEGF belongs to the family of growth factors which include VEGF-A, VEGF-B, VEGF-C, VEGF-D, VEGF-E and Placental growth factor. VEGF-A also exists with different splice variants (VEGF 121, 145, 165, 189 and 206). Different cell surface receptors for VEGF are expressed in endothelial cells. VEGF is regarded to be the major factor for development of new vessels both in physiological and pathological angiogenesis. VEGFs not only stimulate the proliferation of endothelial cells, but they are also responsible for migration, vascular permeability and invasiveness during the angiogenic process. Production of high levels of VEGF is reported in cystic fluid and also around necrotic tissue in GBM patients (Brat and Van Meir, 2004).

Other than VEGF, HIF-1 also stimulates the expression of other angiogenic growth factors which include placental growth factor, basic fibroblast growth factor (bFGF), early growth factor, platelet growth factor Beta (PDGF-β), angiopoietin-1 (Ang1) and-2 (Ang-2). Along with the receptors for vascular proliferation, the endothelial cells express several receptor tyrosine kinases like Tie-1 and Tie-2 which regulate vessel remodeling, maturation and endothelial survival (Nawroth et al., 1993). Ang-1 facilitates the stabilization of new blood vessels and prevents leakiness, whereas in response to availability of VEGF, Ang-2 causes vascular remodeling and growth of new blood vessels. In the absence of Ang-2, regression of vessels occurs (Holash et al., 1999). The levels of angiopoetins and Tie-2 are greatly elevated in GBM samples indicating profuse tumor vascularity and invasiveness (Reiss et al., 2005).

Another potent growth factor, TGF-β and its receptor are highly expressed in gliomal tissues. These growth factors are activated by several proteases and integrins in the hypoxic microenvironment. TGF-beta regulates angiogenesis by activating several growth factors and their receptors including bFGF, PDGF, PDGFR, and EGFR. TGF-B affects angiogenesis by stimulating tumor cells to secrete VEGF and integrins which facilitates the motility of endothelial cells within the glioblastoma tumor.

Glioma cell migration and invasion depends on HIF-1 induced extracellular matrix proteases. Matrix metaloproteases (MMPs) play a major role in extracellular matrix (ECM) degradation and facilitate proliferation and migration of endothelial cells to produce new blood vessels. MMPs also modulate several growth factors and cytokines which affect the endothelial and tumor cell migration ultimately inducing angiogenesis. Lolmede et.al., 2003 reported that several MMPs, including MMP-1, MMP-1, MMP-7 and MMP-9, are activated by HIF-1 dependent pathways (Lolmede et al., 2003). HIF-1 activates TGF-β2, which further regulates the activity of MMPs resulting in suppression of tissue inhibitor of metalloproteases (TIMPs) (Wick et al., 2001). The level of MMP-1 expression is upregulated in several cancers and activates the expression of MMP2 in gliomal cells. Tumor prognosis and vascularity are directly related to the expression of MMPs in gliomas.

Tumor hypoxia can activate the pSTAT3 pathway which triggers the downstream expression of HIF-1α. In gliomas, several immunosuppressive cytokines, including TGF-β, soluble colony stimulating factor-1 (sCSF-1), chemokine ligand 2 (CCL2) and galectin expression, are induced by HIF during hypoxia. Macrophages (microglia) are the dominant infiltrating cells in gliomas. These macrophages become tumor-associated macrophages (TAM) when exposed to the hypoxic tumor microenvironment. The TAMS contribute towards tumor angiogenesis and invasion by activating the STAT3 pathway ultimately resulting in immuno-suppression and tumor supportive phenotypes. HIF -1 promotes expansion of CD133 positive glioma cancer stem cells (gCSCs) which play a role in immuno-suppression. Up-regulation of expression of macrophage migration inhibitory factor genes (MIFs) in glial cells is associated with glioma and promotes tumor angiogenesis and immunosuppression (Bacher et al., 2003).

2.4 Hypoxia as the therapeutic target

Since hypoxia modulates the glioma progression and metastasis, it can be targeted to minimize hypoxic effects on tumor cells. Several HIF-1 inhibiting agents have been used to inhibit the growth and spread of tumor cells (Jensen, 2009). Although activation of HIF-1 induces tumorgenesis, it is also necessary for normal cellular function including physiological angiogenesis, growth and survival. Therefore it is not wise to inhibit the activity of HIF-1 completely using anti-HIF agents. Several strategies have been developed to express therapeutic proteins under hypoxic conditions under the control of an HRE containing promoter (Ruan and Deen, 2001).

HIF-1 binds to the region of HRE elements and activates gene expression. An expression vector using hypoxia inducible cytosine deaminase has been used for cancer in a pro-drug activation strategy (Wang et al., 2005). During hypoxia, cytosine deaminase is expressed and converts a non-toxic 5-fluorcytosine to the highly toxic chemotherapeutic agent 5-fluoruracil. Several researchers are using this approach to activate enzymes required for apoptosis or tissue protection by the process of pro-drug activation (Binley et al., 1999, Ruan et al., 1999, Shibata et al., 2000, Cao et al., 2001). Along with hypoxia regulated expression, tissue-specific expression may increase the possibilities to turn on genes in a regulated and tissue-specific manner. McKie EA (1998) used a GFAP promoter to target astrocytes for expression of transgenes as a potential treatment strategy for glioblastoma (McKie et al., 1998). Hypoxia could be used to switch on a foreign gene in glioma cells or in astrocytes. We have designed an hypoxia-regulated, astrocyte-specific vector which will lead to gene expression only in hypoxic astrocytes while restricting expression in normoxia and other cell types.

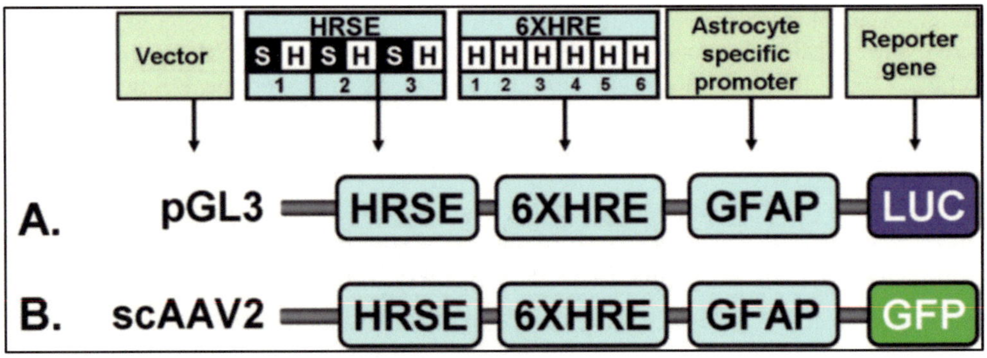

Fig. 2. Construction of hypoxia-regulated astrocyte –specific vector. Three copies of neuron restrictive silencer sequence (S) and three copies of hypoxia responsive element (HRE) sequence were alternated in a combination to make hypoxia responsive silencer elements (HRSE). This sequence provides conditional silencing in normoxia and induces gene expression in hypoxia. Similarly 6 copies of HRE sequence were combined together to make 6XHRE for enhanced hypoxic induction. A) Sequences of HRSE, 6XHRE and human glial fibrillary acidic protein (GFAP) promoter are incorporated into pGL3-basic vector to drive luciferase (LUC) gene expression. B) Sequences of HRSE, 6XHRE and human GFAP promoter are incorporated into self complementary Adeno Associated Virus plasmid vector (scAAV) to make scAAV2 virus which drives the green fluorescent protein (GFP) gene.

3. Design and testing of hypoxia-regulated, astrocyte- specific promoter

Astrocyte specific expression in transgenic mice was shown by Lee *et.al.* in 2008 (Lee et al., 2008). Different conserved domains of the GFAP promoter are used to demonstrate astrocytic specific reporter gene expression. A promoter domain designated Gfabc1d (GFAP) consisting of selected subdomains of the GFAP promoter was shown to exhibit region and astrocyte specific transgene expression in the brain of a transgenic rat. Our lab developed an hypoxia regulated vector (Dougherty et al., 2008) in which a hypoxia responsive enhancer was used together with the retinal pigment epithelial cell (RPE65) (Dougherty et al.). This promoter cassette drives cell-specific and hypoxia responsive transgene expression in cell culture. It was used successfully to drive transgene expression of an anti-angiogenic agent to prevent the neovascularization in the mouse eye following laser treatment (personal communication). These positive results lead us to develop another cell-specific promoter to drive gene expression in astrocytes during hypoxia.

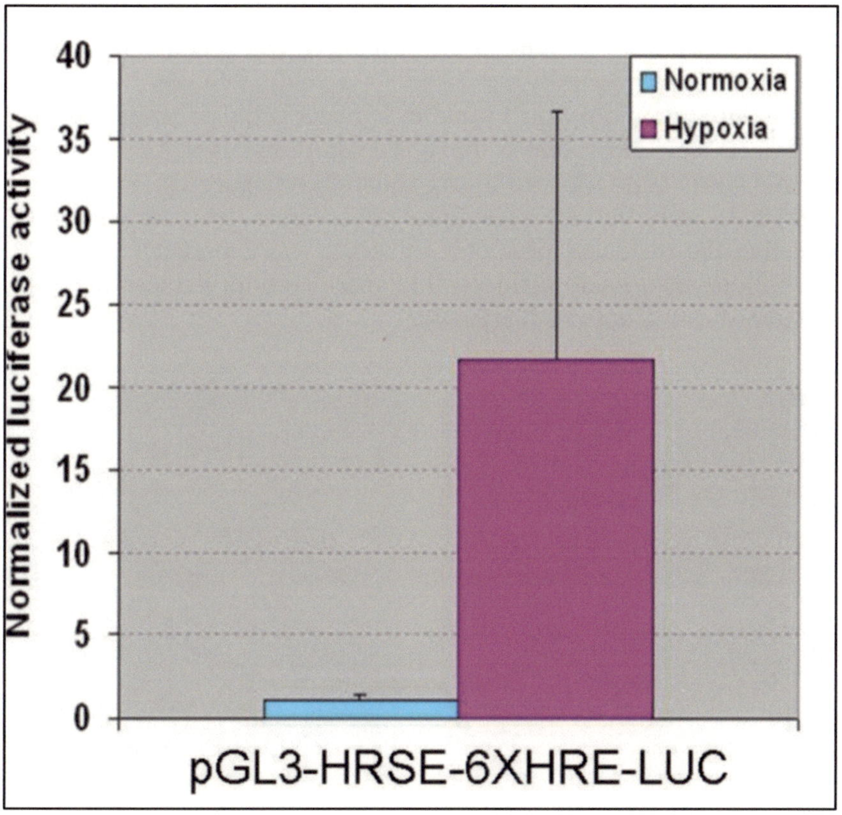

Fig. 3. Hypoxia responsive luciferase expression controlled by the regulated promoter in astrocytes. pGL3-HRSE-6XHRE-Luc plasmid was transfected to rat primary astrocytes. The transfected cells were exposed to either 0.5 % hypoxia or normoxia. After 40hrs of hypoxic or normoxic exposure, for testing the activity of the promoter, luciferase gene expression was measured using Promega's Dual Glow luciferase assay kit (DLA). The activity of regulated promoter showed more than 15-fold induction in hypoxia compared to its normoxc counterpart.

We have designed astrocyte-specific promoters in a pGL3 based vector containing hypoxia responsive elements (HREs), silencer domains and the human GFAP promoter that provide both cell specificity and hypoxia inducible expression as well as normoxic silencing. The human GFAP promoter in a plasmid vector was a generous gift from Dr. Brenner (University of Alabama, Birmingham, AL). The promoter element was amplified and ligated to a pGL3 basic vector to drive the luciferase reporter gene. This construct was named pGL3-GFAP-Luc and is referred to as the unregulated plasmid vector. The addition of 6 copies of the HRE element (Dougherty et al., 2008) will be a target for HIF-1 to bind to and hence turn on gene expression during hypoxia. Incorporation of a silencer element (HRSE) (Dougherty et al., 2008) to the HRE will prevent the expression of the transgene in normoxia and maximize the expression of the transgene in hypoxia. The newly constructed plasmid pGL3-HRSE-6XHRE-GFAP-Luc is referred to as regulated plasmid vector **(Figure 2A).**

Rat primary astrocytes and other cell lines were transfected with the plasmids using lipofectamine. After 40 hours of hypoxic or normoxic exposure, the dual luciferase assay was performed to measure the activity of the promoters. Our preliminary results show that the GFAP promoter was modestly activated (< 3 fold), whereas the regulated GFAP promoter was induced by more than 15-fold in hypoxia and was tissue specific **(Figure 3)**. Promoter constructs were incorporated into a self-complementary Adeno Associated Virus (scAAV) plasmid vector and produced in large quantities **(Figure 2B)**. Vector specificity and hypoxia regulation were tested in cultures of primary rat astrocytes. Our results demonstrated that the regulated promoter construct was completely silenced in aerobic conditions in cultures of primary astrocyte. Hypoxic-exposure induced high levels of GFP expression in transduced astrocytes **(Figure 4)**.

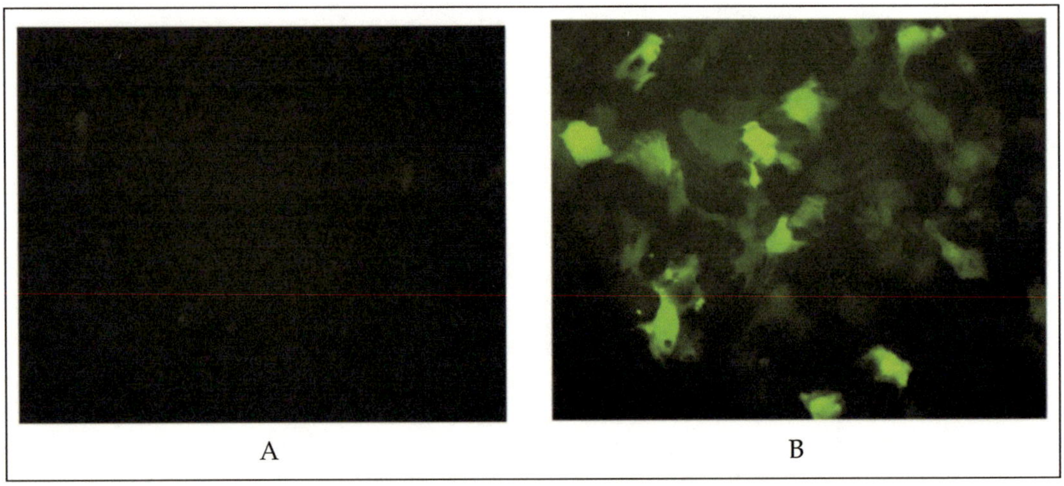

Fig. 4. Hypoxia responsive GFP expression from the regulated vector. scAAV2-HRSE-6XHRE-GFAP-GFP virus vector was transduced tinto primary rat astrocytes (1 X 10^3 viral particles per cell). After 3 days of transduction, the cells were exposed to either 0.5% hypoxia or normoxia for 6 days. In normoxia, the transduced astrocytes do not express GFP (A) whereas in hypoxia, the transduced astrocytes show high level induction of the promoter by expressing GFP (B).

4. Vector choice and route of delivery

Although current therapeutic interventions provide improvements in glioma therapy, these treatments do not result in long term cures. Development of gene therapy could be a potential strategy for long term treatment of GBM. Glioma is an ideal target for gene therapy because, unlike other solid tumors, it rarely metastasizes outside the CNS. Over 30 clinical trials using gene therapy vectors have been initiated with more than 400 glioma patients enrolled worldwide.

The major requirement of gene therapy is to develop vectors which are safe and efficient to deliver the therapeutic genes to a targeted cell type. Several viral and non-viral vectors are being used to transfer genes in both experimental models and clinical research applications. Although non-viral methods have advantages over the viral methods in terms of their large scale production and low host immunogenicity, low levels of transfection and expression of the gene limit their use. Mostly viral vectors have been used as vehicles to carry exogenous genes into human cells since they bind to the host cell and introduce genetic material into the cytoplasm or nucleus as a part of their replication cycle. Viruses used in glioma gene therapy generally fall into two categories: replication incompetent viruses (from which all or most of its genome has been removed) and replication competent viruses (where select viral genes are deleted or mutated so that viruses can replicate and lyse tumor cells selectively) to minimize toxicity and retain gene delivery efficiency (Iwami et al., 2010). Adenoviruses (AdV) or retrovirus (RVs) have both been used in clinical trials to treat gliomas.

Expression of a therapeutic protein depends on choice of vector and the route of delivery. There are several possible routes of delivery including systemic administration, stereotactic injection, intratumoral injection, intramuscular injection, and facial vein injection. Liposomal delivery of HSV-tk has been used to target gliomas using cationic liposomes carrying the human interferon beta gene (Yoshida et al., 2004) in a clinical trial. Adeno viral mediated HSV TK along with the pro-drug ganciclovier was used to treat human glioma (Immonen et al., 2004). Lenti-viral mediated transfer of GAS1 (Lopez-Ornelas et al., 2011) to human gliomas has been used to arrest cell proliferation, cause apoptosis and inhibit tumor growth. A combinational therapy using baculovirus-mediated expression of p53 along with sodium butyrate was also tested to treat human glioblastoma (Guo et al., 2011). AAV is one of the preferred vectors for gene therapy since it is less immunogenic and has an increased rate of transduction efficiency. Research using a variety of serotypes or mutations in the vector capsids has led to better vectors to target specific cell types for expression of the therapeutic protein. It may be preferable to produce a regulated or modest amount of transgene expression (McCarty et al., 2003) in a greater number of cells rather than overproduction in a small number of cells.

Despite its limited capacity in harboring larger size genes, development of the scAAV genome advances AAV gene therapy due to increased transduction efficiency. The scAAV genome is proven to be very suitable for both dividing and non-dividing cells in transgenic mice (Choi et al., 2006). The scAAV has also been used to target both neurons and glia using either intrathalamic or intraventricular injection (Chen et al., 1998, Chen et al., 1999). AAV mediated HSV-tk was targeted in mice bearing human glioma in conjunction with ganciclovir administration (Mizuno et al., 1998). Intramuscular injection of AAV has been used to deliver angiostatin to suppress glioma growth in nude mice (Ma et al., 2002).

Similarly AAV-8 was used to deliver soluble VEGF receptor to the CNS to trap the VEGF in orthotopic brain tumor models of GBM (Harding et al., 2006).

AAV mediated expression of the c-terminal fragment of the human telomerase reverse transcriptase gene (hTERTC27) has proven to be highly effective to reduce tumor growth in human glioblastoma xenografts mouse model (Ng et al., 2007). A chimeric AAV capsid was developed to enhance glioma cell transduction (Maguire et al., 2010). Stereotaxic injections of different AAV serotypes into the striatum of rat brain are reported to enhance glial delivery of the therapeutic protein. Intravenous or intracisternal injection of scAAV2 vectors have been used to study global distribution and dispersion of AAV in a mouse brain (Fu et al., 2003). Although several serotypes of AAV were used, it has been reported that AAV5 and AAV9 appears to best for enhanced glial transduction (Foust et al., 2009, Markakis et al., 2010).

5. Gene therapy strategies for glioma

An extensive range of genes and their signaling pathways contribute to glioma development and the level of severity. It may not be appropriate to consider only one gene or factor for prevention of glioma in a therapeutic strategy. Combinational therapy and pro-drug activation are now being used along with chemotherapy and radiation therapy. The most effective gene therapy strategy in use both in experimental and clinical gene therapy trials employs HSV-tk. While it may prevent the tumor growth initially, HSV-tk cannot reduce glioma growth at a later stage due to its dependence for cell killing on gap junctions between tumor cells. Ultimately a more effective strategy for cell killing may involve developing vectors which can target the local tumor environment.

5.1 Use of cytotoxic or suicidal approach

The suicidal gene therapy approach has been the most generally used in gene therapy clinical trials for glioma. The HSV-tk method which requires a pro-drug to elicit its effect is extensively employed for this purpose. HSV-tk enhances the sensitivity of transduced tumor cells towards the non toxic pro-drug ganciclovir, acyclovir or valaciclovier and then metabolizes the pro-drug into a cytotoxic agent which acts as a potent inhibitor of DNA replication (Tiberghien, 1994, Tiberghien et al., 1994). Several vectors have been used to drive expression of HSV-tk for killing of tumor cells. The effectiveness of suicidal gene therapy mediated by HRE cre/lox driving HSV-tk has been evaluated in a model of tumor xenografts implanted in nude mice (Greco et al., 2006). In a similar strategy a hypoxia regulated expression vector was used to drive the expression of cytosine deaminase gene which activates another pro-drug 5-fluorocytosine to form the highly toxic 5-fluoruracil (Chen et al., 2005, Wang et al., 2005). This cytotoxic compound was able to significantly kill glioblastoma cells in a hypoxia-dependent manner while exerting no toxicity on normal cells. Hypoxia regulated carboxyl esterase expression has been generated using an adeno viral based gene expression system, resulting in conversion of a pro-drug Irinotecan (CPT-11) to its active cytotoxic metabolite which is capable of killing glioma cells (Matzow et al., 2007). Based upon the above evidence of the feasibility of employing hypoxia regulated gene expression in a suicide gene therapy strategy, our vector may be highly applicable for delivering therapeutic genes in astrocytes for control over tumor growth.

5.2 Gene targets involving cell cycle arrest and apoptosis

Transfer of cell cycle genes could be a good strategy for blocking glioma growth (Fueyo et al., 2001). The E2F family of transcription factors contributes to the regulation of cell cycle and cell death genes in glioma. It has been shown that over expression of E2F-1 enhances the anti-glioma effect through increasing apoptosis in human glioma cells (Mitlianga et al., 2002). Another important strategy may be to induce cell cycle arrest and prevent the proliferation of the tumor cells. Soluble form of Gas1 protein is being used by lenti-viral gene transfer methods to arrest the cell cycle (Lopez-Ornelas et al., 2011), (Zamorano et al., 2003), (Zamorano et al., 2004) and preventing the proliferation of glioma cells in nude mice. Hypoxia regulated expression of these proteins has been proposed as a viable approach that can be applied to tumor killing.

The tumor cytokines TNF alpha and IFN beta are very good candidates for inducing apoptosis in hypoxic glioma cells when the respective genes are incorporated into our hypoxia regulated vector. The secretable form of trimeric Tumor Necrosis Factor-Related Apoptosis-Inducing Ligand (TRAIL) has been employed for to targeting gliomas and inducing apoptosis in glioblastoma (Jeong et al., 2009) and TRAIL therefore is also an excellent candidate for incorporation into a regulated gene therapy vector. Overexpression of bone morphogenetic protein (BMP4) was employed to induce apoptosis in glioma stem cells (Zhou et al., 2011) and therefore BMP4 represents a good candidate for enhancing tumor killing. Numerous studies have demonstrated detailed mechanisms by which BMP4 acts to induce BAX and inhibit BCl2 as well as Bcl-X family members. Glioma cells exhibit low endoplasmic reticulum (ER) stress. It is possible that over-expression of ER stress factors could be effective for inducing apoptosis in glioma. ER stress induces C/EBP homologous protein (CHOP) which is a key regulator for cellular apoptosis (Eom et al., 2010). Regulated expression of CHOP would also be valid for inducing apoptosis in tumor cells (Kim et al., 2011).

Gliomas can be targeted by overexpression of micro RNAs (miR). It has been demonstrated that miRs also play an important role in regulation of oncogenes and/or tumor suppressor genes at the post-transcriptional and/or translational level. Oligonucleotides mimicking miR-451 are used to inhibit cell growth, induce G0/G1 phase arrest and enhance apoptosis in different glioma cell lines. Targeting miR-451 also decreases the expression levels of Akt1, CyclinD1, MMP-2, MMP-9 and Bcl-2 genes while increasing expression of the tumor suppressor genes p27 in dose dependent manner (Nan et al., 2010). Adenoviral mediated co-expression of shRNAs for miR-221 and 221 have been used to induce apoptosis in tumor cells (Wang et al., 2011). Mir-34a was overexpressed in a p53 mutant glioma cell line with resulting induction of apoptosis.

Inhibition of MMPs may be a valuable strategy for suppressing glioma growth in regulated manner through induction of apoptosis. In a previous study siRNA mediated downregulation of urokinase-type plasminogen activator receptor (uPAR) and matrix metalloproteinase-9 (MMP-9) were employed to activate caspase-9 mediated apoptosis in glioma (Gondi et al., 2008). It is reported that miR-21 is involved in regulation of genes for glioma cell proliferation, migration and invasion through activation of several MMPs. Downregulation of miR-21 may be an effective strategy for blocking the expression of MMPs and for activating tissue inhibitor of metalloproteinases in glioma cells (Gabriely et al., 2008).

5.3 Anti angiogenic approach

Tumor hypoxia is implicated as a major stimulus for the growth of new blood vessels in tumor angiogenesis through inducing expression of most potent angiogenic factor VEGF. Tumor angiogenesis facilitates the invasion of tumor cells into normal tissue. Inhibiting pro-angiogenic factors such as VEGF, targeting VEGF receptors and over expressing endogenous anti angiogenic factors holds promise as a good strategy to prevent tumor angiogenesis. Since HIF-1α mediates increased tumor aggressiveness in hypoxia, direct inhibition of HIF-1α with siRNA may be effectively used to suppress glioma cell growth and reduce tumor invasiveness in a glioma model (Fujiwara et al., 2007). Targeting of VEGF signaling pathways and their receptors would provide an efficient treatment for glioma angiogenesis. Regulated expression of endogenous anti angiogenic factors (endostatin, angiostatin, pigment epithelial derived factor (PEDF), thrombospondin-1) could be beneficial in conjunction with other chemotherapeutic agents. Intra-arterial delivery of plasmids carrying the endostatin gene results in an 80% reduction in tumor volume, a 40% decrease in tumor angiogenesis and increases the survival time of up to 47% in a rat model of solitary intracerebral 9L tumors (Barnett et al., 2004). Co-delivery of a angiostatin-endostatin fusion gene and soluble VEGF receptor (sFLT-1) by a sleeping beauty transposon completely inhibited tumor growth and enhanced the survival of animals in an experimental GBM model (Ohlfest et al., 2005). AAV mediated delivery of angiostatin was used to treat the malignant brain tumor in a C6 glioma/Wistar rat model with a resulting inhibition of tumor growth and enhanced time of animal survival (Ma et al., 2002).

Antisense TGF-beta and soluble VEGF receptors have been exploited to reduce glioma gowth (Harding et al., 2006). Overall it has been seen that glioma can evade anti angiogenic therapy by up-regulating alternative signaling pathways such as the ILK-1 pathway (Verpelli et al., 2010). Targeting both TGF-beta and VEGF pathways simultaneously shows promise for an improved treatment strategy. Over-expression of PEDF could also be exploited using our regulated vector and in this case the likely results would include activities that are neuroprotective and anti-angiogenic (Zhang et al., 2007). Over expression of PEDF has recently been shown to inhibit tumor malignancy in a rodent glioma model (Guan et al., 2004).

6. Future directions for development of hypoxia regulated anti glioma treatment

Gene therapy strategies have been broadly applied to treat all forms of glioma. Although expression of suicidal genes in tumor cells is effective to a degree in clinical trials, there is a risk that the suicidal genes can express in normal cells with detrimental effects. Use of cell type specific or cancer cell specific promoters may have advantages over universal promoters by restricting gene expression to the desired cells without damaging other cells collaterally. The use of vectors driving hypoxia-regulated astrocyte-specific expression of genes could be an effective strategy to target tumor cell apoptosis, cell cycle arrest and inhibition of key regulators for tumor angiogenesis.

One of the advantages of a hypoxia regulated promoter is it can restrict the expression of genes to hypoxic astrocytes within and in close proximity to the tumor core while avoiding production of the therapeutic protein in neighboring normal cells which may occur when universal promoters are employed. Until now, surgical removal of tumor tissue in combination with radiotherapy has been a relatively effective strategy for treating glioma. However one of the major problems is the recurrence of the tumor which is associated with ROS induced HIF-1 expression. Upon recurrence of glioma the enhanced HIF-1 levels desensitize glioma cells to further treatment. The regulated vector could be employed to resensitize the tumor cells to be more responsive to chemotherapy. Some oncogenes induce HIF-1 in tumor cells in the absence of hypoxia (Lim et al., 2004). Our vector can be used to respond to HIF expression specifically in glial cells should HIF-1 be activated by any of the oncogenes.

Chapter summary

- The hypoxic microenvironment is known to play a major role in several diseases including age related macular degeneration, cardiac and cerebral ischemia, glioma, and other cancers.
- Many endogenous genes that are induced during hypoxia are activated by the binding of the transcription factor HIF-1α to a hypoxia regulated enhancer (HRE) region in their promoter domain.
- For effective gene therapy, there is a great need for a vector that can be regulated according to the local tissue microenvironment.
- By taking advantage of hypoxia for regulating foreign gene expression, a hypoxia regulated vector including hypoxia regulated enhancer could be exploited to modify the cells that reside within the target tissue.
- Gliomas are the most common brain tumors in the central nervous system and the majority of malignant gliomas arise from neoplastic transformation of resident astrocytes.
- Our hypoxia-regulated, astrocyte-specific vector has the capacity to restrict its expression to astrocytes and can be expressed only in the hypoxic microenvironment thus remaining inactive both under hypoxic and normoxic conditions in other cells.
- A variety of therapeutic gene products could be delivered by our hypoxia-regulated promoter to prevent abnormal angiogenesis and induce apoptosis in tumor cells leading to prevention of invasion and infiltration of the glioma into surrounding tissue.
- One of the major problems in surgical removal of tumor tissue is the recurrence of glioma and the enhanced HIF-1 levels desensitize glioma cells to further treatment. The regulated vector could be employed to resensitize the tumor cells to be more responsive to chemotherapy.

As a combinational therapeutic strategy our hypoxia regulated promoter could be employed for expressing therapeutic genes encoding an anti-angiogenic factor in addition to a tumor suppressor gene. The scope and applications of our hypoxia –regulated gene therapy are shown in figure 5. Our strategy of hypoxia-regulated gene therapy may obviate the need for radiation therapy and chemotherapy and may be beneficial in terms of preventing tumor growth as well as eradication of residual cancer cells in instances where a glioma is removed surgically.

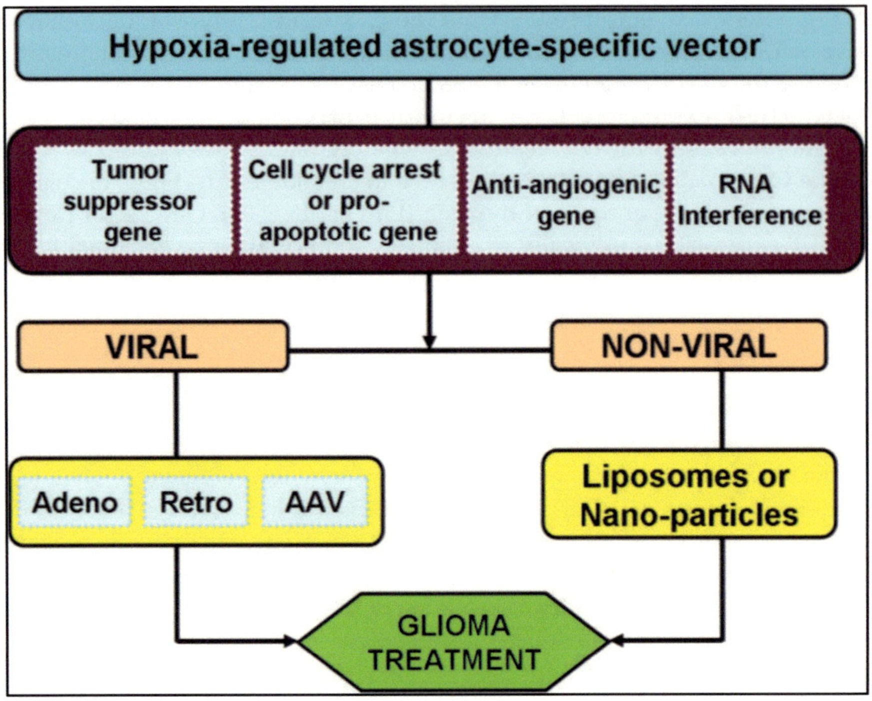

Fig. 5. Strategy for hypoxia-regulated astrocyte-specific gene therapy to treat glioma. The regulated-promoter can be applied to drive expression of genes responsible for tumor suppressor, cell cycle arrest, pro-apoptotic and inhibition of pro-angiogenic processes in astrocytes . The plasmid vectors can be packaged into either viral (Adeno, Retro and AAV) vectors or non-viral liposomes or nano-particles as a potential glioma treatment strategy.

7. References

Bacher M, Schrader J, Thompson N, Kuschela K, Gemsa D, Waeber G, Schlegel J (Up-regulation of macrophage migration inhibitory factor gene and protein expression in glial tumor cells during hypoxic and hypoglycemic stress indicates a critical role for angiogenesis in glioblastoma multiforme. Am J Pathol 162:11-17.2003).

Bar EE, Lin A, Mahairaki V, Matsui W, Eberhart CG (Hypoxia increases the expression of stem-cell markers and promotes clonogenicity in glioblastoma neurospheres. Am J Pathol 177:1491-1502.2010).

Barnett FH, Scharer-Schuksz M, Wood M, Yu X, Wagner TE, Friedlander M (Intra-arterial delivery of endostatin gene to brain tumors prolongs survival and alters tumor vessel ultrastructure. Gene Ther 11:1283-1289.2004).

Binley K, Iqball S, Kingsman A, Kingsman S, Naylor S (An adenoviral vector regulated by hypoxia for the treatment of ischaemic disease and cancer. Gene Ther 6:1721-1727.1999).

Brat DJ, Van Meir EG (Vaso-occlusive and prothrombotic mechanisms associated with tumor hypoxia, necrosis, and accelerated growth in glioblastoma. Lab Invest 84:397-405.2004).

Cao YJ, Shibata T, Rainov NG (Hypoxia-inducible transgene expression in differentiated human NT2N neurons--a cell culture model for gene therapy of postischemic neuronal loss. Gene Ther 8:1357-1362.2001).

Chen G, Song L, Zhu X, Zhang X, Zhang C, Wang T, Tang J (Effect of adeno-associated virus-mediated transfer of low density lipoprotein receptor gene on treatment of hypercholesterolemia. Sci China C Life Sci 41:435-441.1998).

Chen H, McCarty DM, Bruce AT, Suzuki K (Oligodendrocyte-specific gene expression in mouse brain: use of a myelin-forming cell type-specific promoter in an adeno-associated virus. J Neurosci Res 55:504-513.1999).

Chen JK, Hu LJ, Wang J, Lamborn KR, Kong EL, Deen DF (Hypoxia-induced BAX overexpression and radiation killing of hypoxic glioblastoma cells. Radiat Res 163:644-653.2005).

Choi VW, McCarty DM, Samulski RJ (Host cell DNA repair pathways in adeno-associated viral genome processing. J Virol 80:10346-10356.2006).

Dougherty CJ, Smith GW, Dorey CK, Prentice HM, Webster KA, Blanks JC (Robust hypoxia-selective regulation of a retinal pigment epithelium-specific adeno-associated virus vector. Mol Vis 14:471-480.2008).

Eom KS, Kim HJ, So HS, Park R, Kim TY (Berberine-induced apoptosis in human glioblastoma T98G cells is mediated by endoplasmic reticulum stress accompanying reactive oxygen species and mitochondrial dysfunction. Biol Pharm Bull 33:1644-1649.2010).

Evans SM, Jenkins KW, Jenkins WT, Dilling T, Judy KD, Schrlau A, Judkins A, Hahn SM, Koch CJ (Imaging and analytical methods as applied to the evaluation of vasculature and hypoxia in human brain tumors. Radiat Res 170:677-690.2008).

Evans SM, Judy KD, Dunphy I, Jenkins WT, Hwang WT, Nelson PT, Lustig RA, Jenkins K, Magarelli DP, Hahn SM, Collins RA, Grady MS, Koch CJ (Hypoxia is important in the biology and aggression of human glial brain tumors. Clin Cancer Res 10:8177-8184.2004a).

Evans SM, Judy KD, Dunphy I, Jenkins WT, Nelson PT, Collins R, Wileyto EP, Jenkins K, Hahn SM, Stevens CW, Judkins AR, Phillips P, Geoerger B, Koch CJ (Comparative measurements of hypoxia in human brain tumors using needle electrodes and EF5 binding. Cancer Res 64:1886-1892.2004b).

Foust KD, Nurre E, Montgomery CL, Hernandez A, Chan CM, Kaspar BK (Intravascular AAV9 preferentially targets neonatal neurons and adult astrocytes. Nat Biotechnol 27:59-65.2009).

Fu H, Muenzer J, Samulski RJ, Breese G, Sifford J, Zeng X, McCarty DM (Self-complementary adeno-associated virus serotype 2 vector: global distribution and broad dispersion of AAV-mediated transgene expression in mouse brain. Mol Ther 8:911-917.2003).

Fueyo J, Gomez-Manzano C, Liu TJ, Yung WK (Delivery of cell cycle genes to block astrocytoma growth. J Neurooncol 51:277-287.2001).

Fujiwara S, Nakagawa K, Harada H, Nagato S, Furukawa K, Teraoka M, Seno T, Oka K, Iwata S, Ohnishi T (Silencing hypoxia-inducible factor-1alpha inhibits cell migration and invasion under hypoxic environment in malignant gliomas. Int J Oncol 30:793-802.2007).

Gabriely G, Wurdinger T, Kesari S, Esau CC, Burchard J, Linsley PS, Krichevsky AM (MicroRNA 21 promotes glioma invasion by targeting matrix metalloproteinase regulators. Mol Cell Biol 28:5369-5380.2008).

Gondi CS, Dinh DH, Gujrati M, Rao JS (Simultaneous downregulation of uPAR and MMP-9 induces overexpression of the FADD-associated protein RIP and activates caspase 9-mediated apoptosis in gliomas. Int J Oncol 33:783-790.2008).

Greco O, Joiner MC, Doleh A, Powell AD, Hillman GG, Scott SD (Hypoxia- and radiation-activated Cre/loxP 'molecular switch' vectors for gene therapy of cancer. Gene Ther 13:206-215.2006).

Guan M, Pang CP, Yam HF, Cheung KF, Liu WW, Lu Y (Inhibition of glioma invasion by overexpression of pigment epithelium-derived factor. Cancer Gene Ther 11:325-332.2004).

Guo H, Choudhury Y, Yang J, Chen C, Tay FC, Lim TM, Wang S (Antiglioma effects of combined use of a baculovirual vector expressing wild-type p53 and sodium butyrate. J Gene Med 13:26-36.2011).

Harding TC, Lalani AS, Roberts BN, Yendluri S, Luan B, Koprivnikar KE, Gonzalez-Edick M, Huan-Tu G, Musterer R, VanRoey MJ, Ozawa T, LeCouter RA, Deen D, Dickinson PJ, Jooss K (AAV serotype 8-mediated gene delivery of a soluble VEGF receptor to the CNS for the treatment of glioblastoma. Mol Ther 13:956-966.2006).

Holash J, Maisonpierre PC, Compton D, Boland P, Alexander CR, Zagzag D, Yancopoulos GD, Wiegand SJ (Vessel cooption, regression, and growth in tumors mediated by angiopoietins and VEGF. Science 284:1994-1998.1999).

Immonen A, Vapalahti M, Tyynela K, Hurskainen H, Sandmair A, Vanninen R, Langford G, Murray N, Yla-Herttuala S (AdvHSV-tk gene therapy with intravenous ganciclovir improves survival in human malignant glioma: a randomised, controlled study. Mol Ther 10:967-972.2004).

Iwami K, Natsume A, Wakabayashi T (Gene therapy for high-grade glioma. Neurol Med Chir (Tokyo) 50:727-736.2010).

Jensen RL (Brain tumor hypoxia: tumorigenesis, angiogenesis, imaging, pseudoprogression, and as a therapeutic target. J Neurooncol 92:317-335.2009).

Jeong M, Kwon YS, Park SH, Kim CY, Jeun SS, Song KW, Ko Y, Robbins PD, Billiar TR, Kim BM, Seol DW (Possible novel therapy for malignant gliomas with secretable trimeric TRAIL. PLoS One 4:e4545.2009).

Kaynar MY, Sanus GZ, Hnimoglu H, Kacira T, Kemerdere R, Atukeren P, Gumustas K, Canbaz B, Tanriverdi T (Expression of hypoxia inducible factor-1alpha in tumors of patients with glioblastoma multiforme and transitional meningioma. J Clin Neurosci 15:1036-1042.2008).

Kim IY, Kang YJ, Yoon MJ, Kim EH, Kim SU, Kwon TK, Kim IA, Choi KS (Amiodarone sensitizes human glioma cells but not astrocytes to TRAIL-induced apoptosis via CHOP-mediated DR5 upregulation. Neuro Oncol 13:267-279.2011).

Lee Y, Messing A, Su M, Brenner M (GFAP promoter elements required for region-specific and astrocyte-specific expression. Glia 56:481-493.2008).

Lim JH, Lee ES, You HJ, Lee JW, Park JW, Chun YS (Ras-dependent induction of HIF-1alpha785 via the Raf/MEK/ERK pathway: a novel mechanism of Ras-mediated tumor promotion. Oncogene 23:9427-9431.2004).

Lolmede K, Durand de Saint Front V, Galitzky J, Lafontan M, Bouloumie A (Effects of hypoxia on the expression of proangiogenic factors in differentiated 3T3-F442A adipocytes. Int J Obes Relat Metab Disord 27:1187-1195.2003).

Lopez-Ornelas A, Mejia-Castillo T, Vergara P, Segovia J (Lentiviral transfer of an inducible transgene expressing a soluble form of Gas1 causes glioma cell arrest, apoptosis and inhibits tumor growth. Cancer Gene Ther 18:87-99.2011).

Ma HI, Lin SZ, Chiang YH, Li J, Chen SL, Tsao YP, Xiao X (Intratumoral gene therapy of malignant brain tumor in a rat model with angiostatin delivered by adeno-associated viral (AAV) vector. Gene Ther 9:2-11.2002).

Maguire CA, Gianni D, Meijer DH, Shaket LA, Wakimoto H, Rabkin SD, Gao G, Sena-Esteves M (Directed evolution of adeno-associated virus for glioma cell transduction. J Neurooncol 96:337-347.2010).

Markakis EA, Vives KP, Bober J, Leichtle S, Leranth C, Beecham J, Elsworth JD, Roth RH, Samulski RJ, Redmond DE, Jr. (Comparative transduction efficiency of AAV vector serotypes 1-6 in the substantia nigra and striatum of the primate brain. Mol Ther 18:588-593.2010).

Matzow T, Cowen RL, Williams KJ, Telfer BA, Flint PJ, Southgate TD, Saunders MP (Hypoxia-targeted over-expression of carboxylesterase as a means of increasing tumour sensitivity to irinotecan (CPT-11). J Gene Med 9:244-252.2007).

McCarty DM, Fu H, Monahan PE, Toulson CE, Naik P, Samulski RJ (Adeno-associated virus terminal repeat (TR) mutant generates self-complementary vectors to overcome the rate-limiting step to transduction in vivo. Gene Ther 10:2112-2118.2003).

McKie EA, Graham DI, Brown SM (Selective astrocytic transgene expression in vitro and in vivo from the GFAP promoter in a HSV RL1 null mutant vector--potential glioblastoma targeting. Gene Ther 5:440-450.1998).

Mitlianga PG, Gomez-Manzano C, Kyritsis AP, Fueyo J (Overexpression of E2F-1 leads to bax-independent cell death in human glioma cells. Int J Oncol 21:1015-1020.2002).

Mizuno M, Yoshida J, Colosi P, Kurtzman G (Adeno-associated virus vector containing the herpes simplex virus thymidine kinase gene causes complete regression of intracerebrally implanted human gliomas in mice, in conjunction with ganciclovir administration. Jpn J Cancer Res 89:76-80.1998).

Nan Y, Han L, Zhang A, Wang G, Jia Z, Yang Y, Yue X, Pu P, Zhong Y, Kang C (MiRNA-451 plays a role as tumor suppressor in human glioma cells. Brain Res 1359:14-21.2010).

Nawroth PP, Waldherr R, Zhang YM, Lin J, Bierhaus A, Lu J, Riedesel J, Zu EJ, Kasperk C, Ziegler R (Mechanism of endothelial cell activation. Transplant Proc 25:2052-2053.1993).

Ng SS, Gao Y, Chau DH, Li GH, Lai LH, Huang PT, Huang CF, Huang JJ, Chen YC, Kung HF, Lin MC (A novel glioblastoma cancer gene therapy using AAV-mediated long-term expression of human TERT C-terminal polypeptide. Cancer Gene Ther 14:561-572.2007).

Ohlfest JR, Demorest ZL, Motooka Y, Vengco I, Oh S, Chen E, Scappaticci FA, Saplis RJ, Ekker SC, Low WC, Freese AB, Largaespada DA (Combinatorial antiangiogenic gene therapy by nonviral gene transfer using the sleeping beauty transposon causes tumor regression and improves survival in mice bearing intracranial human glioblastoma. Mol Ther 12:778-788.2005).

Reiss Y, Machein MR, Plate KH (The role of angiopoietins during angiogenesis in gliomas. Brain Pathol 15:311-317.2005).

Ruan H, Deen DF (Use of hypoxia-regulated gene expression in tumor-specific gene therapy. Curr Opin Investig Drugs 2:839-843.2001).

Ruan H, Wang J, Hu L, Lin CS, Lamborn KR, Deen DF (Killing of brain tumor cells by hypoxia-responsive element mediated expression of BAX. Neoplasia 1:431-437.1999).

Seidel S, Garvalov BK, Wirta V, von Stechow L, Schanzer A, Meletis K, Wolter M, Sommerlad D, Henze AT, Nister M, Reifenberger G, Lundeberg J, Frisen J, Acker T (A hypoxic niche regulates glioblastoma stem cells through hypoxia inducible factor 2 alpha. Brain 133:983-995.2010).

Shibata T, Giaccia AJ, Brown JM (Development of a hypoxia-responsive vector for tumor-specific gene therapy. Gene Ther 7:493-498.2000).

Tiberghien P (Use of suicide genes in gene therapy. J Leukoc Biol 56:203-209.1994).

Tiberghien P, Reynolds CW, Keller J, Spence S, Deschaseaux M, Certoux JM, Contassot E, Murphy WJ, Lyons R, Chiang Y, et al. (Ganciclovir treatment of herpes simplex thymidine kinase-transduced primary T lymphocytes: an approach for specific in vivo donor T-cell depletion after bone marrow transplantation? Blood 84:1333-1341.1994).

Verpelli C, Bertani G, Cea V, Patti M, Bikfalvi A, Bello L, Sala C (Anti-angiogenic therapy induces integrin-linked kinase 1 up-regulation in a mouse model of glioblastoma. PLoS One 5:e13710.2010).

Wang D, Ruan H, Hu L, Lamborn KR, Kong EL, Rehemtulla A, Deen DF (Development of a hypoxia-inducible cytosine deaminase expression vector for gene-directed prodrug cancer therapy. Cancer Gene Ther 12:276-283.2005).

Wang X, Han L, Zhang A, Wang G, Jia Z, Yang Y, Yue X, Pu P, Shen C, Kang C (Adenovirus-mediated shRNAs for co-repression of miR-221 and miR-222 expression and function in glioblastoma cells. Oncol Rep 25:97-105.2011).

Wick W, Platten M, Weller M (Glioma cell invasion: regulation of metalloproteinase activity by TGF-beta. J Neurooncol 53:177-185.2001).

Yoshida J, Mizuno M, Wakabayashi T (Interferon-beta gene therapy for cancer: basic research to clinical application. Cancer Sci 95:858-865.2004).

Zamorano A, Lamas M, Vergara P, Naranjo JR, Segovia J (Transcriptionally mediated gene targeting of gas1 to glioma cells elicits growth arrest and apoptosis. J Neurosci Res 71:256-263.2003).

Zamorano A, Mellstrom B, Vergara P, Naranjo JR, Segovia J (Glial-specific retrovirally mediated gas1 gene expression induces glioma cell apoptosis and inhibits tumor growth in vivo. Neurobiol Dis 15:483-491.2004).

Zhang T, Guan M, Xu C, Chen Y, Lu Y (Pigment epithelium-derived factor inhibits glioma cell growth in vitro and in vivo. Life Sci 81:1256-1263.2007).

Zhou Z, Sun L, Wang Y, Wu Z, Geng J, Miu W, Pu Y, You Y, Yang Z, Liu N (Bone morphogenetic protein 4 inhibits cell proliferation and induces apoptosis in glioma stem cells. Cancer Biother Radiopharm 26:77-83.2011).

Part 7

LGI1 in Treatment of Glioma

11

The Tumor Suppressor Function of LGI1

Nadia Gabellini
University of Padova
Italy

1. Introduction

The Leucine rich Glioma Inactivated 1 (LGI1) gene has been related to different pathologies such as epilepsy and cancer. The aim of this chapter is to present the evidences on the tumor suppressor function of LGI1. Initially LGI1 gene was identified at the brake point of a balanced chromosome translocation in a glioblastoma cell line (Chernova et al., 1998). The observation that this rearrangement abolished expression of LGI1 and that expression of LGI1 is absent in most high-grade gliomas lead to the hypothesis that it may function as tumor suppressor.

1.1 Evidences for the tumor suppressor function

The tumor suppressor function was sustained by the re-expression of LGI1 in glioblastoma cells, lacking endogenous expression, LGI1 inhibited cell proliferation and migration (Kunapuli et al., 2003). The role of tumor suppressor was further supported by the identification of several mutations in LGI1 gene associated with gliomas (Barnholtz-Sloan et al., 2008). The tumor suppressor function of LGI1 was supported also by the results of LGI1 expression in neuroblastoma and adenocarcinoma cells, in which endogenous expression is very low or absent. The expression of LGI1 in these cancer cells not only produced a potent inhibition of cell proliferation, as in the case of glioblastoma cells, but also impaired cell survival (Gabellini et al., 2006; Gabellini & Masola, 2009). Moreover a study on malignant esophageal tumors showed a significant downregulation of LGI1 (Peng et al. 2008).

1.2 Induction of apoptosis

Investigations on the mechanism of spontaneous cell death caused by the expression of LGI1 in neuroblastoma cells showed the induction of intrinsic apoptosis, produced by an unbalance of important regulator of mitochondrial membrane permeability, namely of the anti-apoptotic B-cell lymphoma 2 gene (BCL2) and of the pro-apoptotic B-cell lymphoma 2-associated X protein gene (BAX). These studies also pointed out a possible involvement of LGI1 in the negative regulation of essential signaling pathways supporting cell proliferation and survival.

1.3 Regulation of signaling pathways

Consistently with the evidence that LGI1 triggered a mitochondrial pathway of apoptosis, the phosphoinositide 3-kinase (PI3K/AKT) pathway, important regulator of BCL proteins, was blocked by the expression of LGI1 (Gabellini & Masola, 2008). In the case of glioblastoma cells the inhibition of cell proliferation and migration exerted by LGI1 was determined by the inhibition of the extracellular signal-regulated kinase subgroup of the mitogen-activated protein kinases (ERK/MAPK pathway), resulting in the downregulation of matrix metalloproteinase (MMP) genes (Kunapuli et al., 2004). These observations pointed out the possibility that LGI1 might impair trophic signaling because the PI3K/AKT and the ERK/MAPK pathways are activated downstream of tyrosine kinase receptors (RTK) in response to growth factors. This possibility is supported by the homology of the leucine-rich repeats flanked by cysteine rich regions (LRR domains) present in the N-terminal region of LGI1 with the region of mammalian Trk receptors involved in neurotrophin binding (Kobe and Deisenhofer 1994; Kalachikov et al. 2002), however, evidences for LGI1 interaction with RTK receptors are lacking presently.

1.4 Suggested functions

The domain architecture of LGI1 protein includes a leucine-rich repeats flanked by cysteine rich regions (LRR domains) and a seven-bladed beta-propeller domain located in the C-terminal half of the protein (Scheel et al., 2002; Staub et al., 2002). Both LGI1 domains appear to be involved in protein-protein interaction and investigation in this direction revealed important aspects on the function of LGI1. LGI1 was shown to be a ligand of the trans-membrane receptor ADAM metallopeptidase 22 (ADAM22), this receptor is highly expressed in brain, but precise information on its function and signaling are limited at the moment (Fukata et al., 2006). It was also shown that LGI1 forms complexes with voltage gated potassium channels (Kv1.1), which are critical regulators of synaptic transmission (Schulte et al., 2006). Their activity is well characterized and is supposed to control several functions in a variety of cell types. In particular, it was shown that binding of LGI1 prevented channel inactivation by Kv1β and that LGI1 mutations associated with Autosomal Dominant Lateral Temporal Epilepsy (ADLTE) produced a modification of the inactivation properties of the channels that might promote epileptic activity.

1.5 Regulation of potassium channels and apoptosis

The role of LGI1 in the regulation of (Kv1.1) is also in relation with the tumor suppressor function of LGI1, since these channels are important regulator of cell survival. In particular the blockage of channel inactivation determined by binding of LGI1 to regulatory subunit Kv1β, results in an increase of K^+ permeability, which has been shown to enhance apoptosis (Yu et al., 1997). Thus in addition to the inhibition of pro-survival pathways such as the PIK/AKT, LGI1 might induce apoptosis by interfering with Kv channels inactivation. Thus the tumor suppressor function of LGI1 might be related to its pro-apoptotic activity, and the dowregulation or inactivation of LGI1 gene often observed in glioblastoma and other cancer cells might be necessary to suppress apoptosis.

2. LGI1 gene

The first isolation LGI1 gene was achieved by positional cloning of the region rearranged by a balanced translocation t(10;19)(q24;q13) in a glioblastoma cell line (Chernova et al., 1998). LGI1 gene covers 40,274 bp of chromosome 10 in the region q23.33. It consists of 8 exons (Fig. 1). The 5′ UTR preceding the codon for the start methione is located in exon 1 sequence.

Exon 8 includes two stop codons alternatively utilized in two spliced isoforms carrying 3'UTRs of different legth. A minimal promoter region is placed immediately upstream of the Transcriptional Start Site (Sommerville et al., 2000).

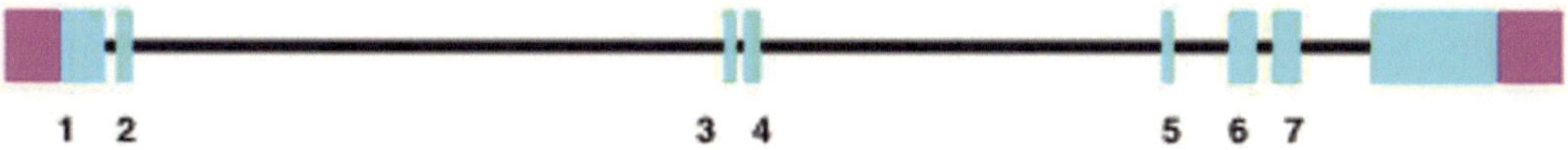

Fig. 1. Organization of LGI1 gene. The coding regions of exons 1-8 are depicted in blue, the untranslated regions (UTR) in pink, introns are shown by black bars.

Processing of the primary LGI1 transcript produces two main isoforms showing tissue specific expression (Chernova et al., 1998; Morante-Redolat et al., 2002). The full length LGI1 mRNA is composed of 2290 bases and corresponds to isoform 1 (RefSeq: NM_005097). Alternative splicing produces the small isoform 2 consisting of 1456 bases including a shorter exon 8.

3. LGI1 protein

The full length LGI1 protein comprises 557 amino acids (64 KDa) and corresponds to isoform 1 (UniProtKB/Swiss-Prot ID: 095970). Isoform 2 is composed of 291 amino acids (Isoform ID: O95970-2); it includes an amino acid sequence variation of residues 280-291 and lacks the C-terminal amino acids stretch (292-557). The domain composition of the full-length protein is shown in Fig.2.

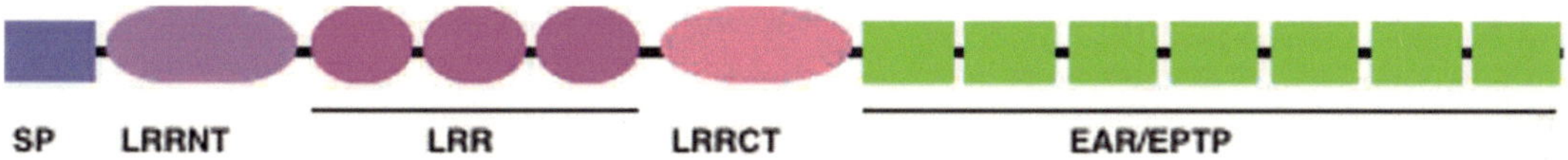

Fig. 2. LGI1 protein (isoform 1).

The N-terminal sequence of LGI1 precursor starts with a cleavable signal peptide (SP, AA: 1-34); the predicted molecular size of the mature protein is 60 KDa. A hydrophobic stretch (amino acids 288-309) was pointed as a possible trans-membrane segment, suggesting that LGI1 might be anchored to the membrane (Chernova et al., 1998). The domain composition of the N-terminal half of LGI1 protein includes three leucine-rich repeats (LRR; AA: 90-113, 114-137 and 138-161) flanked by cysteine-rich leucine-rich repeats (N-terminal LRRNT AA: 41-71 and C-terminal LRRCT AA: 173-222). The C-terminal portion of LGI1 is characterized by the presence of 7 repeats, termed Epilepsy Associated Repeats (EAR; Scheel et al., 2002) or Epitempin (EPTP; Staub et al., 2002) denoted EAR/EPTP repeats (AA: 224-267, 270-313, 316-364, 365-415, 418-462, 463-506, and 509-552).

3.1 Homology

LGI1 is part of a protein family comprising four members (LGI1, LGI2, LGI3, and LGI4) with high sequence homology. The Leucine-Rich repeats flanked by Leucine-rich cysteine-rich domains of LGI protein share the highest identities with that present in cell adhesion proteins and receptors. The structure of LRR domains of LGI1 protein is related to that of

Drosophila protein slit, involved in the development central nervous system for its role in neuronal growth-cone guidance and migration (Battye et al., 2001). The LRR domain of LGI1 is related also to that identified in the extra-cellular region of mammalian Trk receptors, specifically in the region binding neurotrophin (Kobe and Deisenhofer 1994; Kalachikov et al. 2002), suggesting that LGI1 might interfere with ligand binding of Trk receptors. The structure of the EAR/EPTP domain is similar to the ß-propeller domains found in several intracellular and secreted proteins. It was identified by homology among the four paralogous genes LGI1-4, and with the large G protein coupled receptor MASS1/VLGR1, which is mutated in a murine form of audiogenic epilepsy (McMillan et al. 2002). The presence of a similar domain in the integrin α chain receptors (Xiong et al. 2001; Springer 2002) suggests a possible role in cell adhesion. The role suggested for both LRR and EAR/EPTP domains is to provide an interface for protein–protein interaction.

3.2 Cellular localization

The presence of a cleavable signal peptide suggests that LGI1 protein might be addressed to endoplasmic reticulum and localized in the membrane or secreted. Although the presence of the hydrophobic segment initially suggested the it might be associated with the membrane, subsequent studies based on heterologous transfection of the full-length LGI1 cDNA in 293T cells showed the LGI1 protein is secreted (Senechal et al., 2005). However, it was shown also that the short isoform, probably corresponding to isoform 2, is retained within the cell (Sirerol-Piquer et al., 2006).

4. Expression

Northern blot analysis with human tissues detected LGI1 mRNA only in brain and skeletal muscle; two mRNA species were identified (2.4 kb and 1.6 kb) suggesting expression of at least two isoforms. RT-PCR analysis detected LGI1 mRNA also in heart, liver and pancreas although at lower levels (Chernova et al., 1998). High resolution *in situ* hybridization on adult mice brain suggested that LGI1 is primarily expressed in neurons located in specific brain regions. Strong labeling was observed in granule cell layer of the dentate gyrus and in the CA3-CA1 pyramidal cell layers of the hippocampus; weak hybridization signals were observed in the neocortex and limbic region. LGI1 expression is consistently more elevated in the regions implicated in ADLTE (Kalachikov et al., 2002; Herranz-Pérez et al., 2010; Senechal et al., 2005). Subsequent experiments with transgenic mice carrying the GFP reporter gene under the control of regulatory regions of LGI1 gene supported high levels in neurons and revealed LGI1 expression also in glial cells. Strong expression was also identified in the prostate gland, tubules and sympathetic ganglia of the kidney, as well in several glandular tissues as in skin sebaceous glands, in pancreatic islets of Langerhans, endometrium, ovary and testes (Head et al., 2007). The expression profile of LGI1 determined by DNA microarrays, SAGE and EST number (reported by ECgene and Gene Expression Atlas) is in agreement the reported data but extended the expression to pituitary gland, peripheral nerve, B-lymphocytes, eye, lung.

4.1 Expression in tumors

Immunohistochemistry and mRNA analysis showed that LGI1 levels are very low or completely absent in most tumor tissues and in several cancer cell lines including, glioblastoma, neuroblastoma, melanoma and breast, furthermore the decrease of LGI1 expression shows a significant correlation with the grade of malignancy of astrocytic gliomas (Rossi et al., 2005; Besleaga et al., 2003). DNA microarrays, SAGE and EST number suggest low or absent expression in the majority of tumor tissues (see Gabellini, 2007).

5. Glioma

A number of germ line and somatic mutations involved in the initiation and progression of human gliomas have been identified. The most frequent mutations are associated with the tumor suppressor protein p53, which induces cell cycle arrest and apoptosis, with the negative regulator of the cell cycle RB1 and with oncogenic components of the PI3K pathway (Parson et al., 2008; Barnholtz-Sloan et al., 2008). Typical chromosomal alterations occurring in malignant gliomas consist of an increased chromosome 7 copy number, resulting in the amplification of the proto-oncogene for the tyrosine kinase receptor (EGFR; Henn et al. 1986). Other recurrent events are related to the loss of one copy of chromosome 10 and often also the second copy especially of the region 10q23-q26. Loss of heterozygosity in this region is observed in about 80% of glioblastoma multiforme tumors, suggesting the presence of multiple tumor suppressor genes (Karlbom et al., 1993). Indeed this region of chromosome 10 includes the Phosphatase and Tensin Homolog gene (PTEN; 10q23), important tumor suppressor with pro-apoptotic function antagonizing the PI3K pathway (Blanco-Aparicio et al., 2007); the Deleted in Malignant Brain Tumors 1 gene (DMBT1; 10q25-q26; Mollenhauer et al., 1997) and the Leucine-rich, Glioma-Inactivated-1 gene (LGI1; 10q24).

5.1 Alterations of LGI1 gene

The interruption of LGI1 gene by a balanced chromosomal translocation t(10;19)(q24;q13) in the T98G glioma cell line results in the complete loss of LGI1 expression (Chernova et al., 1998). Similar alterations occur also in the A172 glioma cell line and glioblastoma tumors. However, fluorescence *in situ* hybridization study showed that alterations of LGI1 gene are absent in some glioblastoma cell lines (Krex et al., 2002).

5.1.1 Point mutations

The occurrence of point mutations in LGI1 gene has been shown by DNA sequence analysis of brain tumors versus normal brain samples (Barnholtz-Sloan et al., 2008). This study revealed several missense and nonsense tumor-specific mutations, mostly located in the region encoding the N-terminal portion of LGI1 protein including LRR domains and flanking cystein-rich regions (Fig.2). Heterozygous mutations in the human LGI1 gene have been associated with Autosomal Dominant Lateral Temporal Epilepsy (ADLTE), a disorder characterized by partial seizures typically preceded by auditory symptoms (Kalachikov et al., 2002; Morante-Redolat et al., 2002; Michelucci et al., 2009). However, the incidence of malignant brain tumors appears to be unvaried in ADLTE families carrying LGI1 mutations (Brodtkorb et al., 2003), supporting the notion that multiple genetic alterations are necessary for malignant transformation.

5.1.2 Downregulation

Also the downregulation of LGI1 gene expression might be important for malignant transformation. A gradual decline in the expression of LGI1 gene accompanies the malignant progression of gliomas (Besleaga et al., 2003). Northern blot, RT-PCR and immunohystochemistry of various brain tumor samples revealed that in the majority of low-grade tumor such as pilocytic astrocytomas and astrocytomas, defined by the World Health Organization (WHO) grade II, the expression of LGI1 was similar to that of normal brain; in anaplastic astrocytomas (WHO grade III) the levels of LGI1 was consistently lower than in normal tissue, whereas LGI1 expression was absent in 80% of glioblastoma multiforme samples (WHO grade IV). Genetic alterations of the promoter region and epigenetic factors such as methylation of the control regions might determine the differences of LGI1 expression.

5.1.3 Epigenetc factors

The results of tiling array assays (MAUD assay) for the identification of methylated or unmethylated DNA sequences, which can accommodate the entire mouse brain transcriptome, revealed that LGI1 is one of the genes presenting dual methylation pattern of the regulatory regions determining monoallelic expression (Wang et al., 2010). Although mutations of tumor suppressor genes are usually inherited as recessive traits, because both alleles must be inactivated to eliminate gene function, in case of monoallelic expression heterozygous mutations of the ummethylated allele might be sufficient to abolish expression. This explains the dominant inheritance of ADLTE in the presence of heterozygous mutations, furthermore the process of random inactivation of one of the two alleles by methylation accounts for the characteristic incomplete penetrance of this disease.

5.2 Re-expression

The first study supporting the role of tumor suppressor for LGI1 was based on the results of forced expression of LGI1 in glioblastoma cells (Kunapuli et al., 2003). Cells stably expressing LGI1 were obtained by selection of neomycin G418 resistance brought by the plasmid vector in which LGI1 was incorporated. In this study the LGI1 cDNA used for transfection was modified in the region encoding the C-terminal end of LGI1 by the addition of a flag epitope, to allow the detection of the expressed protein in the absence of specific antibodies, which were in preparation. The LGI1 cDNA construct was transfected in the glioblastoma multiforme derived cell line T98G characterized by a chromosomal rearrangement interrupting LGI1 gene t(10;19)(q24;q13) and in the A172 glioma cell lines carrying a reciprocal chromosomal translocation t(10;19)(q26;q13.4), which break up the WDR11 gene (10q25-26) encoding a member of the WD repeat protein family. Both T98G and A172cells lack endogenous LGI1 expression. In addition the U87 cells derived from an astrocitoma and naturally expressing LGI1 were transfected with the same LGI1 construct. T98G and A172 yielded only few clones of stably transfected cells, suggesting that expression of LGI1 affected cell vitality. In contrast cell clones derived from U87 cells grew normally. Variable levels of LGI1 mRNA and protein were detected among the different cell clones, however expression was more elevated in U87 than in T98G and A172 derived cells.

5.2.1 Decline of malignant features

A quantitative cell proliferation assay indicated that the proliferation rate of T98G and A172 cells stably transfected with LGI1 was reduced in comparison with control cells transfected with empty vector; inhibition of cell growth was proportional with the levels of LGI1 expression. In contrast the proliferation rate of U87 derived cells overexpressing LGI1 was similar to that of control cells, suggesting that selection for increased proliferation during malignant transformation operated independently of LGI1 in U87 cells. Also the invasion ability, another feature associated with malignancy, was analyzed in this study. The capability of cells to pass through pores of 8 µm of a coated membrane was evaluated. The majority of the T98G and A172 cell clones stably expressing LGI1 had completely lost their original migration ability; whereas U87 derived cell clones retained the capacity of passage, which was similar to that of control cells. A third characteristic of malignant cells is their capacity to grow without being anchored to a substrate. The ability of cells to grow in an anchorage independent manner was evaluated by counting the number of colonies formed on soft agar. The ability to grow on soft agar was strongly impaired in cell clones expressing LGI1 in comparison with cell transfected with empty vector or with parental T98G and A172 cells whereas the number of colonies formed by U87 cells expressing LGI1 was similar to that of control cells. The results of this study showed that cell proliferation was reduced (≥40%), invasion ability and anchorage-independent growth were almost abolished when LGI1 was re-expressed in glioblastoma cells lacking endogenous LGI1 expression. These results provide a possible explanation for the frequent occurrence of chromosome 10 rearrangements during the transition from low to high-grade gliomas, which might reflect the need of eliminating the tumor suppressor function of LGI1 to allow tumor progression.

6. Neuroblastoma

The function of LGI1 was studied also in a neuronal cell model represented by human neuroblastoma cells. These embryonic cancer cells are pluripotent precursors of the sympathoadrenal nervous system cells deriving from the neuronal crest (see Schwab et al., 2003). The typical alterations of chromoseme 10 observed in glioblastomas are not present in neuroblastoma; instead loss of the chromosome 1p region is frequent in neuroblastomas, as well as the amplification of the proto-oncogene MYCN and alterations of neurotrophin receptors levels (see Schwab, 2004). However, the results of RT-PCR analysis with a series of neuroblastoma cell lines suggested that LGI1 expression was either absent or very weak in the vast majority of the cases, suggesting that LGI1 gene is often downregulated in neuroblastoma cells as well (Rossi et al., 2005). Our results of RT-PCR analysis with two human neuroblastoma cell lines (SH-SY5Y and SK-NBE) employed for transfection experiments described below showed negligible levels of LGI1, especially when compared with expression in human whole brain, which was estimated about 30-fold greater.

6.1 Over-expression in neuroblastoma cells

Human neuroblastoma cells SH-SY5Y and SK-N-BE were transfected with the full-length LGI1 cDNA inserted in the expression vector pcDNA3 and with the empty vector as control (Gabellini et al., 2006). Neomycin G418 selection was performed to obtain stably transfected cell clones. During the procedure it became apparent that cells transfected with LGI1 grew more slowly than control cells. In addition only few cell clones stably transfected with LGI1 came across selection, whereas transfection with pcDNA3 generated a greater number of cell clones, suggesting that expression of LGI1 affected cell survival. A semiquantitative RT-PCR analysis of LGI1 mRNA on cell clones transfected with LGI1 was performed to evaluate the levels of LGI1 expression, a segment of the glyceraldehyde-3-phosphate dehydrogenase (GAPDH) was amplified in parallel reactions to evaluate the relative mRNA content of the samples (Fig. 3).

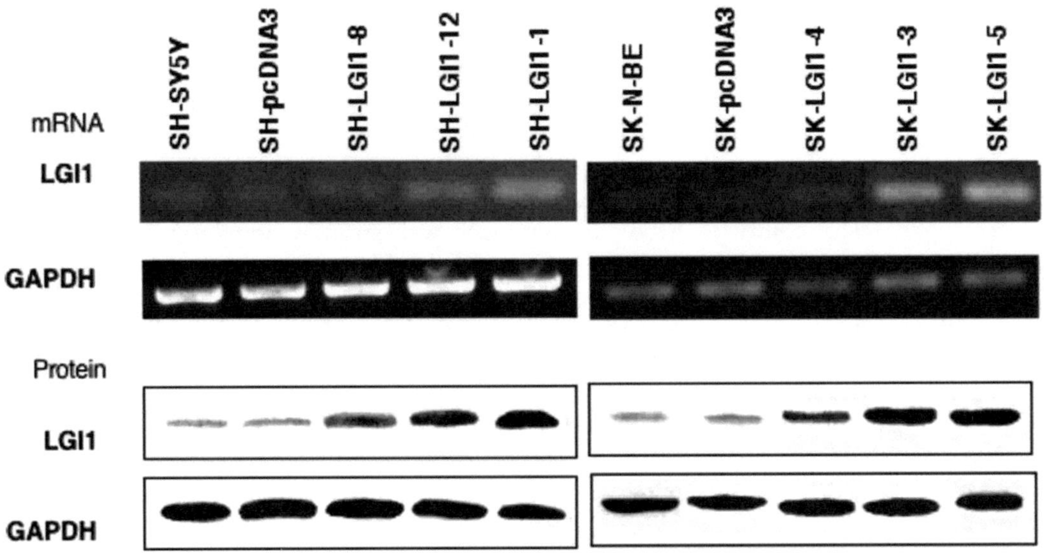

Fig. 3. Evaluation of LGI1 mRNA and protein in the neurobalstoma cells

Three cell clones derived from SH-SY5Y cells, designated SH-LGI1-8, SH-LGI1-12, and SH-LGI1-1, showed LGI1 mRNA levels slightly higher than original or pcDNA3-transfected cells, the latter showed barely detectable levels of LGI1 mRNA. The densitometry values of ethidium bromide stained PCR products were normalized to the corresponding values of GAPDH. The results showed on average 5-, 10- and 20-fold, increase in cell clones SH-LGI1-8, -12, -1, respectively. The levels of LGI1 mRNA in three cell clones SK-LGI1-3, -4, -5, derived from SK-NB-E were 4-, 6- and 8-fold greater than those estimates in control cells. The evaluation of LGI1 protein was performed by Western blot analysis of whole cells using an antibody directed to the N-terminal peptide of LGI1 (Fig. 3). Blots were re-probed with antibodies to GAPDH to normalize the protein content of the samples. The normalized densitometry values of the LGI1 protein (60 KDa) were in good agreement with the mRNA data. Because it was shown that LGI1 protein was secreted in the medium of transfected 293T cells (Senechal et al., 2005), the conditioned medium of neuroblastoma cell clones was concentrated and analyzed by Western blotting, nevertheless LGI1 protein was detected only in the cell lysates. It is possible that in neuroblastoma cells LGI1 protein might be anchored to the extra-cellular site of the plasma membrane, in agreement with the presence of a signal peptide and of a putative trans-membrane segment emerged from its primary structure, and with its immune-localization in secretory vesicle (Morante-Redolat et al. 2002).

6.1.1 Inhibition of cell proliferation

The proliferation rate of neuroblastoma cells over-expressing LGI1 was measured by the BrDU incorporation two days following plating (250 cells/mm^2). The results showed a significant decrease of cell proliferation in all LGI1-transfected cells in comparison with original neuroblastoma cells or with pcDNA3 transfected cells, which showed similar rates. The proliferation of SH-LGI1-8, SH-LGI1-12 and SH-LGI1-1 cell clones was 40%, 70% and 90%, lower than that of control cells, respectively.

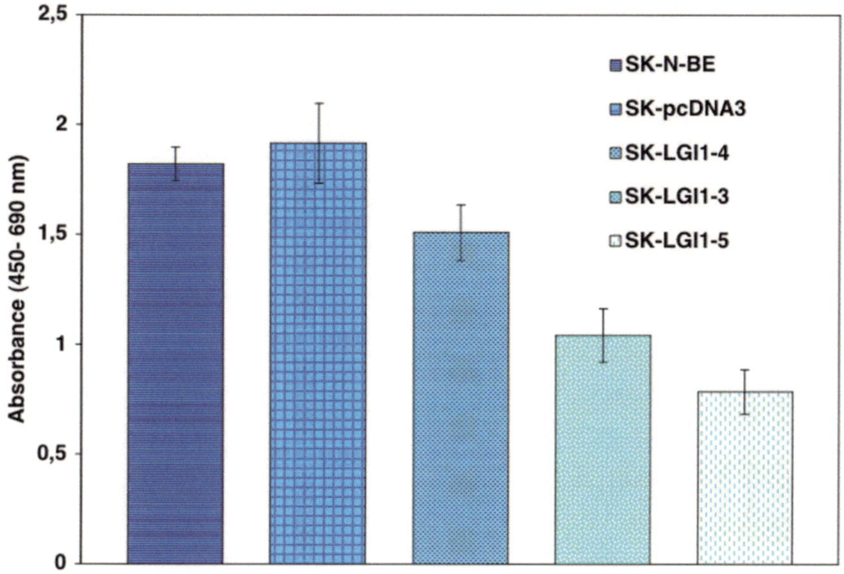

Fig. 4. Decline of cell proliferation

Similarly, the proliferation of LGI1 cell clones derived from SK-N-BE was consistently inhibited when compared to that of control cells. The proliferation rate of SK-LGI1-4, SK-LGI1-3 and SK-LGI1-5 was decreased on average by 20%, 50% and 60%, respectively (Fig. 4). The proliferation rates of SK-LGI1 cell clones and that of pcDNA3 were significantly different from that of control pcDNA3 cells or parental cells (mean ±SD; n=9-12; Student's t test $p<0,0004$). The study revealed a striking correlation between the extent of growth inhibition and the level of LGI1 expression, similarly to what occurred when LGI1 was re-expressed in glioblastoma cells lacking endogenous expression (Section 5.2).

6.1.2 Impaired survival

The viability of SH-SY5Y cell clones was assessed by a cytotoxicity assay based on tetrazolium salt (WST-8). The assays measures dehydrogenase activity of living cells, thus giving an indication of both cell proliferation and cytotoxicity. The results showed that the number of viable SH-LGI1 cells was consistently lower than that of control cells. Four days after plating (250 cells/mm^2) viability of SH-LGI1-8, -12 and -1 cell was 29%, 46% and 60% lower than that of control cells, respectively. In line with the results of BrDU incorporation, this assay showed a direct relation between the levels of LGI1 expression and the decrement of cell viability. The cytotoxic effect of LGI1 became more pronounced when cells were plated at high density (1000/mm^2). In these conditions death of LGI1 cells became morphologically evident already after the second day of culture, while after four days the majority LGI1 cells were dead. In contrast, only a relatively modest decrease of cell viability was measured with control cells transfected with pcDNA3 or parental SH-SY5Y cells, indicating a strong cyotototoxic effect of LGI1 (Gabellini et al., 2006). The lactate dehydrogenase assay (LDH) was also employed to measure effective cell death. The fraction of LDH released in the medium as a consequence of cell death was calculated as percentage of the total LDH activity. The assay was performed 2- and 3- days following plating (1000/mm^2), at these time points the WST8 assay indicated extensive death of LGI1 cells. In accord, the results of LDH assays showed that the percentage of cytoxicity of all LGI1 cell clones was substantially greater than that of control cells. The percentage of SH-LGI1-8 and SH-LGI1-1 cell death was considerably greater than that of pcDNA3 or parental cells (Fig. 5; mean ±SD, n=12-20; Student's t test $p<0,001$). Significant differences between the percentage of cytoxicity of SK-LGI1 and SK-pcDNA3 cells were also detected. Cell death increased in parallel with the levels of LGI1 expression suggesting that the elevated levels of LGI1 affected cell survival. This observation might explain the marked downregulation of LGI1 gene expression observed in neuroblastoma cells.

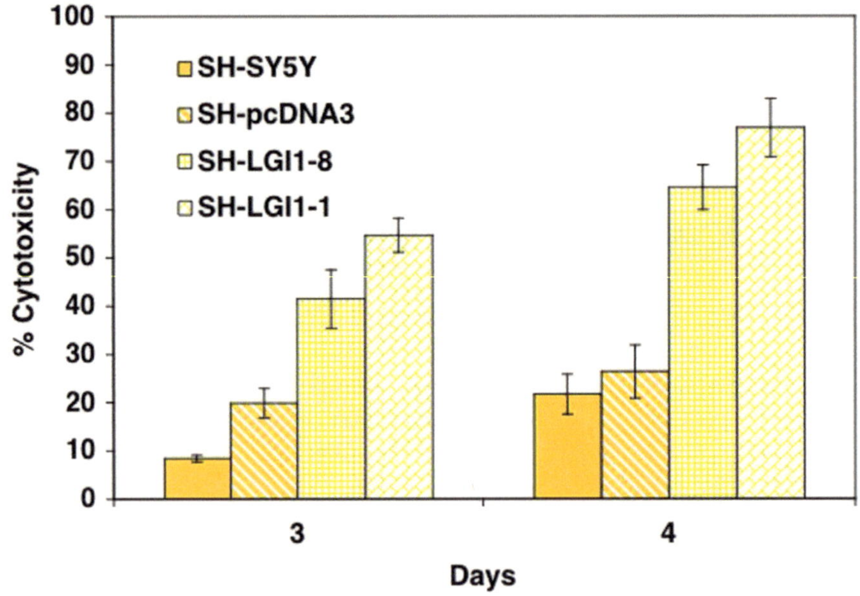

Fig. 5. Increased cell death.

6.1.3 Glioblastoma cell death

Although in the case of glioblastoma cells a quantification of cell death was not performed, it was observed that T98G and A172 stably transfected with LGI1 produced only few cell clones (Kunapuli et al., 2003). Since the levels of LGI1 expression measured in both stably transfected glioblastoma and neuroblastoma cell clones were relatively low, it might be suggested that high levels of LGI1 are not be compatible with the existence of both types of cancer cells.

6.2 Apoptosis

The mode of neuroblastoma cell death induced by the elevation of LGI1 levels was investigated. The evaluation of several apoptotic markers such as activation of caspase-3/7, alteration of the BCL-2 to BAX ratio, release of cytochrome c and AIF from mitochondria, oligonucleosomal DNA fragmentation, phosphatydil serine (PS) exposure and nuclear morphology (Gabellini et. al., 2006). The data reported in the following sections suggests that LGI1 impairs survival of neuroblastoma cells by inducing intrinsic apoptosis. Although inhibition of cell proliferation similarly occurs in glioblastoma and neuroblastoma cells, up to now induction of apoptosis in glioblastoma cells have not been not reported. The results of this study strengthen the tumor suppressor function of LGI1 and outline the possibility that the downregulation of LGI1 gene expression observed in several cancer cells might be necessary to suppress apoptosis.

6.2.1 Activation of caspases–3 -7

The proteolytic activity of caspase-3 and -7, important effectors of apoptosis in mammalian cells (see Hengartner, 2000), was determined by the relative fluorescence (RFLU) emitted by the specific substrate (Z-DEVD-R110) upon cleavage. The RFLU values of SH-LGI1 cells, control SH-SY5Y and SH-pcDNA3 cells were determined each 24 hrs during a period of 4 days after plating 250, 500 or 1000 cells/mm². The average numbers of living cells determined in replicated samples by cytotoxicity assays was used to correct each RFLU value, with the aim to normalize variations of basal caspase activity resulting from variable cell proliferation rates. The caspase-3/7 activity of all cell types increased progressively during the time course at each cell density, however, the RFLU values of all LGI1 cells were significantly higher than those of pcDNA3 cells or original SH-SY5Y cells, (mean ±SD, n=12; Student's t $p < 0{,}0001$).

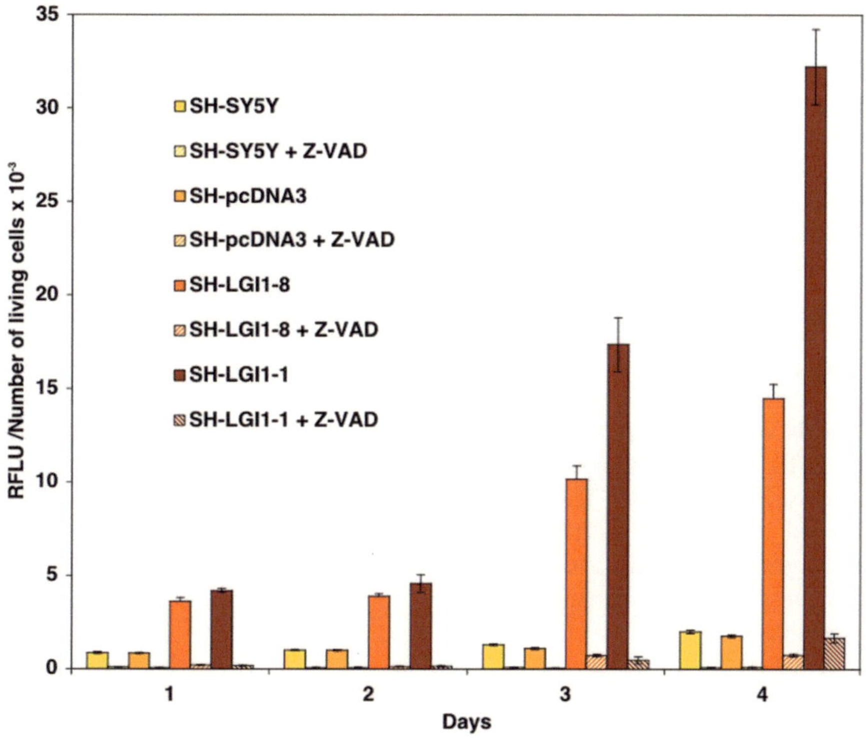

Fig. 6. Enhancement of caspase –3 –7 activity and inhibition by Z-VAD-FMK.

In the conditions of high cell density (1000 cells/mm^2), which showed the greatest cytotoxicity (Fig. 5), caspase-3 -7 activity was on average 4 - 5 fold greater in SH-LGI1 cells than in control cells during the initial two days; and increased up to 10- to 20-fold during the following 2 days in coincidence with the appearance of extensive cell death (Fig. 6). The broad-range caspase inhibitor Z-VAD-FMK blocked caspases -3 -7 in all cell types (~ 90%). The activity of caspase -3 -7 correlated with the extent of cytotoxicity and with the levels of LGI1 expression, suggesting that increased LGI1 levels triggered apoptosis of neuroblastoma cells.

6.2.2 Intrinsic apoptosis

The involvement of caspases linked to death receptor stimulation in the initiation of the apoptotic stimulus was investigated by measuring cytotoxicity and cell proliferation in the presence of the broad caspase inhibitor Z-VAD-FMK. The percentages of cytotoxicity of SH-LGI1 cells were similar to those determined in the absence of the inhibitor, whereas SK-LGI1 cells showed a small decrease. Thus the inhibition of proteases by Z-VAD-FMK substantially failed to prevent cell death. This suggested that apoptosis of neuroblastoma cells might be initiated in the absence of caspase activation, thus involvement of the extrinsic pathway of apoptosis linked to caspase-8 activation by death receptors is unlikely. These evidences suggest that apoptosis of LGI1 cells most likely involves the activation of the intrinsic mitochondrial pathway of apoptosis.

6.2.3 Decreased ratio of BCL-2 to BAX

The relative proportion of the anti-apoptotic BCL2 and of the pro-apoptotic BAX gene products is crucial to control apoptosis. These members of the BCL protein family play an important role in the regulation of mitochondrial outer membrane permeability determining the release of death factors that initiate intrinsic apoptosis (see Reed, 1998; Cory and Adams, 2002). Beside the release of cytochrome c, which stimulates formation of the apoptosome complex and caspase-3 activation, the proteins of the BCL family also control the release of the caspases-independent apoptotic effectors AIF and endonuclease G (Susin et al., 1999; Li et al., 2001). Thus to substantiate the evidence that LGI1 might initiate a mitochondrial pathway of apoptosis we evaluated the expression of BCL-2 and BAX by RT-PCR and Western blot (Fig. 7). The densitometry values of BCL2 and BAX were normalized to the GAPDH value of each sample. The results of the semiquantitative RT-PCR analysis showed that the levels of BCL-2 mRNA were reduced by 30% to 50% in neuroblastoma cells expressing LGI1 when compared with control cells, on the contrary the levels of BAX mRNA increased 2- to 3-fold. The results of Western blot showed that also BAX protein increased in all LGI1 cells (Fig. 7). The amount of BAX protein was directly proportional to that of LGI1 protein, reaching the highest levels in SH-LGI1-1 cells (~10-fold). At the opposite in this cell clone expressing the maximum levels of LGI1, the amount of BCL-2 protein was lowest.

The results indicated that an increase of LGI1 expression even if modest strongly influenced the balance between pro- and anti-apoptotic BCL2 proteins, in favor of pro-apoptotic factors. Because the pro-apoptotic function of BAX is prevented by its heterodimerization with BCL2, the ratio of BCL2 to BAX determines the execution of apoptosis in various cancer cells including neuroblastoma (Lombet et al., 2001). Thus LGI1 appears to stimulate the intrinsic pathway of programmed cell death through the alteration of BCL2 to BAX ratio.

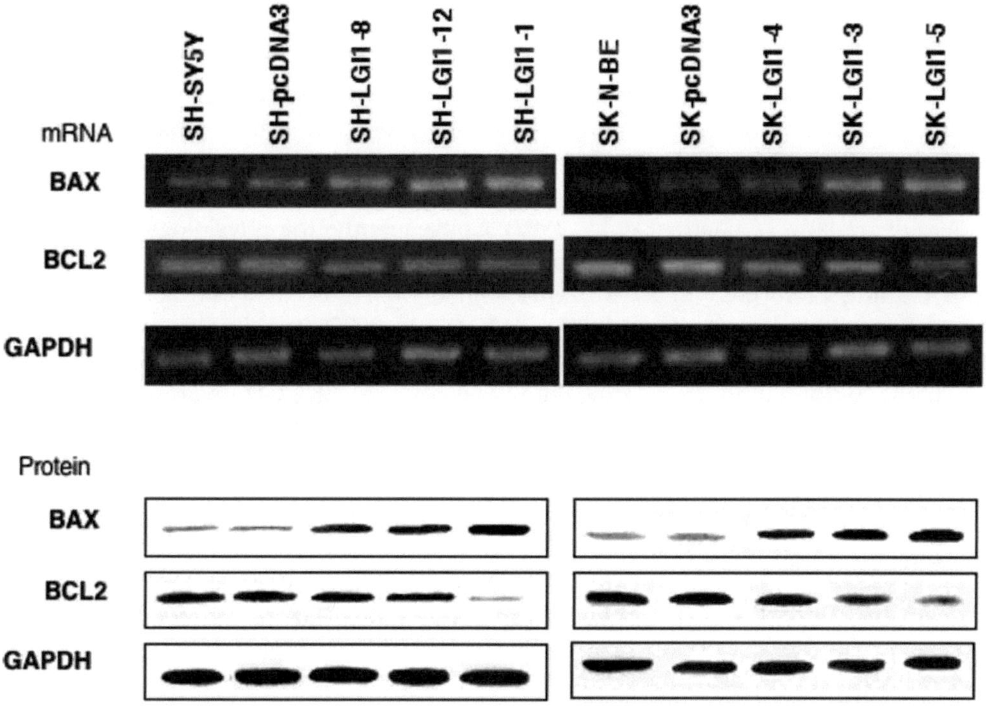

Fig. 7. Alteration of BCL2 and BAX levels by expression of LGI1 in neuroblastoma cells

6.2.4 Release of apoptosis-inducing factors from mitochondria

The shift of BCL-2 to BAX ratio suggested that LGI1 cell death might be triggered by the mitochondrial pathway of apoptosis by the release of cytochrome c and apoptosis inducing factor (AIF); (see Kroemer and Reed, 2000; Martinou and Green, 2001). The amount of cytocrome c released in the cytosol was determined by ELISA assays of cytosolic fractions isolated from neuroblastoma cells cultured for 3 days at high cell density, at what time massive death of LGI1-cells and large activation of caspase 3/7 occurred (Fig. 5, Fig. 6). The amount of cytochrome c in the cytosolic fraction of LGI1 cells was significantly greater than that present in fractions from control cells. A 2.4- to 3.5-fold increase of cytosolic cytochrome c was detected in SH- and SK-LGI1 cells. Consistently with the notion that cytosolic cytochrome c activates caspase-3, the greatest activation of caspases 3/7 in LGI1 cells coincides with the release of cytochrome c. The death effector AIF translocates to the nucleus following transition of mitochondrial membrane permeability, where it induces chromatin condensation and high molecular weight DNA fragmentation ending with apoptosis, independently on caspases activation (Susin et al., 1999; Cregan et al. 2002). The amount of AIF in nuclear fractions of the neuroblastoma cell clones was determined by Westen blot in the same experimental conditions used to determine the release of cytocrome c. The nuclear content of AIF was on average 2- to 4- fold greater in LGI1 cells than in control cells. In agreement with the failure of the caspase inhibitor Z-VAD-FMK to increase cell survival, the observed translocation of AIF in the nucleus might support the apoptotic program, even in the absence of caspases activation.

7. Adenocarcinoma

HeLa cells derive from a human cervical adenocarcinoma and have been shown to contain several copies of the human papillomavirus HPV-18 integrated in their genome (Inagaki et al., 1988). In particular HeLa cells express the viral oncoprotein E6, which in complex with a cellular protein interacts with the tumor suppressor protein p53, to promote its ubiquitin-dependent degradation (Scheffner et al., 1993). Consequently, the physiological function of p53 sustaining cell cycle arrest and apoptosis is inhibited. The results of RT-PCR and Western blotting performed to assed expression of LGI1 revealed the absence of LGI1 mRNA and protein in HeLa cells (Gabellini and Masola, 2009). This finding is in agreement the results of Expressed Sequence Tags (ESTs) in human uterine tumors as well as in normal uterine tissue (information from UniGene). The absence of LGI1 expression has been reported also in mouse uterus (Head et al., 2007). Furthermore, the analysis by a proteomic approach of several Barrett's-related adenocarcinomas compared to normal mucosa samples showed 100% downregulation of LGI1 (Peng et al. 2008).

7.1 Expression in HeLa cells

The robust growth and survival ability together with the absence of endogenous LGI1 expression render HeLa cells an appropriate system to examine the tumor suppressor function of LGI1. We performed stable transfection of HeLa cells with LGI1 cDNA and with empty vector pcDNA3 using the same procedure adopted for neuroblastoma cells. The characterization of stably transfected cell clones expressing LGI1 clearly showed inhibition of cell proliferation and increased of cell death, as in the case of neuroblastoma cells. Again expression of LGI1 modified the balance of BCL2 to BAX in favor of the pro-apoptotic factor (Gabellini and Masola, 2009). Consistently with the downregulation of LGI1 reported in Barrett's-related adenocarcinomas this study supports the role of tumor suppressor of LGI1 in adenocarcinoma-derived cells (Peng et al., 2008), in addition to neuroblastoma and glioblastoma.

7.2 Induction of apoptosis

The activity of the apoptosis effectors caspase-3 and -7 was measured to investigate the mode of cell death caused by the expression of LGI1. The caspase-3 and -7 activity of HeLa cells expressing LGI1 was consistently greater than that of control cells. To strengthen the evidence on the induction of apoptosis of HeLa cell expressing LGI1, the relative amount of BCL2 and BAX expression was assessed by semi-quantitative PCR analysis and Western blotting. The levels of the anti-apoptotic BCL2 decreased whereas those of pro-apoptotic BAX systematically increased in all cell clones expressing LGI1 when compared with control cells, the variations correlated with LGI1 levels. The decreased ratio of BCL2/BAX supports the activation of the intrinsic pathway of apoptosis by the release of apoptogenic molecules from mitochondria of HeLa cells as it occurs in various cancer cell types (Xiong et al., 2003; Lombet et al., 2001; Raisova et al., 2001). In the case of HeLa cells the activity of LGI1 seems to antagonize that of the HPV oncoprotein E6. The latter impedes apoptosis by blocking p53 transcriptional regulation activity, which enhance the expression of BAX and repress that of BCL2 (Scheffneret al., 1993; Miyashita and Reed 1995; Wu et al., 2001). In other words LGI1 might destabilize the equilibrium of BCL2 and BAX in favour of apoptosis. The evidence that LGI1 interferes with central pro-survival pathway phosphoinositide 3-kinase (PI3K)/AKT, discussed in the next section, supports this suggestion because this pathway directly regulates BCL2 and BAX expression (Brunet et al., 2001).

8. Inhibition of the phosphoinositide 3-kinase pathway in neuroblastoma cells

The observation that neuroblastoma cells overexpressing LGI1 required daily changes of growth medium raised the possibility of an increased necessity of fresh serum to sustain survival. Thus the possibility that essential signaling pathways mediating survival stimuli conveyed by serum growth factors might be inhibited by LGI1 was investigated. The PI3K/AKT pathway is a central signaling pathway activated downstream of growth factor receptors. The activation of receptor tyrosine kinase stimulates PI3K to produce the second messengers phosphatidylinositol-3, 4,5-trisphosphate (PIP3), this activates the serine-threonine protein kinase AKT (protein kinase B), which directly regulates key cellular functions including apoptosis. AKT inactivates death signals by phopshorylating pro-apoptotic proteins such as forkhead transcription factors, caspase-9, Bad (Fukunaga et al. 2005; Clerkin et al., 2008). At the same time AKT up-regulates the expression of anti-apoptotic proteins such as BCL-XL and prevents the translocation of BAX to mitochondria (Tsuruta et al., 2002). AKT also up-regulates vascular endothelial growth factor (VEGF) and hypoxia-inducible factor 1 (HIF-1), thus enhancing angiogenesis, tumor growth and metastasis (Jiang and Liu, 2009). Furthermore, AKT prevents apoptosis determined by loss of cell-matrix interactions (anoikis), thus favoring metastasis formation (Wang, 2004).

8.1 Failure of PI3K inhibitors to increase cell death

The possibility that the elevation of LGI1 levels might inhibit trophic signaling through the PI3K/AKT pathway was investigated by measuring the fraction of dead cells in the presence of increasing amounts of the PI3K inhibitors wortmannin (Fig. 8) or LY294002. The results of LDH assays showed that the fraction of control cells death increased proportionally with the concentration of inhibitors to reach a maximum of about 30% at 50 nM wortmannin or 50 μM LY294002.

By contrast, the PI3K inhibitors failed to increase significantly dead of LGI1 cells, which even in the absence of inhibitors was similar to maximum values determined in the presence of the inhibitors with control pcDNA3 cells. The failure of the inhibitors to significantly increase cell death suggested that PI3K pathway was already inhibited by LGI1. This was particularly evident with SH-LGI1-12 cell clones, in which the effects of the inhibitors were completely absent.

8.2 Inhibition of AKT phosphorylation

The blockage of PI3K in LGI1 cells was further investigated by the evaluation of the activating AKT phosphorylation. For this purpose we performed an ELISA assays with two antibodies: one directed to AKT phospho-serine 473 and one to the total AKT protein. Cells were stimulated with 10% serum for 30 minutes to induce AKT phosphorylation, following

16 hours of serum starvation. The results of the quantitative analysis showed a sharp enhancement of AKT phosphorylation in control pcDNA3 cells (about 5-fold), which was abolished by inhibition of PI3K with wortmannin (50 nM), however, significant phosphorylation of AKT was absent in both LGI1 cell clones (Fig. 9).

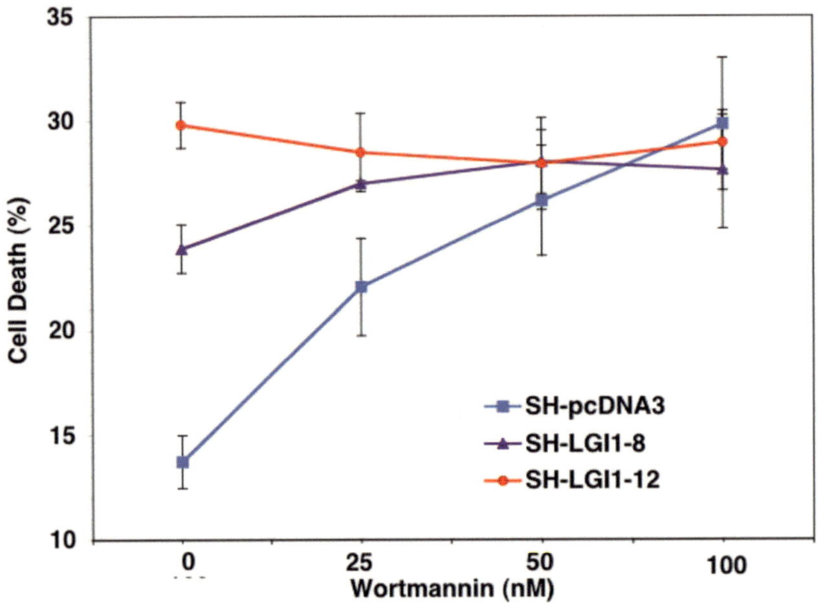

Fig. 8. Effects of PI3K inhibition on neuroblastoma cell death

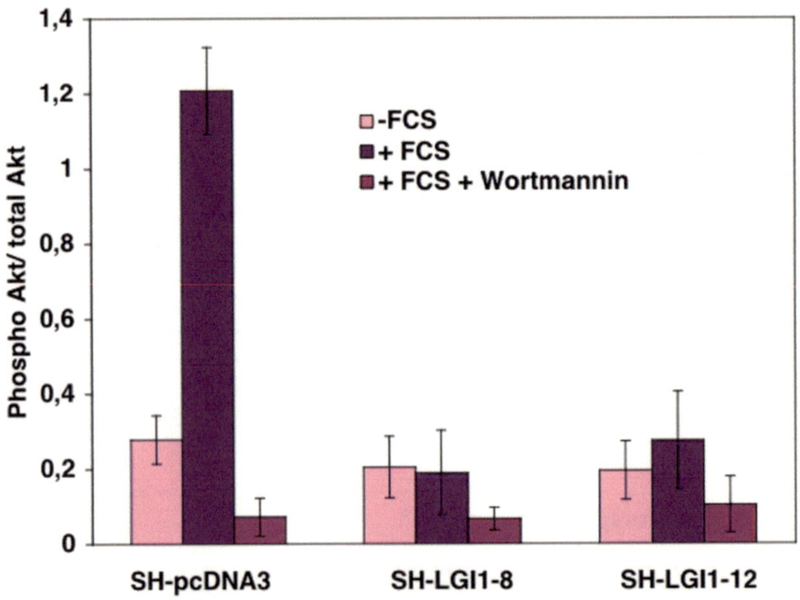

Fig. 9. Quantitative analysis of AKT phosphorylation induced by serum (FCS) in the presence or absence of PI3K inhibitor wormannin

The blockage of the downstream target of PI3K in LGI1 cells was supported by Western blotting of phospho-AKT and total AKT in the same experimental conditions used for ELISA assays. Following serum stimulation phopho-AKT Ser-473 was observed only in control pcDNA3 cells, which was consistently prevented in the presence of the inhibitor wortmannin. AKT failed to be phosphorylated in both LGI1 cell clones in response to serum (Fig. 10).

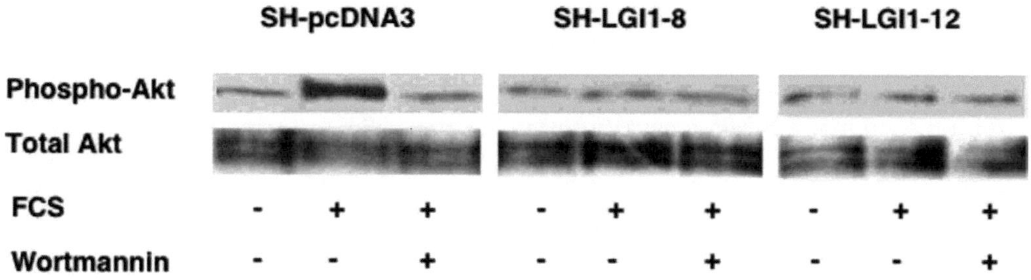

Fig. 10. Western blot analysis of total AKT and phospho-AKT induced by serum (FCS) in the presence or absence of PI3K inhibitor wormannin

The inhibition of the PI3K/AKT pathway in LGI1 cells is in agreement with the evidence that LGI1 triggers an intrinsic pathway of apoptosis, because deficiency of AKT activity shift the balance of mitochondrial factors in favor of apoptosis (Section 6.2.3).

9. Blockage of the MAPK/ERK pathway in glioblastoma cells

Also the mitogen-activated protein kinases (MAPKs) pathway can be activated downstream of tyrosine kinase receptors. This central signaling pathway controls a number of crucial cellular responses such as proliferation, migration and apoptosis. It is divided in at least four segments: the ERK pathway, which is activated downstream of growth factor receptors, and the JNK, p38 and ERK5 pathways, which are activated by stress and also in response to growth factors. Modifications of the MAPKs signaling determined by mutations or altered regulation of the components of this pathway, such as Ras or epidermal growth factor receptor, play an important role in cancerogenesis and metastasis formation (Roberts & Der 2007). In particular, the amplification of the epidermal growth factor receptor (EGFR) is one of the typical genetic alterations occurring in gliomas (Henn et al. 1986). The state of this signaling pathway was investigated in glioblastoma cells re-expressing LGI1, in view of the evidences on the inhibition of cell proliferation and migration ability emerged by the re-expression of LGI1 in glioblasoma cells (section 5.2.1).

9.1 Downregulation of matrix metalloproteinases

Matrix metalloproteinases (MMPs) are involved in the degradation of the extracellular matrix. Their physiological role is particularly important in development, tissue repair, and angiogenesis. MMPs are highly expressed in malignant brain tumors and have been implicated in the malignant developmemt of gliomas (Chintala et al. 1999; VanMeter et al., 2001). The increase of MMPs expression in tumors facilitates metastasis formation and neovascularization. Gene expression profiling of glioblastoma T98G cells re-expressing LGI1 compared with T98G control cell clones lacking LGI1 expression was performed to identify differentially expressed genes and to achieve some indications on the signaling pathway affected by LGI1 (Kunapuli et al. 2004). Oligonucleotide microarray analysis revealed that several genes for extracellular matrix proteins were downregulated in cells re-expressing LGI1. In particular the expression of matrix metalloproteinase -1 and -3 (MMP-1 and MMP-3) showed a significant downregulation, which was substantiated by RT-PCR analysis.

9.2 Inhibition of ERK1/2 phosphorylation

The influence of LGI1 on the activation MAPKs signaling pathways that were shown to control transcription of MMP genes (Westermarck et al., 2001) was investigated in the T98G glioblastoma cell clones (Kunapuli et al. 2004). In particular the phosphorylation status of the extracellular signal protein kinases ERK1/2 was analyzed by Western blot. The levels of phosphorylated ERK1/2 were lower in T98G cells expressing LGI1 than in control cells. Pharmacological treatment with MEK1 inhibitors significantly decreased the levels of ERK1/2 phosphorylation and inhibited the expression of MMP-1/-3 in T98G control cells. Also inhibitors of the p38 MAPK pathway interfered with the expression of MMP-1/-3, however, p38 phosphorylation was not modified significantly by the expression of LGI1. Thus the ERK1/2 pathway was identified as the specific target of inhibition by LGI1, resulting in the reduction of MMPs expression and consequently of the invasive potential of glioblastoma cells (Kunapuli et al. 2004).

9.3 Type-II tumor suppressor

The finding that LGI1 controls the expression of MMPs is consistent with the downregulation of LGI1 expression during the malignant progression of brain tumors. The downregulation of LGI1 might result in the increase of MPP expression supporting tumor growth and metastasis formation. These findings raised the possibility that the tumor suppressor function of LGI1 might impede malignant development, thus it was proposed to function as a type-II tumor suppressor gene (Besleaga et al., 2003).

9.4 Cell specific inhibition of signaling pathways

The re-expression of LGI1 in T98G glioblastoma cells produced a specific inhibition of the ERK1/2 pathway without hindering the PI3/AKT pathway, whereas the PI3K/AKT pathway was inhibited by the expression of LGI1 in neuroblastoma cells (Fig. 11). In neuroblastoma cells the effects of LGI1 on the MAPK/ERK pathway were determined in the same neuroblastoma cell samples employed for the analysis of AKT. Western blot with antibodies directed to phopho-ERK1/2 and to total ERK1/2 was performed to determine the phosphorylation status of ERK1/2. Addition of serum on starved cells induced ERK1/2 phosphorylation about 2-fold in all cell clones independently on the expression of LGI1. This observation confirmed the specificity of the PI3K/AKT pathway inhibition by LGI1 in neuroblastoma cells.

This divergence might depend on the specific activation of signaling pathway linked to growth factor receptors (RTK) in different cancer cells (Fig.11). Further investigations are needed to clarify the mechanism of PI3K/AKT pathway and ERK1/2 pathway inhibition produced by LGI1; this might provide new strategies to control cell survival, proliferation and metastasis formation.

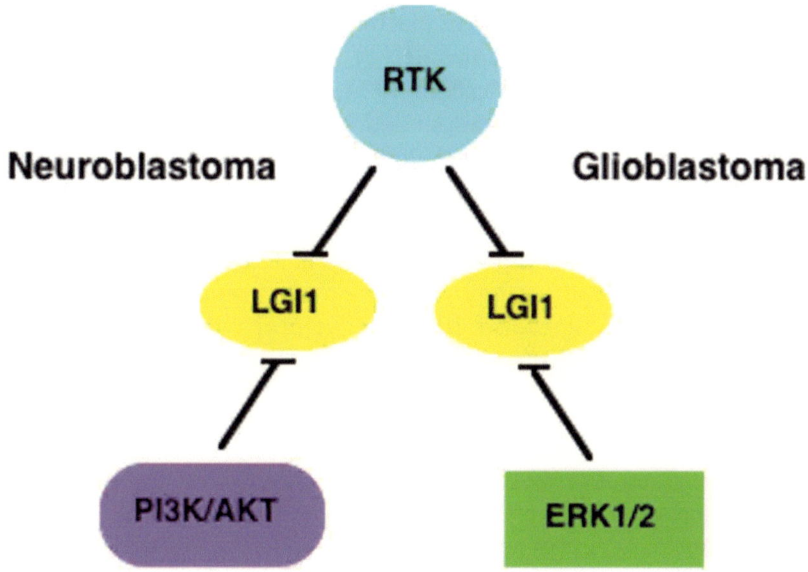

Fig. 11. Inhibition of signaling pathway downstream of RTK by LGI1 in neuroblastoma and glioblastoma cells.

10. Interacting proteins

LGI1 protein includes domains predicted to be involved protein-protein interaction (Section 3). The search for proteins interacting with LGI1 provided important indications on its function. First it was shown to interact with voltage gated potassium channel (Kv1.1) in axonal terminal of CNS neurons (Schulte et al., 2006), then it was described as a ligand for the epilepsy related neuronal receptor ADAM metallopeptidase 22 (Fukata et al., 2006). In contrast with the limited information on the function and signaling of ADAM22, Kv channels are well characterized and their activity is supposed to control a variety of cell functions. The voltage sensitive activity of Kv channels is particularly important in neurons where it controls membrane polarization, axon potential formation, firing properties and neurotransmitters release. However, it is also important in non-excitable cells, because it controls intracellular Ca^{2+} concentration, cell volume and cell survival (O'Grady & Lee, 2005).

10.1 Preclusion of Kv1 channels inactivation by Kvβ1

The membrane protein complex including Kv channels was affinity purified using antibodies to Kv1.1 subunit from rat brain and the protein complex was characterized using a proteomic approach (Schulte et al., 2006). Beside Kv1.1 also the regulatory subunit Kvβ1 and other subunits constituting the channels, plus several other proteins including Lgi1 were co-purified. The interaction of Lgi1 with Kv1.1 was unambiguous demonstrated by reverse co-purification with antibodies to Lgi1. In particular it was shown that Lgi1 co-purified with the Kv1.4 and Kvβ1 subunits. This was further confirmed by the results of immunohistochemitry on mouse brain showing co-localization of Lgi1 and Kv1.1 in the specific brain areas (described in Section 4), with prevalent pre-synaptic localization. To explore the functional role of Lgi1 on Kv channels activity, Kv1.1, Kv1.4, and Kvβ1 subunits, which compose a type of channel capable of inactivation, were expressed in *Xenopus* oocytes and patch-clamp recordings were performed in the presence or absence of Lgi1 co-expression. These experiments demonstrated that Lgi1 clearly reduced channel inactivation, the decay of the recorded currents corresponded to that of channels composed of Kv1.1-Kv1.4 suggesting that Lgi1 prevents channel closure by the Kvβ1 subunit. The expression of LGI1 carrying ADLTE mutations failed to antagonize the inactivation by Kvβ1, suggesting that loss of LGI1 function may enhances channel inactivation by Kvβ1. This study suggested that modifications of the inactivation properties of Kv channels in ADLTE patients carrying LGI1 mutations support epileptic activity. However, the immunohystochemistry analysis revealed that expression of Lgi1 also occurs in neurons that do not express Kv1.1, suggesting that LGI1 might have different functions.

10.2 Increased K^+ permeability and induction of apoptosis

The regulation of Kv channel activity by LGI1 was discussed in the context of epilepsy; however, it might be related also to the tumor suppressor function of LGI1 because these channels are important regulator of cell survival. Indeed the upregulation of Kv1.1 activity was associated with neuronal apoptosis, while the inhibition or downregulation Kv channels with increased cell survival (Hu et al., 2008; Yu et al., 1997). Since it was shown that binding of LGI1 to Kv1β prevents channel inactivation, a deficit of LGI1 would results in a decreased of K^+ permeability and inhibition of apoptosis.

11. LGI1 as a therapeutic target

The discoveries that LGI1 inhibits central signaling pathways that regulate cell proliferation, survival, motility and angiogenesis render LGI1 an attractive therapeutic target. The decline of LGI1 expression in the malignant progression of gliomas and the downregulation of MMP production caused by the re-expression of LGI1 in glioblatoma cells, point out LGI1 as a target for the treatment of malignant brain tumors. However, a better understanding of the mechanisms of apoptosis and of MMP expression regulation is necessary to develop efficacious strategies of intervention.

11.1 Future directions

Gene therapy to achieve the re-expression of LGI1 might be a useful approach to treat malignant brain tumors with downregulated expression of LGI1, however, because gliomas are genetically heterogeneous, the determination of the genetic alterations that characterize each tumor is required to create effective strategies. An important mechanism of carcinogenesis tumor invasion, and metastasis operative in cancer cells is gene silencing by DNA hypermethylation of tumor suppressor genes. Epigenetic therapy to reduce promoter methylation might become suitable to re-express LGI1 in malignant brain tumors when an appropriate technology will be developed.

12. Conclusion

Several evidences supporting the tumor suppressor role of LGI1 have been presented here. The discovery of chromosomal rearrangements leading to loss of LGI1 expression in glioblastoma cells, mutations in LGI1 gene specifically associated with gliobastoma and the downregulation of LGI1 expression in several tumors all point out a role of LGI1 in tumor suppression. Furthermore the findings that re-expression of LGI1 in glioblastoma cells impaired cell growth and migration ability through inhibition of the ERK1/2 pathway, with consequent downregulation of MMPs expression, support a role in the suppression of metastasis formation and tumor vascularization. This is in line with the downregulation of LGI1 expression observed in the malignant progression of gliomas. The findings that increased expression of LGI1 impaired growth and survival of neuroblastoma cells further strengthen the tumor suppressor role of LGI1. The involvement of LGI1 in the negative regulation of the PI3K/AKT pathway supporting cell proliferation and survival explains the mechanism of spontaneous cell death triggered by the elevation of LGI1 levels in neuroblatoma cells. The activation of intrinsic apoptosis triggered by LGI1 is consistent with a blockage of AKT activity, which regulates Bcl-2 family members involved in the control of mitochondrial membrane permeability. Furthermore, the interaction of LGI1 protein with voltage gated potassium channels (Kv1.1) shown to prevent channel inactivation by Kv1β subunit, provides an additional link with apoptosis since these channels are important regulators of cell survival. Because suppression of apoptosis in cancer cells is one of the main strategies to achieve the survival advantage required for malignant progression, it is feasible that alterations of LGI1 gene or downregulation of expression often observed in cancer cells might be required to suppress apoptosis through the inhibition of survival pathways linked to growth factor receptors and of Kv channels activity.

13. Chapter summary

- Alterations of LGI1 gene occur in some glioblastomas.
- Downregulation of LGI1 gene is associated with the malignant progression of gliomas.
- Downregulation of LGI1 gene occurs in several other tumors.
- Re-expression of LGI1 gene in glioblastoma cells, lacking endogenous LGI1 expression, decreases cell proliferation and invasiveness through the inhibition of the MAPK/ERK1-2 pathway and downregulation of MMP production.
- Overexpression of LGI1 in neuroblastoma cells, in which endogenous LGI1 expression is downregulated, impairs proliferation and induces apoptosis through the inhibition of the PI3K/AKT pathway.
- The pro-apoptotic function of LGI1 is also linked to the upregulation of Kv channels activity through the blockage of the negative regulator Kv beta subunit.
- The downregulation or inactivation of LGI1 gene often observed in tumor cells might be related to the suppression of apoptosis, beside enhancement of cell proliferation and invasion.

14. References

Barnholtz-Sloan, J.; Sloan, A.E.; Land, S. & Kupsky, W. Monteiro AN. (2008) Somatic alterations in brain tumors. *Oncology Reports.* Vol.20, No.1, pp203-210. ISSN 1021335X

Battye, R.; Stevens, A.; Perry, R.L. & Jacobs, J.R. (2001) Repellent signaling by Slit requires the leucine-rich repeats. *Journal of Neuroscience*. Vol.21, No.12, pp.4290-4298. ISSN 02706474

Besleaga, R.; Montesinos-Rongen, M.; Perez-Tur, J.; Siebert, R.& Deckert, M. (2003) Expression of the LGI1 gene product in astrocytic gliomas: downregulation with malignant progression. *Virchows Archiv*. Vol.443, No.4, pp.561-564. ISSN 09456317

Blanco-Aparicio, C.; Renner, O.; Leal, J.F. & Carnero, A. PTEN, more than the AKT pathway. (2007) *Carcinogenesis*. Vol. 28. No,7. pp.1379-1386. ISSN 01433334

Brodtkorb, E.; Nakken, K.O. & Steinlein, O.K. (2003) No evidence for a seriously increased malignancy risk in LGI1-caused epilepsy. *Epilepsy Research*. Vol.56, No.2-3, pp205-208. ISSN 09201211

Brunet, A.; Datta, S.R. & Greenberg, M.E. (2001) Transcription-dependent and -independent control of neuronal survival by the PI3K-Akt signaling pathway. *Current Opinion in Neurobiology*. Vol.11, No.3, pp.297-305. ISSN 09594388

Chernova, O.B.; Somerville, R.P. & Cowell, J.K. (1998). A novel gene, LGI1, from 10q24 is rearranged and downregulated in malignant brain tumors. *Oncogene*. Vol.17, No.22, pp. 2873-2881. ISSN 09509232

Chintala, S.K.; Tonn, J.C. & Rao, J.S. (1999) Matrix metalloproteinases and their biological function in human gliomas. *International Journal of Developmental Neuroscience*. Vol.17, No.5-6, pp.495-502 ISSN 07365748

Clerkin, J.S.; Naughton, R.; Quiney, C. & Cotter, T.G. (2008) Mechanisms of ROS modulated cell survival during carcinogenesis. *Cancer Letters*. Vol.266, No.1, pp.30-36. ISSN 03043835

Cory, S. & Adams, J.M. (2002) The BCL2 family: regulators of the cellular life-or-death switch. *Nature Review Cancer*. Vol.2, No.9, pp.647-656. ISSN 1474175X

Cregan, S.P.; Fortin, A.; MacLaurin, J.G.; Callaghan, S.M.; Cecconi, F.; Yu, S.W.; Dawson, T.M.; Dawson, V.L.; Park, D,S,; Kroemer, G. & Slack, R,S. (2002) Apoptosis-inducing factor is involved in the regulation of caspase-independent neuronal cell death. *Journal of Cell Biology*. Vol.158, No.3, pp.507-517. ISSN 00219525

Fukata, Y.; Adesnik, H.; Iwanaga, T.; Bredt, D.S.; Nicoll, R.A. & Fukata, M. (2006) Epilepsy-related ligand/receptor complex LGI1 and ADAM22 regulate synaptic transmission. *Science*. Vol.313, No.5794, pp.1792-1795. ISSN 00368075

Fukunaga, K.; Ishigami, T. & Kawano, T. (2005) Transcriptional regulation of neuronal genes and its effect on neural functions: expression and function of forkhead transcription factors in neurons. *Journal of Pharmacological Sciences*. Vol.98, No.3, pp.205-211. ISSN 13478613

Gabellini, N. & Masola, V. (2008) LGI1 affects survival of neuroblastoma cells by inhibiting signaling through Phosphoinositide 3-Kinase. *Current Signal Transduction Therapy*. Vol.3, No.2, pp.129-132. ISSN 15743624

Gabellini, N. & Masola, V. (2009) Expression of LGI1 impairs proliferation and survival of HeLa Cells. *International Journal of Cell Biology*. 2009:417197. ISSN 16878876

Gabellini, N. (July 2007). LGI1 (Leucine-rich, Glioma Inactivated protein 1 precursor), In: *Atlas Genetics and Cytogenetics in Oncology and Haematology*. Available from http://AtlasGeneticsOncology.org/Genes/LGI1ID311ch10q23.html

Gabellini, N.; Masola, V.; Quartesan, S.; Oselladore, B.; Nobile, C.; Michelucci, R.; Curtarello, M.; Parolin, C. & Palù, G. (2006) Increased expression of LGI1 gene triggers growth inhibition and apoptosis of neuroblastoma cells. *Journal of Cellular Physiology*. Vol.207, No.3, pp711-721. ISSN 00219541

Head, K.; Gong, S.; Joseph, S.; Wang, C.; Burkhardt, T.; Rossi, M.R.; LaDuca, J.; Matsui, S.; Vaughan, M.; Hicks, D.G.; Heintz, N.& Cowell, J.K. (2007) Defining the expression pattern of the LGI1 gene in BAC transgenic mice. *Mammalian Genome* Vol.18, No.5, pp.328-337. ISSN 09388990

Hengartner, M.O. . (2000) The biochemistry of apoptosis. *Nature*. Vol. 407, No.6805, pp.770-776.

Henn, W. ; Blin, N. & Zang, K.D. Polysomy of chromosome 7 is correlated with overexpression of the erbB oncogene in human glioblastoma cell lines. (1986). *Human Genetics*. Vol.74, No.1, pp. 104-106. ISSN 03406717

Herranz-Pérez, V.; Olucha-Bordonau, F.E.; Morante-Redolat, J.M. & Pérez-Tur, J. (2010) Regional distribution of the leucine-rich glioma inactivated (LGI) gene family transcripts in the adult mouse brain. *Brain Research*. Vol.1307, pp.177-194. ISSN 00068993

Hu, C.L.; Zeng, X.M.; Zhou, M.H.; Shi, Y.T.; Cao, H. & Mei, Y.A. (2008) Kv 1.1 is associated with neuronal apoptosis and modulated by protein kinase C in the rat cerebellar granule cell. *Journal of Neurochemistry*. Vol.106, No.3, pp.1125-3117. ISSN 00223042

Inagaki, Y.; Tsunokawa, Y.; Takebe, N.; Nawa, H.; Nakanishi, S.; Terada, M. & Sugimura, T. (1988) Nucleotide sequences of cDNAs for human papillomavirus type 18 transcripts in HeLa cells. *Journal of virology*. Vol.62, No.5, pp.1640-1646. ISSN 0022538X

Jiang, B.H. & Liu, L.Z. (2009) PI3K/PTEN signaling in angiogenesis and tumorigenesis. *Advanced Cancer Research*. Vol.102, pp19-65. ISSN 0065-230X

Kalachikov, S.; Evgrafov, O.; Ross, B.; Winawer, M.; Barker-Cummings, C.; Martinelli Boneschi, F.; Choi, C.; Morozov, P.; Das, K.; Teplitskaya, E.; Yu, A.; Cayanis, E.; Penchaszadeh, G.; Kottmann, A.H.; Pedley, T.A.; Hauser, W.A.; Ottman, R. & Gilliam, T.C. (2002) Mutations in LGI1 cause autosomal-dominant partial epilepsy with auditory features. *Nature Genetics*. Vol.30, No.3, pp.335-341. ISSN 10614036

Karlbom, A.E. ; James, C.D. ; Boethius, J.; Cavenee, W.K.; Collins, V.P.; Nordenskjöld, M. & Larsson, C. (1993) Loss of heterozygosity in malignant gliomas involves at least three distinct regions on chromosome 10. *Human Genetics* Vol.92, No.2, pp. 169-174. ISSN 03406717

Kobe, B. & Deisenhofer, J. (1994) The leucine-rich repeat: a versatile binding motif. *Trends in Biochemical Sciences*. Vol.19, No.10, pp.415-421. ISSN 09680004

Krex, D.; Hauses, M.; Appelt, H.; Mohr, B.; Ehninger, G.; Schackert, H.K. & Schackert, G. (2002) Physical and functional characterization of the human LGI1 gene and its possible role in glioma development. *Acta Neuropathologica*. Vol.103, No.3, pp.255-266. ISSN 00016322

Kroemer, G. & Reed, J.C. (2000) Mitochondrial control of cell death. *Nature Medicine*. Vol.6, No.5, pp.513-519. ISSN 10788956

Kunapuli, P.; Chitta, K.S. & Cowell, J.K. (2003) Suppression of the cell proliferation and invasion phenotypes in glioma cells by the LGI1 gene. *Oncogene*. Vol.22, No.26, pp.3985-3991. ISSN 09509232

Kunapuli,P.; Kasyapa, C.S.; Hawthorn, L. & Cowell,J.K. (2004) LGI1, a Putative Tumor Metastasis Suppressor Gene, Controls in Vitro Invasiveness and Expression of

Matrix Metalloproteinases in Glioma Cells through the ERK1/2 Pathway. *Journal of Biological Chemistry*. Vol. 279, No. 22, pp. 23151–23157. ISSN 00219285

Li, L.Y.; Luo, X. & Wang, X. (2001) Endonuclease G is an apoptotic DNase when released from mitochondria. *Nature*. Vol.412, No.6842, pp.95-99. ISSN 00280836

Lombet, A.; Zujovic, V.; Kandouz, M.; Billardon, C.; Carvajal-Gonzalez, S.; Gompel, A. & Rostène, W. (2001) Resistance to induced apoptosis in the human neuroblastoma cell line SK-N-SH in relation to neuronal differentiation. Role of Bcl-2 protein family. *European journal of biochemistry*. Vol.268, No.5, pp1352-1362. ISSN 0014-2956

Martinou, J.C. & Green, D.R. (2001) Breaking the mitochondrial barrier. *Nature Reviews Molecular Cell Biology*. Vol.2, No.1, pp.63-67. ISSN 14710072

McMillan, D.R.; Kayes-Wandover, K.M.; Richardson, J.A. & White, P.C. (2002) Very large G protein-coupled receptor-1, the largest known cell surface protein, is highly expressed in the developing central nervous system. *Journal of Biological Chemistry*. Vol.277, No.1, pp.785-792. ISSN 00219285

Michelucci, R.; Pasini, E.; & Nobile, C. (2009) Lateral temporal lobe epilepsies: clinical and genetic features. *Epilepsia*. Vol.50 Suppl. 5, pp.52-54. ISSN 00139580

Miyashita, T.& Reed, J.C. (1995) Tumor suppressor p53 is a direct transcriptional activator of the human bax gene. *Cell*. Vol.80, No.2, pp.293-299. ISSN 00928674

Mollenhauer, J.; Wiemann, S.; Scheurlen, W.; Korn, B.; Hayashi, Y.; Wilgenbus, K.K.; von Deimling, A. & Poustka, A. (1997) DMBT1, a new member of the SRCR superfamily, on chromosome 10q25.3-26.1 is deleted in malignant brain tumors. *Nature Genetics*. Vol.17, No.1, pp.32-39. ISSN 10614036

Morante-Redolat, J.M.; Gorostidi-Pagola, A; Piquer-Sirerol, S.; Sáenz, A.; Poza, J.J.; Galán, J.; Gesk, S.; Sarafidou, T.; Mautner, V.F.; Binelli, S.; Staub, E.; Hinzmann, B.; French, L.; Prud'homme, J.F.; Passarelli, D.; Scannapieco, P.; Tassinari, C.A.; Avanzini, G.; Martí-Massó, J.F.; Kluwe, L.; Deloukas, P.; Moschonas, N.K.; Michelucci, R.; Siebert, R.; Nobile, C.; Pérez-Tur, J. & López de Munain, A. (2002) Mutations in the LGI1/Epitempin gene on 10q24 cause autosomal dominant lateral temporal epilepsy. *Human Molecular Genetics*. Vol.11, No.9, pp. 1119-1128. ISSN 09646906

O'Grady, S.M. & Lee, S.Y. (2005) Molecular diversity and function of voltage-gated (Kv) potassium channels in epithelial cells. *The International Journal of Biochemistry & Cell Biology*. Vol.37, No.8, pp.1578–1594. ISSN 13572725

Parsons, D.W.; Jones, S,; Zhang, X.; Lin, J.C.; Leary. R.J.; Angenendt, P.; Mankoo, P.; Carter, H,; Siu. I.M. ; Gallia, G.L.; Olivi, A. ; McLendon, R, ; Rasheed, B.A.; Keir, S.; Nikolskaya, T,; Nikolsky, Y. ; Busam, D.A.; Tekleab, H.; Diaz, L.A. Jr; Hartigan, J.; Smith, D.R.; Strausberg, R.L.; Marie, S.K.; Shinjo, S.M.; Yan, H.; Riggins, G.J.; Bigner, D.D.; Karchin, R.; Papadopoulos, N.; Parmigiani, G.; Vogelstein, B,; Velculescu, V.E. & Kinzler, K.W. (2008) An integrated genomic analysis of human glioblastoma multiforme. *Science*. Vol.321, No.5897, pp.1807-1812. ISSN 00368075

Peng, D.; Sheta, E.A.; Powell, S.M.; Moskaluk, C.A.; Washington, K.; Goldknopf, I..L. & El-Rifai, W. (2008) Alterations in Barrett's-related adenocarcinomas: a proteomic approach. *International Journal of Cancer*. Vol.122, No.6, pp.1303-1310. ISSN 00207136

Raisova, M.; Hossini, A.M.; Eberle, J.; Riebeling, C.; Wieder, T.; Sturm, I.; Daniel, P.T.; Orfanos, C.E. & Geilen, C.C. (2001) The Bax/Bcl-2 ratio determines the susceptibility of human melanoma cells to CD95/Fas-mediated apoptosis. Journal of Investigative Dermatology. Vol.117, No.2, pp.333-340. ISSN 0022202X

Reed, J.C. (1998) Bcl-2 family proteins. *Oncogene*. Vol.17, No.25, pp3225-3236. ISSN 09509232

Roberts PJ, Der CJ. (2007) Targeting the Raf-MEK-ERK mitogen-activated protein kinase cascade for the treatment of cancer. *Oncogene*. Vol.26, No.22, pp.3291-3310. ISSN 09509232

Rossi, M.R.; Huntoon, K. & Cowell, J.K. (2005) Differential expression of the LGI and SLIT families of genes in human cancer cells. *Gene*. Vol.15, No.356, pp85-90. ISSN 03781119

Scheel, H.; Tomiuk, S. & Hofmann, K. A. common protein interaction domain links two recently identified epilepsy genes. (2002) *Human Molecular* Genetics. Vol.11, No.15, pp.1757-1762. ISSN 09646906

Scheffner, M.; Huibregtse, J.M.; Vierstra, R.D. & Howley, P.M. (1993) The HPV-16 E6 and E6-AP complex functions as a ubiquitin-protein ligase in the ubiquitination of p53. *Cell*. Vol.75, No.3, pp.495-505. ISSN 00928674

Schulte, U.; Thumfart, J.O.; Klöcker, N.; Sailer, C.A.; Bildl, W.; Biniossek, M.; Dehn, D.; Deller, T.; Eble, S.; Abbass, K.; Wangler, T.; Knaus, H.G.& Fakler, B. (2006) The epilepsy-linked Lgi1 protein assembles into presynaptic Kv1 channels and inhibits inactivation by Kvbeta1. *Neuron*. Vol.49, No.5, pp 697-706. ISSN 08966273

Schwab, M. (2004) MYCN in neuronal tumors. *Cancer Letters*. Vol.204, No.2, pp.179-187. ISSN 03043835

Schwab, M.; Westermann, F.; Hero, B. & Berthold F. (2003) Neuroblastoma: biology and molecular and chromosomal pathology. *The Lancet oncology*. Vol.4, No.8, pp.472-480. ISSN 14702045

Senechal, K.R.; Thaller, C. & Noebels, J.L.ADPEAF mutations reduce levels of secreted LGI1, a putative tumor suppressor protein linked to epilepsy. (2005) *Human Molecular Genetics*. Vol.14, No.12, pp.1613-1620. ISSN 09646906

Sirerol-Piquer, M.S.; Ayerdi-Izquierdo, A.; Morante-Redolat, J.M.; Herranz-Pérez, V.; Favell, K.; Barker, P.A. & Pérez-Tur, J. (2006) The epilepsy gene LGI1 encodes a secreted glycoprotein that binds to the cell surface. *Human Molecular Genetics*. Vol.15, No.23, pp.3436-3445. ISSN 09646906

Somerville, R.P.; Chernova, O.; Liu, S.; Shoshan, Y. & Cowell, J.K. Identification of the promoter, genomic structure, and mouse ortholog of LGI1. (2000) *Mammalian Genome*. Vol.11, No.8, pp.622-627. ISSN 09388990

Springer, T.A. (2002) Predicted and experimental structures of integrins and beta-propellers. *Current Opinion in Structural Biology*. Vol.12, No.6, pp.802-813. ISSN 0959440X

Staub, E.; Pérez-Tur, J.; Siebert, R.; Nobile, C.; Moschonas, N.K.; Deloukas, P. & Hinzmann; B. (2002) The novel EPTP repeat defines a superfamily of proteins implicated in epileptic disorders. *Trends in Biochemical Sciences*. Vol.27, No.9, pp.441-444. ISSN 09680004

Susin, S.A.; Lorenzo, H.K.; Zamzami, N.; Marzo, I.; Snow, B.E.; Brothers, G.M.; Mangion, J.; Jacotot, E.; Costantini, P.; Loeffler, M.; Larochette, N.; Goodlett, D.R.; Aebersold, R.; Siderovski, D.P.; Penninger, J.M. & Kroemer, G. (1999) Molecular characterization of mitochondrial apoptosis-inducing factor. *Nature*. Vol.397, No.6718, pp.441-446. ISSN 00280836

Tsuruta, F.; Masuyama, N. & Gotoh, Y. (2002) The phosphatidylinositol 3-kinase (PI3K)-Akt pathway suppresses Bax translocation to mitochondria. *Journal of Biological Chemistry*. Vol.277, No.16, pp.14040-14047. ISSN 00219285

VanMeter, T.E.; Rooprai, H.K.; Kibble, M.M.; Fillmore, H.L.; Broaddus, W.C. and Pilkington, G.J. (2001) The role of matrix metalloproteinase genes in glioma invasion: co-dependent and interactive proteolysis. *Journal of Neuro-oncololy*. Vol.53, No.2; pp.213-235. ISSN 0167-594X

Wang, J.; Valo, Z.; Bowers, C.W.; Smith, D.D.; Liu, Z. & Singer-Sam, J. (2010) Dual DNA methylation patterns in the CNS reveal developmentally poised chromatin and monoallelic expression of critical genes. *PLoS One*. Vol.5, No.11, e.13843. ISSN 19326203

Wang, L.H. (2004) Molecular signaling regulating anchorage-independent growth of cancer cells. *Mount Sinai Journal of Medicine*. Vol.71, No.6, pp.361-367. ISSN 0027-2507

Westermarck, J.; Li, S.P.; Kallunki, T.; Han, J. & Kähäri, V.M. (2001) p38 mitogen-activated protein kinase-dependent activation of protein phosphatases 1 and 2A inhibits MEK1 and MEK2 activity and collagenase 1 (MMP-1) gene expression. *Molecular and Cellular Biology*. Vol.21, No.7, pp.2373-2383. ISSN 02707306

Wu, Y.; Mehew, J.W.; Heckman, C.A.; Arcinas, M. & Boxer, L.M. (2001) Negative regulation of bcl-2 expression by p53 in hematopoietic cells. *Oncogene*. Vol.20, No.2, pp. 240-251. ISSN 09509232

Xiong, J.; Chen, J.; Chernenko, G.; Beck, J.; Liu, H.; Pater, A. & Tang, S.C. (2003) Antisense BAG-1 sensitizes HeLa cells to apoptosis by multiple pathways. *Biochemical and Biophysical Research Communications*. Vol.312, No.3, pp.585-591. ISSN 0006291X

Xiong, J.P.; Stehle, T.; Diefenbach, B.; Zhang, R.; Dunker, R.; Scott, D.L.; Joachimiak, A.; Goodman, S.L. & Arnaout, M.A. (2001) Crystal structure of the extracellular segment of integrin alpha Vbeta3. *Science*. Vol.294, No.5541, pp.339-345. ISSN 00368075

Yu, S.P.; Yeh, C.H.; Sensi, S.L.; Gwag, B.J.; Canzoniero, L.M.; Farhangrazi, Z.S.; Ying, H.S.; Tian, M.; Dugan, L.L. & Choi, D.W. (1997) Mediation of neuronal apoptosis by enhancement of outward potassium current. *Science*. Vol.278, No.5335, pp.114-117. ISSN 00368075

Part 8

Antioxidant Adaptive Response in Glioma

12

Antioxidant Adaptive Response of Malignant Glioma Related to Resistance to Antitumor Treatment

Tomohiro Sawa and Takaaki Akaike
Department of Microbiology, Graduate School of Medical Sciences, Kumamoto University
Japan

1. Introduction

Glioblastomas are the most frequent and most malignant nervous system tumors [Stewart & Kleihues, 2003]. Despite technological advances in surgical treatment and new regimens of radiotherapy combined with chemotherapy, the median survival of patients with these tumors is approximately 1 year, and only 3% of patients survive more than 3 years [Stupp et al., 2005]. Glioblastomas have been traditionally defined as two clinically and cytogenetically distinct diseases: the primary or de novo glioblastomas and the secondary glioblastomas. The latter commonly appear in younger people (median age at onset ~45 years) as low-grade gliomas and possess aberrations in genes encoding platelet-derived growth factor receptor (*PDGFR*) and *TP53* [Stewart & Kleihues, 2003]. Primary glioblastomas occur more frequently (>80% of cases) and develop rapidly in older people (median age at onset ~60 years); survival of patients with such tumors is short, less than 3 months [Stewart & Kleihues, 2003]. The genetic profile of primary glioblastomas includes amplification and overexpression of the gene encoding epidermal growth factor receptor (*EGFR*), mutations of the phosphatase and tensin homolog (*PTEN*) gene, $p16^{INK4A}$ deletions, and loss of chromosome 10 [Stewart & Kleihues, 2003]. Several inhibitors that target *EGFR* or its downstream signaling cascade including Akt and mTOR have been evaluated for potential application in glioblastoma treatment [Krakstad & Chekenya, 2010]. Recent clinical trials of *EGFR* inhibitors, however, showed no therapeutic benefit [Prados et al., 2006; Rich et al., 2004].

Chemotherapy plays an important role in combined treatment of gliomas, whereas it appears to fail in a significant clinical outcome. This may be largely due to drug resistance of malignant gliomas developed [Lu & Shervington, 2008; Sarkaria, et al, 2008; Frosina, 2009; Bleau et al., 2009]. Multiple mechanisms may be involved in the development of drug resistance in gliomas, including DNA repair enzyme activities, particularly O^6-methylguanine methyltransferase for alkylating agents, overexpression of antiapoptotic proteins such as Bcl-2 or Bcl-X_L and ABC transporters that efflux anticancer drugs. Clarification of mechanisms for glioma drug resistance may provide us an important insight for the development of promising strategies for the treatment of gliomas.

A number of studies have suggested that heme oxygenase-1 (HO-1) expression occurs in various types of tumors, both animal models and human cancers including glioblastomas

[Fang et al., 2004a; Hara et al., 1996]. HO is a rate-limiting enzyme that catalyzes the initial step of heme degradation in which oxidative cleavage of the porphyrin ring results in generation of biliverdin, carbon monoxide (CO), and free iron [Maines, 1988; Schacter, 1988]. Cytosolic biliverdin reductase then reduces the biliverdin to form the potent antioxidant bilirubin. Three mammalian HO isoforms have been identified: HO-1, HO-2, and HO-3. Among them, HO-1 is a member (HSP-32) of the heat shock protein family, and HO-1 expression is triggered by various stress-inducing stimuli including hypoxia [Motterlini et al., 2000], heavy metals [Keyse & Tyrrell, 1989; Mitani et al., 1993], UV irradiation [Keyse & Tyrrell, 1989], and reactive oxygen species (ROS) and nitric oxide (NO) [Doi et al., 1999; Foresti et al., 1997]. Because of the antioxidant and cytoprotective nature of HO products, elevated HO-1 expression in glioblastomas may be a key component of cellular adaptation to oxidative stress and toxic insults induced by chemotherapeutic agents [Fang et al., 2004b]. The fact that HO-1 expression is related to resistance of glioma cells to oxidative stress and anticancer agents indicates that the pathways involved in regulating HO-1 expression in gliomas may be molecular targets for treatment. This chapter describes the mechanisms and regulation of HO-1 expression and the adaptive response of glioma cells. The chapter pays particular attention to the adaptive response signaling that is mediated by 8-nitroguanosine 3′,5′-cyclic monophosphate (8-nitro-cGMP), a newly discovered nitrated nucleotide that functions as an endogenous inducer of the response [Akaike et al., 2010; Fujii et al., 2010; Sawa et al., 2007; Zaki et al., 2009]. Also discussed is the potential application of HO inhibitors as a new class of chemotherapeutic and chemosensitizing agents.

2. Antioxidant adaptive response mediated by a nitrated cyclic nucleotide

The antioxidant adaptive response to oxidative stress is a critically important mechanism that allows aerobic organisms to maintain redox homeostasis. The Keap1 (Kelch-like ECH-associated protein 1)/Nrf2 (nuclear factor-erythroid 2-related factor 2) system plays a key role in adaptation to oxidative stress and toxic insults of electrophilic compounds (including many chemotherapeutic agents) by inducing antioxidant and cytoprotective enzymes such as HO-1.

2.1 The Keap1/Nrf2 system as a sensor of oxidants and electrophiles

Keap1 contains reactive cysteine residues that can serve as sensing moieties for oxidants and electrophiles [Dinkova-Kostova et al., 2005; Itoh et al., 2004; Sekhar et al., 2010]. Various electrophiles called Nrf2 inducers, both naturally occurring and synthetic, have reportedly reacted with Keap1 cysteine residues.

Keap1, which exists as dimers inside cells, comprises five distinct domains: (i) the N-terminal region (NTR, amino acids 1-60); (ii) the BTB (Bric-a-brac, Tramtrack, Broad-complex) domain (amino acids 61-178), which is an evolutionarily conserved protein-protein interaction motif that occurs in actin-binding proteins and zinc finger transcription factors and participates in binding to Rbx1-bound Cullin 3 (Cul3) [Dinkova-Kostova et al., 2005] and formation of homodimers [Zipper & Mulcahy, 2002]; (iii) the intervening region (IVR, amino acids 179-321), which is a central linker domain, especially rich in cysteine, that also takes part in binding toRbx1-bound Cul3 [A. Kobayashi et al., 2004]; (iv) the Kelch repeat domain (amino acids 322-608), which mediates binding to the Nef2 domain of Nrf2 [M.

Kobayashi et al., 2002]; and (v) the C-terminal region (CTR, amino acids 609-625). Site-directed mutagenesis assays have revealed that three cysteine residues, Cys151, Cys273, and Cys288, play critical roles in the Keap1-Nrf2 complex interaction [D.D. Zhang & Hannink, 2003]. Cys151, located in the BTB domain, is probably the major site that is directly alkylated by chemopreventive agents that work by activating the antioxidant response element (ARE) through Nrf2 [Eggler et al., 2007]. This modification of Cys151 leads to conformational changes in the BTB domain via perturbation of the homodimerization site and results in switching ubiquitination from Nrf2 to Keap1, thereby facilitating translocation of Nrf2 to the nucleus and its accumulation there [Eggler et al., 2005]. Cys273 and Cys288, which are located in the IVR domain of Keap1, are essential for stability of the Nrf2-Keap1 complex and maintenance of Nrf2 homeostasis [Wakabayashi et al., 2004]. ARE inducers, via conformational changes in Keap1—i.e., covalent modification or oxidation of cysteine thiol groups in the IVR region of Keap1—make Keap1 incapable of binding to Nrf2 and thereby facilitate nuclear translocation of Nrf2.

Nrf2, a member of the cap'n'collar family of basic region leucine zipper transcription factors, has a crucial role in regulating several stress-responsive genes, including HO-1 [Dinkova-Kostova et al., 2005; Bloom & Jaiswal, 2003; Itoh et al., 2004; Zhu et al., 2005]. Under basal conditions, transcriptional activity of Nrf2 is negatively regulated by the Nrf2-binding partner Keap1, a cysteine-rich cytoplasmic protein [Dinkova-Kostova et al., 2005; Sekhar et al., 2010; Surh et al., 2009; Zhao et al., 2010]. Keap1, serving as a substrate adaptor protein for a Cul3-dependent ubiquitin ligase complex, targets Nrf2 for ubiquitination and proteasomal degradation [Dinkova-Kostova et al., 2005; Sekhar et al., 2010; Surh et al., 2009; Zhao et al., 2010]. During oxidative stress, chemical modification of one or more cysteine residues of Keap1 facilitates Nrf2 dissociation, which leads to nuclear translocation of Nrf2. After migration to the nucleus, Nrf2 forms heterodimers with small musculoaponeurotic fibrosarcoma (sMaf) proteins and then binds to the cis-acting ARE [Motohashi & Yamamoto, 2007]. The result is transcriptional activation of a battery of genes that encode various phase II detoxifying or antioxidant enzymes, such as glutathione *S*-transferase (GST), NAD(P)H:quinone oxidoreductase (NQO1), and HO-1, as well as other cytoprotective proteins [Nguyen et al., 2003] .

2.2 Nitrated guanine nucleotide as an endogenous electrophile that activates the Keap1/Nrf2 system

Both NO and ROS are critically involved, via Nrf2-dependent mechanisms, as endogenous inducers of HO-1 expression in gliomas. 8-Nitro-cGMP is a nitrated nucleotide that was identified as a second messenger in NO and ROS signaling in induction of an adaptive response mediated by the Keap1/Nrf2 system [Akaike et al., 2010; Fujii et al., 2010; Ihara et al., 2011b; Sawa et al., 2007, 2011; Zaki et al., 2009]. 8-Nitro-cGMP also functions in extracellular signal-regulated kinase pathways in neurons [Kurauchi et al., 2011]. Formation of 8-nitro-cGMP can be triggered in rat C6 glioma cells by treatment with a chemical NO donor (*S*-nitroso-*N*-acetylpenicillamine or treatment with inflammatory stimuli (lipopolysaccharide plus pro-inflammatory cytokines) that activate endogenous NO production via expression of inducible NO synthase [Fujii et al., 2010]. Under these conditions, ROS production is also increased and depends on both NADPH oxidase and mitochondria [Ahmed et al., 2011a]. Pharmacological studies have suggested that 8-nitro-cGMP is formed from its precursor 8-nitroguanosine 5′-triphosphate by means of catalytic action of soluble guanylate cyclase [Fujii et al., 2010; Ihara et al., 2011a]. So far, guanine nitration has been identified in various biological systems including lungs of mice suffering from viral pneumonia [Akaike et al., 2003], lungs of patients with idiopathic pulmonary fibrosis and lung cancer [Terasaki et al., 2006], and urine from cigarette smokers [Sawa et al., 2006].

Activation of the Keap1/Nrf2-mediated adaptive response by 8-nitro-cGMP involves a unique post-translational modification of the cysteine residues of Keap1 [Akaike et al., 2010; Fujii et al., 2010; Sawa et al., 2007; Zaki et al., 2009]. 8-Nitro-cGMP is the first known endogenously formed electrophilic nucleotide [Akaike et al., 2010; Fujii et al., 2010; Saito et al., 2008; Sawa et al., 2007; Zaki et al., 2009]. Because of its electrophilic characteristics, 8-nitro-cGMP reacts with cysteine residues in proteins, particularly residues with low pK_a values that facilitate deprotonation of those residues to form a cysteine thiolate anion [Ahmed et al., 2011b; Akaike et al., 2010; Sawa et al., 2010]. Reaction of 8-nitro-cGMP with the thiolate anion results in cGMP adduction to the cysteine residue, a process called "protein *S*-guanylation" (Fig. 1) [Sawa et al., 2007]. Keap1 was identified as a possible target during 8-nitro-cGMP-induced protein *S*-guanylation in cells [Fujii et al., 2010; Sawa et al., 2007; Zaki et al., 2009]. In fact, Keap1 *S*-guanylation was clearly demonstrated when rat C6 glioma cells were treated with lipopolysaccharide plus pro-inflammatory cytokines [Fujii et al., 2010]. Mass spectrometry revealed that Keap1 *S*-guanylation in rat C6 cells occurred predominantly at Cys434 [Fujii et al., 2010]. X-ray crystallographic analysis suggested that the Cys434 residue is located at blade 3 and is exposed to the outer surface of the β-propeller structure [Lo et al., 2006; Padmanabhan et al., 2006].

With regard to the mechanism of how *S*-guanylation of Cys434 causes Nrf2 activation, two possibilities present themselves. One is that *S*-guanylation of Cys434 may weaken Keap1 binding to the ETGE and DLG motifs of Nrf2, because Cys434 is located close to the Nrf2-binding region of the DC domain. The alternative possibility is that Cys434 modification may affect the integrity of the entire Keap1-Nrf2 complex. Fitting the atomic DC domain model into the overall Keap1 homodimer structure obtained via single-particle electron microscopy showed that the globular part of the Keap1 cherry-bob structure was bulkier than the DC domain, which suggests that the external DC domain surface is wrapped with the other part of Keap1, perhaps the IVR between the BTB and DC domains [Ogura et al., 2010]. Thus, *S*-guanylation may cause disruption of the globular structure incorporating the DC domain, which would disturb the entire structure and result in reduced ubiquitin ligase activity of the Cul3-Keap1 complex.

Among genes regulated by Nrf2, HO-1 has been regarded as conferring important protection against oxidative stress [T.J. Chen et al., 2006; Y.C. Chen et al., 2006; Konorev et al., 2002]. HO-1 may induce cytoprotective responses through various mechanisms including (i) reducing prooxidant levels (heme) [Jeney et al., 2002]; (ii) raising antioxidant levels (bilirubin) [Baranano et al., 2002]; (iii) generating the antiapoptotic CO [Brouard et al., 2000]; (iv) inducing ferritin, which detoxifies and removes free ferric ions [Balla et al., 1992]; and (v) blocking overstimulation of an immune response [Lee & Chau, 2002]. We found that 8-nitro-cGMP increased Nrf2 accumulation in the nucleus and HO-1 expression in rat C6 glioma cells (Fig. 2) [Fujii et al., 2010]. Treatment with 8-nitro-cGMP caused C6 cells to become resistant to cell death induced by oxidative stress related to hydrogen peroxide exposure [Fujii et al., 2010]. Therefore, 8-nitro-cGMP conceivably participates in an antioxidant signaling pathway involved in cytoprotection or adaptive responses to ROS and oxidative stress.

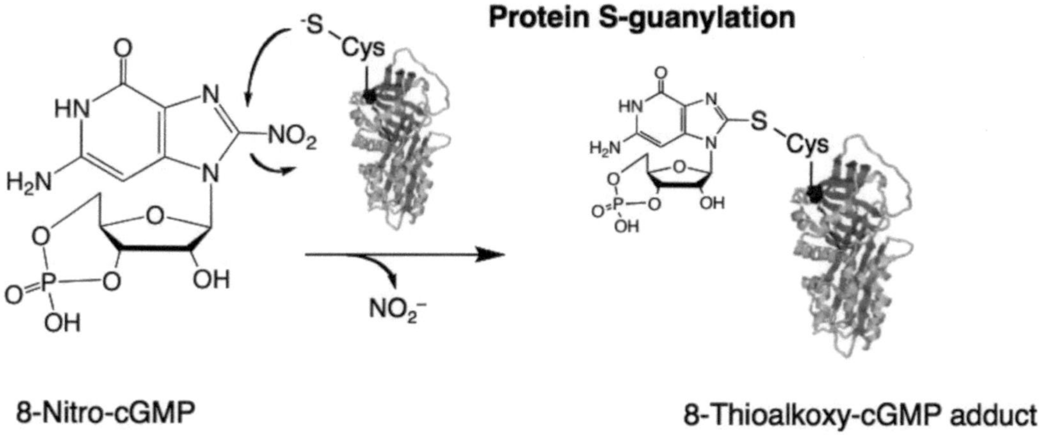

Fig. 1. Schematic representation of protein *S*-guanylation induced by 8-nitro-cGMP. The nucleophilic protein thiolate anions attack the C8 of 8-nitro-cGMP, which results in adduction of cGMP moieties to cysteine residues in proteins, with concomitant release of a nitrite anion.

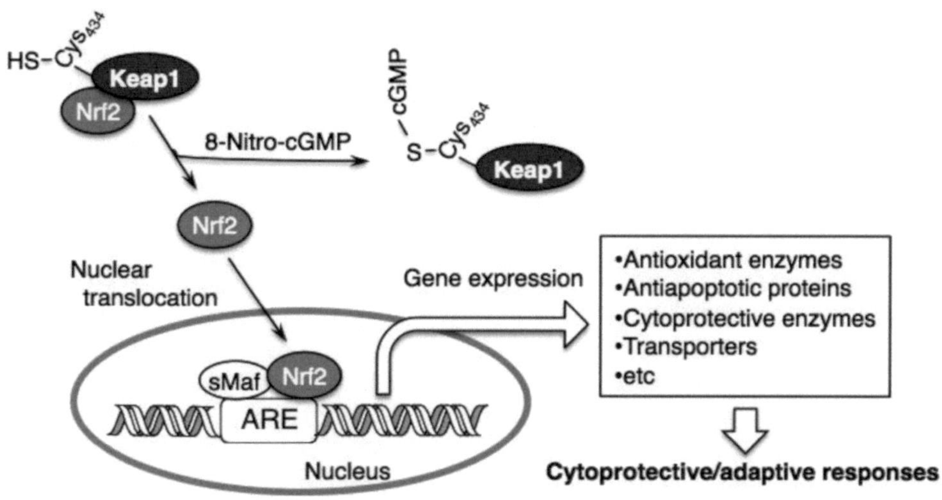

Fig. 2. 8-Nitro-cGMP-mediated cytoprotection as a result of *S*-guanylation of Keap1. *S*-Guanylation of Keap1 facilitates dissociation of Nrf2 from Keap1 and leads to translocation of Nrf2 to the nucleus. In the nucleus, Nrf2 forms a heterodimer with sMaf proteins, thereby inducing expression of various cytoprotective enzymes.

3. Genetic regulation of the Keap1/Nrf2 system in cancer cells

Hypermethylation of the promoter CpG island is an epigenetic mechanism that leads to gene silencing [Warnecke & Bestor, 2000]. Quite recently, promoter methylation of the *KEAP1* gene was found in malignant gliomas [Muscarella et al., 2011]. A strong inverse correlation was discovered between methylation levels and *KEAP1* mRNA transcript in tumor tissue [Muscarella et al., 2011], which suggests the occurrence of *KEAP1* gene silencing in gliomas. The reduction in *KEAP1* expression caused by promoter methylation may contribute to constitutive Nrf2 stabilization and subsequent activation of an antioxidant response in gliomas, as seen in certain cancer cells such as those in the lung [Wang et al., 2008] and prostate [P. Zhang et al., 2010]. Inactivation of Keap1 functions by somatic mutations causing amino acid substitutions has been found in cancer cells in the breast, lung, gallbladder, and liver [Shibata et al., 2008a; Singh et al., 2006; Taguchi et al., 2011]. Also, mutations in the *NRF2* gene that are related to the reduction in Keap1-Nrf2 interaction were identified in human cancers of the lung, head and neck, and esophagus [Shibata et al., 2008b; Taguchi et al., 2011]. Such mutations in the *KEAP1* and *NRF2* genes, however, have not yet been found in gliomas and hence warrant further investigation.

4. HO-1 as a target for chemosensitization: The therapeutic potential of HO inhibitors

Many antitumor agents, such as cisplatin, doxorubicin, mitomycin C, vinblastine, and arsenic trioxide, produce cytotoxic effects via generation of ROS and/or electrophilic actions, which lead to oxidative stress [Dilda & Hogg, 2007; Fang et al., 2007; Simizu et al., 1998]. Hence, those antitumor agents activate Nrf2-dependent HO-1 induction, either by direct actions or by indirect means, i.e., by augmenting the intrinsic signaling cascade mediated by endogenous inducers including 8-nitro-cGMP, as mentioned above. Tumor cells subsequently become resistant to treatment with those antitumor agents. That the HO-1-dependent antioxidant system would be a potential target for chemosensitization is therefore conceivable. The following discussion will cover the effects of disrupting the HO-1-dependent antioxidant system on chemosensitivity, with particular attention to HO inhibitors as new chemosensitizers.

Knockdown of HO-1 or its master regulator Nrf2 is a straightforward approach to disrupting the HO-1 antioxidant system. We found that knockdown of HO-1 by means of small interfering RNA (siRNA) resulted in the induction of apoptosis in SW480 human colon cancer cells in culture [Fang et al., 2003]. Liu et al. [2011] reported that Nrf2 knockdown effectively led to suppressed HO-1 expression and enhanced sensitization to arsenic trioxide-induced apoptosis in cultured human glioma cells U251MG and A172. Quite recently, HO-1 expression was found to be regulated post-transcriptionally by microRNA (miRNA). Beckman et al. [2011], by using an HO-1 reporter assay, found that a combination of two miRNAs (miR-377 and miR-217) markedly reduced HO-1 expression. Mature miRNAs are ~21-22 nucleotides long and affect post-translational expression of genes by interacting with complementary target sites in the 3′-untranslated region of the mRNA [Jackson & Standart, 2007]. The exact molecular mechanisms used by miRNAs to mediate translational repression are still being studied intensively; however, modulation of HO-1 activity by miRNAs may be an alternative strategy for sensitizing tumor cells to chemotherapy.

Direct inhibition of HO-1 enzyme activity may be an alternative approach for disruption of the HO-1-mediated antioxidant system in tumor cells. Metalloporphyrins are a class of compounds in which various metals such as cobalt, zinc, manganese, chromium, or tin replace the central iron in heme [Drummond, 1987]. These metalloporphyrins can act as competitive inhibitors of the HO reaction because they bind inefficiently to molecular oxygen, so HO is prevented from degrading the metalloporphyrins [Drummond, 1987].

Antitumor and chemosensitizing effects of metalloporphyrin-type HO inhibitors such as zinc protoporphyrin (ZnPP) and cobalt protoporphyrin have been demonstrated in cultured tumor cells and in animal models [Doi et al., 1999; Fang et al., 2003, 2004b; Liu et al., 2011; Tanaka et al., 2003]. Combining chemotherapeutic agents such as camptothecin, doxorubicin, arsenic trioxide, gemcitabine, and imatinib, as well as irradiation, with ZnPP or related inhibitors may lead to improved antitumor treatment [Fang et al., 2004b; Gleixner et al., 2009; Liu et al., 2011; Mayerhofer et al., 2008; Miyake et al., 2010].

Polyethylene glycol-conjugated ZnPP (PEG-ZnPP) is a water-soluble derivative of ZnPP (Fig. 3) [Sahoo et al., 2002]. PEG-ZnPP accumulates in solid tumor tissues after intravenous injection because of its unique ability to form micelles in aqueous media [Fang et al., 2003; Sahoo et al., 2002]. As evidenced by accumulation of PEG-ZnPP in tumors, tumor-targeted inhibition of HO activity may be achieved by using PEG-ZnPP, which induces apoptosis in solid tumors via induction of oxidative stress [Fang et al., 2003]. Potent synergistic activity was also observed when PEG-ZnPP was combined with antitumor agents [Fang et al., 2004b]. This combined treatment was tolerated well, with no evident signs of severe toxicity and no dose-limiting toxicity so far. These observations point to new applications of PEG-ZnPP in combination therapy with various anticancer agents as well as irradiation.

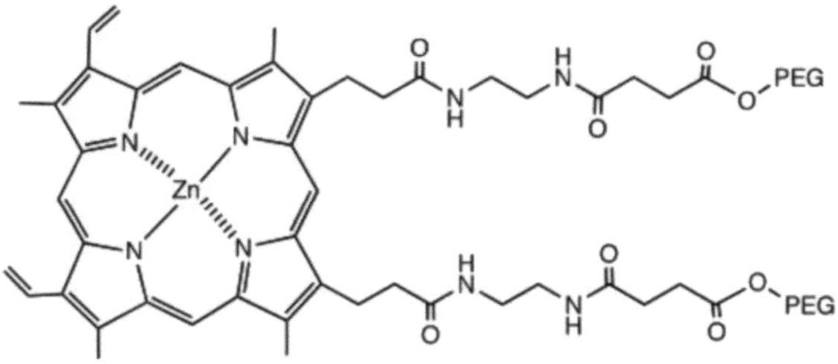

PEG-ZnPP (metalloporphyrin-type inhibitor)

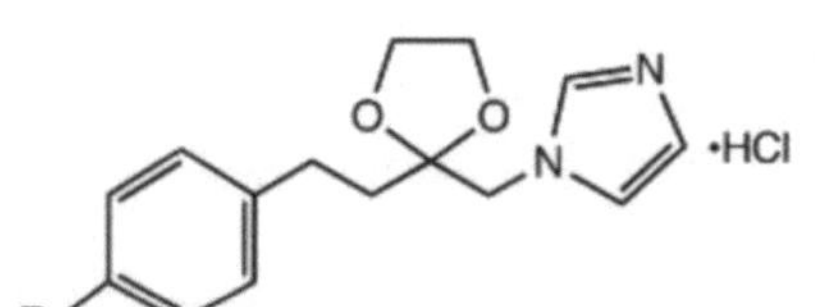

2-[2-(4-Bromophenyl)ethyl]-2-[(1*H*-imidazol-1-yl)methyl]-1,3-dioxolane hydrochloride (imidazole-dioxolane-type inhibitor)

Fig. 3. Chemical structures of HO inhibitors used in combination with anticancer agents to treat tumors.

In addition to the metalloporphyrin-type HO inhibitors, non-porphyrin-based HO inhibitors have been developed (Fig. 3). Azalanstat, an imidazole-dioxolane compound, was produced as such an HO inhibitor [Vlahakis et al., 2005]. With azalanstat as the lead compound, so far more than 100 imidazole-based compounds have been synthesized and their HO inhibitory activities evaluated [Kinobe et al., 2006; Roman et al., 2007; Vlahakis et al., 2005]. Some of these compounds are quite selective for HO-1, with selectivity indices greater than 300 relative to HO-2, a constitutive isoform of HO [Kinobe et al., 2008]. One recent study showed that the imidazole-based compound OB-24 exhibited potent antitumor activity in a hormone-refractory prostate cancer model, especially in combination with paclitaxel [Alaoui-Jamali et al., 2009], which suggests that additional investigations of this type of HO inhibitor and possible uses for tumor chemosensitization are warranted.

Chapter summary

- Drug resistance is a major cause of treatment failure in patients with malignant gliomas.
- Multiple mechanisms may be involved in the development of drug resistance in gliomas, including augmented DNA repair enzyme activities, overexpression of antiapoptotic proteins and ABC transporters, whereas detailed mechanisms remain unknown.
- Heme oxygenase-1 (HO-1), a rate-limiting enzyme for heme degradation, may contribute to the development of chemoresistance in gliomas, via inducing gene expression of antioxidant, antiapoptotic, cytoprotective enzymes and drug transporters.
- Nitric oxide, reactive oxygen species, and their down stream electrophilic second messengers such as nitrated cyclic nucleotide play crucial roles in HO-1 expression via activation of redox-sensitive transcriptional factor (Nrf2).
- HO inhibitors exhibit potential to sensitize tumor cells against chemotherapy.

5. Conclusion

This chapter describes induction mechanisms of the antioxidant adaptive response in gliomas. Nrf2 stabilization may be induced by post-translational cysteine modification of Keap1, which is a repressor of Nrf2, under conditions of excess production of NO and ROS. 8-Nitro-cGMP is a newly discovered second messenger for NO and ROS signaling that can induce *S*-guanylation of Keap1 in glioma cells. *KEAP1* gene silencing via promoter methylation is an alternative mechanism that may contribute to constitutive Nrf2 stabilization. Activation of Nrf2 signaling leads to the expression of genes encoding phase II detoxifying or antioxidant enzymes as well as other cytoprotective proteins. Among these enzymes, HO-1 is known as a strong antioxidant and antiapoptotic enzyme that protects cells from oxidative stress-related injury. Many studies have shown that inhibition of HO-1 activity, by using either siRNA or HO-1 inhibitors, is a promising strategy for chemosensitization of cancer cells. In addition to direct antioxidant actions of HO-1, which support cancer cell growth as discussed in this chapter, HO-1 expression may contribute to the growth of gliomas by facilitating neovascularization via a vascular endothelial growth factor-dependent mechanism [Morita et al., 2009; Nishie et al., 1999]. HO-1 expression is also correlated with progression of gliomas, possibly through FoxP3-mediated T cell immune suppression [Deininger et al., 2000; El Andaloussi & Lesniak, 2007]. Improved understanding of the mechanisms mediating the Keap1/Nrf2-HO-1 antioxidant response and regulation by 8-nitro-cGMP and its downstream signaling cascade is necessary for development of chemotherapeutic drugs that will target malignant gliomas.

6. Acknowledgment

We thank J.B. Gandy for excellent editing of the manuscript.

7. References

Ahmed, K.A., Sawa, T., Ihara, H., Kasamatsu, S., Yoshitake, J., Rahaman, M.M., Okamoto, T., Fujii, S. & Akaike, T. (2011a). Regulation by mitochondrial superoxide and NADPH oxidase of cellular formation of nitrated cyclic GMP: potential implications for ROS signaling. *Biochem. J.*, in press.

Ahmed, K.A., Sawa, T. & Akaike, T. (2011b). Protein cysteine *S*-guanylation and electrophilic signal transduction by endogenous nitro-nucleotides. *Amino Acids,* Vol. 162, No. 8, pp. 123-130.

Akaike, T., Fujii, S., Sawa, T. & Ihara, H. (2010). Cell signaling mediated by nitrated cyclic guanine nucleotide. *Nitric Oxide,* Vol. 23, No. 3 pp. 166-174.

Akaike, T., Okamoto, S., Sawa, T., Yoshitake, J., Tamura, F., Ichimori, K., Miyazaki, K., Sasamoto, K. & Maeda, H. (2003). 8-Nitroguanosine formation in viral pneumonia and its implication for pathogenesis. *Proc. Natl. Acad. Sci. USA*, Vol. 100, No. 2, pp. 685-690.

Alaoui-Jamali, M.A., Bismar, T.A., Gupta, A., Szarek, W.A., Su, J., Song, W., Xu, Y., Xu, B., Liu, G., Vlahakis, J.Z., Roman, G., Jiao, J. & Schipper, H.M. (2009). A novel experimental heme oxygenase-1-targeted therapy for hormone-refractory prostate cancer. *Cancer Res.*, Vol. 69, No. 20, pp. 8017-8024.

Balla, G., Jacob, H.S., Balla, J., Rosenberg, M., Nath, K., Apple, F., Eaton, J.W. & Vercellotti, G.M. (1992). Ferritin: a cytoprotective antioxidant strategem of endothelium. *J. Biol. Chem.*, Vol. 267, No. 25, pp. 18148-18153.

Baranano, D.E., Rao, M., Ferris, C.D. & Snyder, S.H. (2002). Biliverdin reductase: a major physiologic cytoprotectant. *Proc. Natl. Acad. Sci. USA*, Vol. 99, No. 25, pp. 16093-16098.

Beckman, J.D., Chen, C., Nguyen, J., Thayanithy, V., Subramanian, S., Steer, C.J. & Vercellotti, G.M. (2011). Regulation of heme oxygenase-1 protein expression by miR-377 in combination with miR-217. *J. Biol. Chem.*, Vol. 286, No. 5, pp. 3194-3202.

Bleau, A.M., Huse, J.T. & Holland, E.C. (2009). The ABCG2 resistance network of glioblastoma. *Cell Cycle* 8; 2936-44.

Bloom, D.A. & Jaiswal, A.K. (2003). Phosphorylation of Nrf2 at Ser^{40} by protein kinase C in response to antioxidants leads to the release of Nrf2 from INrf2, but is not required for Nrf2 stabilization/accumulation in the nucleus and transcriptional activation of antioxidant response element-mediated NAD(P)H:quinone oxidoreductase-1 gene expression. *J. Biol. Chem.*, Vol. 278, No. 45, pp. 44675-44682.

Brouard, S., Otterbein, L.E., Anrather, J., Tobiasch, E., Bach, F.H., Choi, A.M. & Soares, M.P. (2000). Carbon monoxide generated by heme oxygenase 1 suppresses endothelial cell apoptosis. *J. Exp. Med.*, Vol. 192, No. 7, pp. 1015-1026.

Chen, T.J., Jeng, J.Y., Lin, C.W., Wu, C.Y. & Chen, Y.C. (2006). Quercetin inhibition of ROS-dependent and -independent apoptosis in rat glioma C6 cells. *Toxicology*, Vol. 223, No. 1-2, pp. 113-126.

Chen, Y.C., Chow, J.M., Lin, C.W., Wu, C.Y. & Shen, S.C. (2006). Baicalein inhibition of oxidative-stress-induced apoptosis via modulation of ERKs activation and induction of HO-1 gene expression in rat glioma cells C6. *Toxicol. Appl. Pharmacol.*, Vol. 216, No. 2, pp. 263-273.

Deininger, M.H., Meyermann, R., Trautmann, K., Duffner, F., Grote, E.H., Wickboldt, J. & Schluesener, H.J. (2000). Heme oxygenase (HO)-1 expressing macrophages/microglial cells accumulate during oligodendroglioma progression. *Brain Res.*, Vol. 882, No. 1-2, pp. 1-8.

Dilda, P.J. & Hogg, P.J. (2007). Arsenical-based cancer drugs. *Cancer Treat. Rev.*, Vol. 33, No. 6, pp. 542-564.

Dinkova-Kostova, A.T., Holtzclaw, W.D. & Kensler, T.W. (2005). The role of Keap1 in cellular protective responses. *Chem. Res. Toxicol.*, Vol. 18, No. 12, pp. 1779-1791.

Doi, K., Akaike, T., Fujii, S., Tanaka, S., Ikebe, N., Beppu, T., Shibahara, S., Ogawa, M. & Maeda, H. (1999). Induction of haem oxygenase-1 nitric oxide and ischaemia in experimental solid tumours and implications for tumour growth. *Br. J. Cancer.*, Vol. 80, No. 12, pp. 1945-1954.

Drummond, G.S. (1987). Control of heme metabolism by synthetic metalloporphyrins. *Ann. NY Acad. Sci.*, Vol. 514, pp. 87-95.

Eggler, A.L., Liu, G., Pezzuto, J.M., van Breemen, R.B. & Mesecar, A.D. (2005). Modifying specific cysteines of the electrophile-sensing human Keap1 protein is insufficient to disrupt binding to the Nrf2 domain Neh2. *Proc. Natl. Acad. Sci. USA*, Vol. 102, No. 29, pp. 10070-10075.

Eggler, A.L., Luo, Y., van Breemen, R.B. & Mesecar, A.D. (2007). Identification of the highly reactive cysteine 151 in the chemopreventive agent-sensor Keap1 protein is method-dependent. *Chem. Res. Toxicol.*, Vol. 20, No. 12, pp. 1878-1884.

El Andaloussi, A. & Lesniak, M.S. (2007). $CD4^+CD25^+FoxP3^+$ T-cell infiltration and heme oxygenase-1 expression correlate with tumor grade in human gliomas. *J. Neurooncol.*, Vol. 83, No. 2, pp. 145-152.

Fang, J., Akaike, T. & Maeda, H. (2004a). Antiapoptotic role of heme oxygenase (HO) and the potential of HO as a target in anticancer treatment. *Apoptosis*, Vol. 9, No. 1, pp. 27-35.

Fang, J., Nakamura, H. & Iyer, A.K. (2007). Tumor-targeted induction of oxystress for cancer therapy. *J. Drug Target.*, Vol. 15, No. 7-8, pp. 475-486.

Fang, J., Sawa, T., Akaike, T., Akuta, T., Sahoo, S.K., Khaled, G., Hamada, A. & Maeda, H. (2003). In vivo antitumor activity of pegylated zinc protoporphyrin: targeted inhibition of heme oxygenase in solid tumor. *Cancer Res.*, Vol. 63, No. 13, pp. 3567-3574.

Fang, J., Sawa, T., Akaike, T., Greish, K. & Maeda, H. (2004b). Enhancement of chemotherapeutic response of tumor cells by a heme oxygenase inhibitor, pegylated zinc protoporphyrin. *Int. J. Cancer.*, Vol. 109, No. 1, pp. 1-8.

Foresti, R., Clark, J.E., Green, C.J. & Motterlini, R. (1997). Thiol compounds interact with nitric oxide in regulating heme oxygenase-1 induction in endothelial cells. Involvement of superoxide and peroxynitrite anions. *J. Biol. Chem.*, Vol. 272, No. 29, pp. 18411-18417.

Frosina, G. (2009). DNA repair and resistance of gliomas to chemotherapy and radiotherapy. *Mol Cancer Res* 7; 989-99.

Fujii, S., Sawa, T., Ihara, H., Tong, K.I., Ida, T., Okamoto, T., Ahtesham, A.K., Ishima, Y., Motohashi, H., Yamamoto, M. & Akaike, T. (2010). The critical role of nitric oxide signaling, via protein *S*-guanylation and nitrated cyclic GMP, in the antioxidant adaptive response. *J. Biol. Chem.*, Vol. 285, No. 31, pp. 23970-23984.

Gleixner, K.V., Mayerhofer, M., Vales, A., Gruze, A., Hormann, G., Cerny-Reiterer, S., Lackner, E., Hadzijusufovic, E., Herrmann, H., Iyer, A.K., Krauth, M.T., Pickl, W.F., Marian, B., Panzer-Grumayer, R., Sillaber, C., Maeda, H., Zielinski, C. & Valent, P. (2009). Targeting of Hsp32 in solid tumors and leukemias: a novel approach to optimize anticancer therapy. *Curr. Cancer Drug Targets*, Vol. 9, No. 5, pp. 675-689.

Hara, E., Takahashi, K., Tominaga, T., Kumabe, T., Kayama, T., Suzuki, H., Fujita, H., Yoshimoto, T., Shirato, K. & Shibahara, S. (1996). Expression of heme oxygenase and inducible nitric oxide synthase mRNA in human brain tumors. *Biochem. Biophys. Res. Commun.*, Vol. 224, No. 1, pp. 153-158.

Ihara, H., Ahmed, K.A., Ida, T., Kasamatsu, S., Kunieda, K., Okamoto, T., Sawa, T. & Akaike, T. (2011a). Methodological proof of immunocytochemistry for specific identification of 8-nitroguanosine 3',5'-cyclic monophosphate formed in glia cells. *Nitric Oxide* 25; 169-75.

Ihara, H., Sawa, T., Nakabeppu, Y. & Akaike, T. (2011b). Nucleotides function as endogenous chemical sensors for oxidative stress signaling. *J. Clin. Biochem. Nutr.*, Vol. 48, No. 1, pp. 33-39.

Itoh, K., Tong, K.I. & Yamamoto, M. (2004). Molecular mechanism activating Nrf2-Keap1 pathway in regulation of adaptive response to electrophiles. *Free Radic. Biol. Med.*, Vol. 36, No. 10, pp. 1208-1213.

Jackson, R.J. & Standart, N. (2007). How do microRNAs regulate gene expression? *Sci. STKE*, Vol. 2007, No. 367, p. re1.

Jeney, V., Balla, J., Yachie, A., Varga, Z., Vercellotti, G.M., Eaton, J.W. & Balla, G. (2002). Pro-oxidant and cytotoxic effects of circulating heme. *Blood*, Vol. 100, No. 3, pp. 879-887.

Keyse, S.M. & Tyrrell, R.M. (1989). Heme oxygenase is the major 32-kDa stress protein induced in human skin fibroblasts by UVA radiation, hydrogen peroxide, and sodium arsenite. *Proc. Natl. Acad. Sci. USA*, Vol. 86, No. 1, pp. 99-103.

Kinobe, R.T., Dercho, R.A. & Nakatsu, K. (2008). Inhibitors of the heme oxygenase–carbon monoxide system: on the doorstep of the clinic? *Can. J. Physiol. Pharmacol.*, Vol. 86, No. 9, pp. 577-599.

Kinobe, R.T., Vlahakis, J.Z., Vreman, H.J., Stevenson, D.K., Brien, J.F., Szarek, W.A. & Nakatsu, K. (2006). Selectivity of imidazole-dioxolane compounds for in vitro inhibition of microsomal haem oxygenase isoforms. *Br. J. Pharmacol.*, Vol. 147, No. 3, pp. 307-315.

Kobayashi, A., Kang, M.I., Okawa, H., Ohtsuji, M., Zenke, Y., Chiba, T., Igarashi, K. & Yamamoto, M. (2004). Oxidative stress sensor Keap1 functions as an adaptor for

Cul3-based E3 ligase to regulate proteasomal degradation of Nrf2. *Mol. Cell. Biol.*, Vol. 24, No. 16, pp. 7130-7139.

Kobayashi, M., Itoh, K., Suzuki, T., Osanai, H., Nishikawa, K., Katoh, Y., Takagi, Y. & Yamamoto, M. (2002). Identification of the interactive interface and phylogenic conservation of the Nrf2-Keap1 system. *Genes Cells*, Vol. 7, No. 8, pp. 807-820.

Konorev, E.A., Kotamraju, S., Zhao, H., Kalivendi, S., Joseph, J. & Kalyanaraman, B. (2002). Paradoxical effects of metalloporphyrins on doxorubicin-induced apoptosis: scavenging of reactive oxygen species versus induction of heme oxygenase-1. *Free Radic. Biol. Med.*, Vol. 33, No. 7, pp. 988-997.

Krakstad, C. & Chekenya, M. (2010). Survival signalling and apoptosis resistance in glioblastomas: opportunities for targeted therapeutics. *Mol. Cancer*, Vol. 9, p. 135.

Kurauchi, Y., Hisatsune, A., Isohama, Y., Sawa, T., Akaike, T., Shudo, K. & Katsuki, H. (2011). Midbrain dopaminergic neurons utilize nitric oxide/cyclic GMP signaling to recruit ERK that links retinoic acid receptor stimulation to up-regulation of BDNF. *J. Neurochem.*, Vol. 116, No. 3, pp. 323-333.

Lee, T.S. & Chau, L.Y. (2002). Heme oxygenase-1 mediates the anti-inflammatory effect of interleukin-10 in mice. *Nat. Med.*, Vol. 8, No. 3, pp. 240-246.

Liu, Y., Liang, Y., Zheng, T., Yang, G., Zhang, X., Sun, Z., Shi, C. & Zhao, S. (2011). Inhibition of heme oxygenase-1 enhances anti-cancer effects of arsenic trioxide on glioma cells. *J. Neurooncol*, Vol. 104, No. 2, pp. 449-458.

Lo, S.C., Li, X., Henzl, M.T., Beamer, L.J. & Hannink, M. (2006). Structure of the Keap1:Nrf2 interface provides mechanistic insight into Nrf2 signaling. *EMBO J.*, Vol. 25, No. 15, pp. 3605-3617.

Lu, C. & Shervington, A. (2008). Chemoresistance in gliomas. *Mol Cell Biochem* 312; 71-80.

Maines, M.D. (1988). Heme oxygenase: function, multiplicity, regulatory mechanisms, and clinical applications. *FASEB J.*, Vol. 2, No. 10, pp. 2557-2568.

Mayerhofer, M., Gleixner, K.V., Mayerhofer, J., Hoermann, G., Jaeger, E., Aichberger, K.J., Ott, R.G., Greish, K., Nakamura, H., Derdak, S., Samorapoompichit, P., Pickl, W.F., Sexl, V., Esterbauer, H., Schwarzinger, I., Sillaber, C., Maeda, H. & Valent, P. (2008). Targeting of heat shock protein 32 (Hsp32)/heme oxygenase-1 (HO-1) in leukemic cells in chronic myeloid leukemia: a novel approach to overcome resistance against imatinib. *Blood*, Vol. 111, No. 4, pp. 2200-2210.

Mitani, K., Fujita, H., Fukuda, Y., Kappas, A. & Sassa, S. (1993). The role of inorganic metals and metalloporphyrins in the induction of haem oxygenase and heat-shock protein 70 in human hepatoma cells. *Biochem. J.*, Vol. 290 (Pt 3), pp. 819-825.

Miyake, M., Fujimoto, K., Anai, S., Ohnishi, S., Nakai, Y., Inoue, T., Matsumura, Y., Tomioka, A., Ikeda, T., Okajima, E., Tanaka, N. & Hirao, Y. (2010). Inhibition of heme oxygenase-1 enhances the cytotoxic effect of gemcitabine in urothelial cancer cells. *Anticancer Res.*, Vol. 30, No. 6, pp. 2145-2152.

Morita, K., Lee, M.S. & Her, S. (2009). Possible relation of hemin-induced HO-1 expression to the upregulation of VEGF and BDNF mRNA levels in rat C6 glioma cells. *J. Mol. Neurosci.*, Vol. 38, No. 1, pp. 31-40.

Motohashi, H. & Yamamoto, M. (2007). Carcinogenesis and transcriptional regulation through Maf recognition elements. *Cancer Sci.*, Vol. 98, No. 2, pp. 135-139.

Motterlini, R., Foresti, R., Bassi, R., Calabrese, V., Clark, J.E. & Green, C.J. (2000). Endothelial heme oxygenase-1 induction by hypoxia. Modulation by inducible nitric-oxide synthase and *S*-nitrosothiols. *J. Biol. Chem.*, Vol. 275, No. 18, pp. 13613-13620.

Muscarella, L.A., Barbano, R., D'Angelo, V., Copetti, M., Coco, M., Balsamo, T., la Torre, A., Notarangelo, A., Troiano, M., Parisi, S., Icolaro, N., Catapano, D., Valori, V.M., Pellegrini, F., Merla, G., Carella, M., Fazio, V.M. & Parrella, P. (2011). Regulation of KEAP1 expression by promoter methylation in malignant gliomas and association with patient's outcome. *Epigenetics*, Vol. 6, No. 3, pp. 317-325.

Nguyen, T., Sherratt, P.J. & Pickett, C.B. (2003). Regulatory mechanisms controlling gene expression mediated by the antioxidant response element. *Annu. Rev. Pharmacol. Toxicol.*, Vol. 43, pp. 233-260.

Nishie, A., Ono, M., Shono, T., Fukushi, J., Otsubo, M., Onoue, H., Ito, Y., Inamura, T., Ikezaki, K., Fukui, M., Iwaki, T. & Kuwano, M. (1999). Macrophage infiltration and heme oxygenase-1 expression correlate with angiogenesis in human gliomas. *Clin. Cancer Res.*, Vol. 5, No. 5, pp. 1107-1113.

Ogura, T., Tong, K.I., Mio, K., Maruyama, Y., Kurokawa, H., Sato, C. & Yamamoto, M. (2010). Keap1 is a forked-stem dimer structure with two large spheres enclosing the intervening, double glycine repeat, and C-terminal domains. *Proc. Natl. Acad. Sci. USA*, Vol. 107, No. 7, pp. 2842-2847.

Padmanabhan, B., Tong, K.I., Ohta, T., Nakamura, Y., Scharlock, M., Ohtsuji, M., Kang, M.I., Kobayashi, A., Yokoyama, S. & Yamamoto, M. (2006). Structural basis for defects of Keap1 activity provoked by its point mutations in lung cancer. *Mol. Cell*, Vol. 21, No. 5, pp. 689-700.

Prados, M.D., Lamborn, K.R., Chang, S., Burton, E., Butowski, N., Malec, M., Kapadia, A., Rabbitt, J., Page, M.S., Fedoroff, A., Xie, D. & Kelley, S.K. (2006). Phase 1 study of erlotinib HCl alone and combined with temozolomide in patients with stable or recurrent malignant glioma. *Neuro-oncol.*, Vol. 8, No. 1, pp. 67-78.

Rich, J.N., Reardon, D.A., Peery, T., Dowell, J.M., Quinn, J.A., Penne, K.L., Wikstrand, C.J., Van Duyn, L.B., Dancey, J.E., McLendon, R.E., Kao, J.C., Stenzel, T.T., Ahmed Rasheed, B.K., Tourt-Uhlig, S.E., Herndon, J.E., 2nd, Vredenburgh, J.J., Sampson, J.H., Friedman, A.H., Bigner, D.D. & Friedman, H.S. (2004). Phase II trial of gefitinib in recurrent glioblastoma. *J. Clin. Oncol.*, Vol. 22, No. 1, pp. 133-142.

Roman, G., Riley, J.G., Vlahakis, J.Z., Kinobe, R.T., Brien, J.F., Nakatsu, K. & Szarek, W.A. (2007). Heme oxygenase inhibition by 2-oxy-substituted 1-(1*H*-imidazol-1-yl)-4-phenylbutanes: effect of halogen substitution in the phenyl ring. *Bioorg. Med. Chem.*, Vol. 15, No. 9, pp. 3225-3234.

Sahoo, S.K., Sawa, T., Fang, J., Tanaka, S., Miyamoto, Y., Akaike, T. & Maeda, H. (2002). Pegylated zinc protoporphyrin: a water-soluble heme oxygenase inhibitor with tumor-targeting capacity. *Bioconjug. Chem.*, Vol. 13, No. 5, pp. 1031-1038.

Saito, Y., Taguchi, H., Fujii, S., Sawa, T., Kida, E., Kabuto, C., Akaike, T. & Arimoto, H. (2008). 8-Nitroguanosines as chemical probes of the protein *S*-guanylation. *Chem. Commun. (Camb.)*, No. 45, pp. 5984-5986.

Sarkaria, J.N., Kitange, G.J., James, C.D., Plummer, R., Calvert, H., Weller, M. & Wick, W. (2008). Mechanisms of chemoresistance to alkylating agents in malignant glioma. *Clin Cancer Res* 14; 2900-8.

Sawa, T., Arimoto, H. & Akaike, T. (2010). Regulation of redox signaling involving chemical conjugation of protein thiols by nitric oxide and electrophiles. *Bioconjug. Chem.*, Vol. 21, No. 7, pp. 1121-1129.

Sawa, T., Ihara, H. & Akaike, T. (2011). Antioxidant effect of a nitrated cyclic nucleotide functioning as an endogenous electrophile. *Curr. Top. Med. Chem.*, in press.

Sawa, T., Tatemichi, M., Akaike, T., Barbin, A. & Ohshima, H. (2006). Analysis of urinary 8-nitroguanine, a marker of nitrative nucleic acid damage, by high-performance liquid chromatography-electrochemical detection coupled with immunoaffinity purification: association with cigarette smoking. *Free Radic. Biol. Med.*, Vol. 40, No. 4, pp. 711-720.

Sawa, T., Zaki, M.H., Okamoto, T., Akuta, T., Tokutomi, Y., Kim-Mitsuyama, S., Ihara, H., Kobayashi, A., Yamamoto, M., Fujii, S., Arimoto, H. & Akaike, T. (2007). Protein *S*-guanylation by the biological signal 8-nitroguanosine 3',5'-cyclic monophosphate. *Nat. Chem. Biol.*, Vol. 3, No. 11, pp. 727-735.

Schacter, B.A. (1988). Heme catabolism by heme oxygenase: physiology, regulation, and mechanism of action. *Semin. Hematol.*, Vol. 25, No. 4, pp. 349-369.

Sekhar, K.R., Rachakonda, G. & Freeman, M.L. (2010). Cysteine-based regulation of the CUL3 adaptor protein Keap1. *Toxicol. Appl. Pharmacol.*, Vol. 244, No. 1, pp. 21-26.

Shibata, T., Kokubu, A., Gotoh, M., Ojima, H., Ohta, T., Yamamoto, M. & Hirohashi, S. (2008a). Genetic alteration of Keap1 confers constitutive Nrf2 activation and resistance to chemotherapy in gallbladder cancer. *Gastroenterology*, Vol. 135, No. 4, pp. 1358-1368.e1-4.

Shibata, T., Ohta, T., Tong, K.I., Kokubu, A., Odogawa, R., Tsuta, K., Asamura, H., Yamamoto, M. & Hirohashi, S. (2008b). Cancer related mutations in *NRF2* impair its recognition by Keap1-Cul3 E3 ligase and promote malignancy. *Proc. Natl. Acad. Sci. USA*, Vol. 105, No. 36, pp. 13568-13573.

Simizu, S., Takada, M., Umezawa, K. & Imoto, M. (1998). Requirement of caspase-3(-like) protease-mediated hydrogen peroxide production for apoptosis induced by various anticancer drugs. *J. Biol. Chem.*, Vol. 273, No. 41, pp. 26900-26907.

Singh, A., Misra, V., Thimmulappa, R.K., Lee, H., Ames, S., Hoque, M.O., Herman, J.G., Baylin, S.B., Sidransky, D., Gabrielson, E., Brock, M.V. & Biswal, S. (2006). Dysfunctional KEAP1-NRF2 interaction in non-small-cell lung cancer. *PLoS Med.*, Vol. 3, No. 10, p. e420.

Stewart, B.W. & Kleihues, P. (Eds.). (2003). *World Cancer Report*, IARC Press, ISBN, Lyon.

Stupp, R., Mason, W.P., van den Bent, M.J., Weller, M., Fisher, B., Taphoorn, M.J., Belanger, K., Brandes, A.A., Marosi, C., Bogdahn, U., Curschmann, J., Janzer,

R.C., Ludwin, S.K., Gorlia, T., Allgeier, A., Lacombe, D., Cairncross, J.G., Eisenhauer, E. & Mirimanoff, R.O. (2005). Radiotherapy plus concomitant and adjuvant temozolomide for glioblastoma. *N. Engl. J. Med.*, Vol. 352, No. 10, pp. 987-996.

Surh, Y.J., Kundu, J.K., Li, M.H., Na, H.K. & Cha, Y.N. (2009). Role of Nrf2-mediated heme oxygenase-1 upregulation in adaptive survival response to nitrosative stress. *Arch. Pharm. Res.*, Vol. 32, No. 8, pp. 1163-1176.

Taguchi, K., Motohashi, H. & Yamamoto, M. (2011). Molecular mechanisms of the Keap1-Nrf2 pathway in stress response and cancer evolution. *Genes Cells*, Vol. 16, No. 2, pp. 123-140.

Tanaka, S., Akaike, T., Fang, J., Beppu, T., Ogawa, M., Tamura, F., Miyamoto, Y. & Maeda, H. (2003). Antiapoptotic effect of haem oxygenase-1 induced by nitric oxide in experimental solid tumour. *Br. J. Cancer*, Vol. 88, No. 6, pp. 902-909.

Terasaki, Y., Akuta, T., Terasaki, M., Sawa, T., Mori, T., Okamoto, T., Ozaki, M., Takeya, M. & Akaike, T. (2006). Guanine nitration in idiopathic pulmonary fibrosis and its implication for carcinogenesis. *Am. J. Respir. Crit. Care Med.*, Vol. 174, No. 6, pp. 665-673.

Vlahakis, J.Z., Kinobe, R.T., Bowers, R.J., Brien, J.F., Nakatsu, K. & Szarek, W.A. (2005). Synthesis and evaluation of azalanstat analogues as heme oxygenase inhibitors. *Bioorg. Med. Chem. Lett.*, Vol. 15, No. 5, pp. 1457-1461.

Wakabayashi, N., Dinkova-Kostova, A.T., Holtzclaw, W.D., Kang, M.I., Kobayashi, A., Yamamoto, M., Kensler, T.W. & Talalay, P. (2004). Protection against electrophile and oxidant stress by induction of the phase 2 response: fate of cysteines of the Keap1 sensor modified by inducers. *Proc. Natl. Acad. Sci. USA*, Vol. 101, No. 7, pp. 2040-2045.

Wang, R., An, J., Ji, F., Jiao, H., Sun, H. & Zhou, D. (2008). Hypermethylation of the Keap1 gene in human lung cancer cell lines and lung cancer tissues. *Biochem. Biophys. Res. Commun.*, Vol. 373, No. 1, pp. 151-154.

Warnecke, P.M. & Bestor, T.H. (2000). Cytosine methylation and human cancer. *Curr. Opin. Oncol.*, Vol. 12, No. 1, pp. 68-73.

Zaki, M.H., Fujii, S., Okamoto, T., Islam, S., Khan, S., Ahmed, K.A., Sawa, T. & Akaike, T. (2009). Cytoprotective function of heme oxygenase 1 induced by a nitrated cyclic nucleotide formed during murine salmonellosis. *J. Immunol.*, Vol. 182, No. 6, pp. 3746-3756.

Zhang, D.D. & Hannink, M. (2003). Distinct cysteine residues in Keap1 are required for Keap1-dependent ubiquitination of Nrf2 and for stabilization of Nrf2 by chemopreventive agents and oxidative stress. *Mol. Cell. Biol.*, Vol. 23, No. 22, pp. 8137-8151.

Zhang, P., Singh, A., Yegnasubramanian, S., Esopi, D., Kombairaju, P., Bodas, M., Wu, H., Bova, S.G. & Biswal, S. (2010). Loss of Kelch-like ECH-associated protein 1 function in prostate cancer cells causes chemoresistance and radioresistance and promotes tumor growth. *Mol. Cancer Ther.*, Vol. 9, No. 2, pp. 336-346.

Zhao, C.R., Gao, Z.H. & Qu, X.J. (2010). Nrf2-ARE signaling pathway and natural products for cancer chemoprevention. *Cancer Epidemiol.*, Vol. 34, No. 5, pp. 523-533.

Zhu, H., Itoh, K., Yamamoto, M., Zweier, J.L. & Li, Y. (2005). Role of Nrf2 signaling in regulation of antioxidants and phase 2 enzymes in cardiac fibroblasts: protection against reactive oxygen and nitrogen species-induced cell injury. *FEBS Lett.*, Vol. 579, No. 14, pp. 3029-3036.

Zipper, L.M. & Mulcahy, R.T. (2002). The Keap1 BTB/POZ dimerization function is required to sequester Nrf2 in cytoplasm. *J. Biol. Chem.*, Vol. 277, No. 39, pp. 36544-36552.

Part 9

TRP Channels in Glioma Therapy

13

Ionic Channels in the Therapy of Malignant Glioma

Xia Ding[1,2], Hua He[3], Yicheng Lu[3,*] and Yizheng Wang[1,*]
[1]*Lab of Neural Signal Transduction, Institute of Neuroscience, Shanghai Institute for Biological Sciences, State Key Laboratory of Neuroscience,*
[2]*The Graduate School, Chinese Academy of Sciences, Shanghai,*
[3]*Department of Neurosurgery, Changzheng Hospital, Second Military Medical University; Shanghai Institute of Neurosurgery, Shanghai,*
China

1. Introduction

Glioma is among the deadliest tumors worldwide. Despite its relative low onset incidence, glioma, especially malignant glioma, causes high mortality. Due to the utmost aggressiveness of tumor cells, malignant glioma is almost incurable by conventional therapeutic approaches. Finding new molecular targets, which are responsible for tumor progression, can amplify our understanding about malignant glioma and targeting these molecules combining with conventional approaches may ameliorate the therapeutic outcome for patients with malignant glioma.

Intracellular ions are fundamentally essential for cell behavior and ionic channels have been known to play versatile roles in numerous physiological and pathological processes. As for glioma biology is concerned, many types of ionic channels such as Ca^{2+}, K^+, Na^+ and Cl^- channels are involved in glioma cell proliferation, survival, invasion and also glioma angiogenesis. In this chapter, we are going to discuss the implications of ionic channels in the therapy of malignant glioma. Our recent work has indicated the role of one type of Ca^{2+} channels, namely the transient receptor potential (TRP) channel in human glioma progression. We thus are going to discuss the roles of Ca^{2+} channels in glioma cell biology as well as the possibility of Ca^{2+} channels to be therapeutic targets in glioma treatment.

Calcium (Ca^{2+}) is the second messenger for signal transduction to direct many cellular processes and Ca^{2+} channels play critical roles in controlling cell behavior, such as neurotransmitter release and muscle contraction. In recent years, the roles of Ca^{2+} channels in tumor cell biology have undergone intensive study. Many types of Ca^{2+} channels have abnormal expression in tumor cells compared to their corresponding normal cells and they also have specific functions in tumor cell proliferation, survival and invasion, making them appropriate candidate targets in tumor therapy. It has now become clear that TRP channels and voltage-gated Ca^{2+} channels participate in the progression of human glioma, some TRP

---

* Corresponding Authors

channel proteins are highly expressed in malignant glioma and function as essential regulators of glioma cell proliferation. The potential of these channels to be anti-glioma target will be highlighted in this chapter.

2. Difficulties in treating malignant glioma

Glioma is the most common form of brain tumor. It accounts for about half of all the brain tumors (Central Brain Tumor Registry of the United States [CBTRUS], 2008). According to the histological features, glioma has three major types: astrocytoma, oligodendroglioma and oligoastrocytoma (Huse & Holland, 2010). The World Health Organization classifies glioma as I to IV grade. As for astrocytoma, grade I is the pilocytic astrocytoma, grade II is the diffuse astrocytoma, grade III is anaplastic astrocytoma, and grade IV is glioblastoma multiforme (GBM) (Wen & Kesari, 2008). Grade I and II are low-grade glioma, high-grade glioma including grade III and IV are usually regarded as malignant glioma. GBM is the most common type of malignant glioma. It accounts for approximately 60 to 70% of all malignant glioma (Wen & Kesari, 2008). Histologically, GBM has several characteristics: nuclear atypia, enriched mitosis, necrosis and microvascular enrichment (Behin et al., 2003). GBM can be either original or secondary and secondary GBM develops from low-grade glioma.

GBM is extremely lethal, despite advances in therapy approaches, patients with GBM have very short survival time, averaging approximately 12 to 15 months (Wen & Kesari, 2008). Current therapeutic approaches for GBM include surgery resection, irradiation therapy and chemotherapy. However, all these approaches have very limited improvement on patients' survival, largely due to the intrinsic nature of GBM tumor cells, which are highly proliferative, invasive and often drug resistant. Finding new and specific drug targets for GBM challenges basic research. Current GBM drugs mainly targets DNA synthesis and DNA damage repair processes, for example, DNA alkylating agents (Temozolomide, 1,3-Bis(2-chloroethyl)-1-nitrosourea, BCNU, CCNU) and DNA topoisomerase inhibitors (Irinotecan, topotecan) (Brandes et al., 2001; Stupp et al., 2005). Accumulating evidences support the notion that intracellular ions, and especially ionic channels play important roles in the malignant behavior of glioma cells and it is possible that targeting the glioma-related ionic channels could suppress tumor cell growth. In the following, we are going to discuss the rationale and practice of this channel-targeting strategy.

3. Intracellular ions and ionic channels are fundamental for biological behavior of cells

Intracellular ions provide the basic environment for cellular activity and are required for maintaining enzyme activity, protein folding, cytoskeleton dynamics, cellular adhesion and cellular excitability (Berridge et al., 2003; Kunzelmann, 2005). Because of the important role of intracellular ions, ionic channels are of especial importance to cells. They play versatile roles in cellular activity, such as action potential generation, muscle contraction and neurotransmitter release. Among all the ionic channels, Ca^{2+}, K^+, Na^+ and Cl^- channels are four types of channels that receive the most attention. Extensive studies have reported their roles in both physiological and pathological processes. For example, Ca^{2+} channels in neuronal plasticity and cell apoptosis (Burgoyne, 2007), K^+ channels in regulating neuronal excitability and epilepsy (Lee & Cui, 2010; Zhang et al., 2010), Na^+ channels in action potential initiation and pain sensory (Cregg et al., 2010), Cl^- channels in regulating cell volume (Duran et al., 2010). More and more evidence have also shown these four types of ionic channels to be important for cell proliferation, migration and survival, suggesting that they might serve as potential targets in tumor therapy. Indeed, ionic channels play important roles in a wide variety of malignant tumors, including in the breast (S. Yang et al., 2009), colon (House et al., 2010), liver (Holzer, 2011), stomach (Holzer, 2011), oesophagus (Holzer, 2011), ovary (S.L. Yang et al., 2009), prostate (Flourakis et al., 2010), endometrium (Wang et al., 2007), lung (S.H. Jang, et al., 2010), skin (Bode et al., 2009) and brain (Ding et al., 2010).

The following parts of the chapter will discuss the above four types of ionic channels in glioma cell biology and implications of these channels in glioma therapy (Table 1). Schematic topology of each channel is summarized in Table 2.

4. Involvement of Ca^{2+} signaling and Ca^{2+} channels in GBM progression

The seminal role of intracellular Ca^{2+} in cell behavior has been well established. Ca^{2+} is a critical second messenger for signal transduction and Ca^{2+} signaling is required for gene expression, cell proliferation, cell migration, cell survival, cytoskeleton dynamics, fertilization, axonal growth cone turning and so on (Berridge, 2003). Intracellular Ca^{2+} signaling consists of many Ca^{2+} signaling apparatus, including receptors/channels, transducers, Ca^{2+} effectors, Ca^{2+}-sensitive enzymes, Ca^{2+} pumps and Ca^{2+} exchangers (Roderick & Cook, 2008). Many of these Ca^{2+} signaling apparatus are involved in regulating glioma behavior. For example, the Ca^{2+}-permeable α-amino-3-hydroxy-5-methyl-4-isoxazolepropionate (AMPA)-type glutamate receptors are expressed in GBM cells and can be activated to mediate extracellular Ca^{2+} entry (Ishiuchi et al., 2002). Overexpression of the AMPA receptors facilitates tumor cell proliferation and migration. One of the Ca^{2+}-sensitive enzymes is the Ca^{2+}-activated protease calpain, which is required for GBM cell invasion (H.S. Jang et al., 2010).

In the intricate network of Ca^{2+} signaling, Ca^{2+} channels are essential contributors to Ca^{2+} signaling transduction in response to different stimuli. Different types of Ca^{2+} channels are activated to initiate specific Ca^{2+} signaling pathways to allow cells to respond to stimuli. As for GBM cells are concerned, Ca^{2+} channels are involved in cell survival, proliferation, invasion and tumor angiogenesis. These GBM-related Ca^{2+} channels now include the transient receptor potential (TRP) channels and voltage-gated Ca^{2+} channels (VGCC).

4.1 TRP channels

TRP channels were first discovered in the fly visual system and participate in light sensing. TRP channel family is now known to be a large family containing 28 members in mammals (Montell, 2005; Ramsey et al., 2006). TRP channel family encompasses seven subfamilies with respect to channel structure similarity, these seven subfamilies include TRPC (Canonical), TRPV (Vanilloid), TRPM (Melastatin), TRPA (Ankyrin), TRPN (Nompc), TRPP (Polycystin) and TRPML (Mucolipdin) (Montell, 2005; Ramsey et al., 2006). All of the TRP family members have six transmembrane domains and the pore region is located between the fifth and sixth transmembrane domains. Both the N- and C-terminals are located intracellularly. Functional TRP channels are formed as homotetramers or heterotetramers of different TRP members. They are non-selective cation channels and are primarily permeable to Ca^{2+} and Na^{+}, some are also permeable to Mg^{2+}. TRP channels were found to functionally express in diverse tissues. These channels participate in a variety of physiological and pathological processes, such as neuronal survival (Jia et al., 2007), axon guidance (Li et al., 2005), pain sensory (Cortright et al., 2007), endothelial permeability (Ahmmed & Malik, 2005), pathogenesis of certain renal disease (Reiser et al., 2005; Winn et al., 2005; Heeringa et al., 2009), cardiovascular disease (Kuwahara et al., 2006; Onohara et al., 2006) and so on. The functions of many TRP channels still remain to be explored. The glioma-related TRP channels now include the TRPC, TRPV and TRPM channels.

4.1.1 Implication of TRPC channels in glioma progression and therapy

TRPC channels are the first mammalian TRP subfamily to be discovered and share the highest homology with fly TRP (about 30-40% in protein sequence identity) (Montell, 2005). In mammalian cells, TRPC channels contain seven members from TRPC1 to TRPC7 (Vazquez et al., 2004). TRPC channels can be activated by receptor-operated pathway, store-operated pathway, mechanical stretch, membrane trafficking, oxidative stress and Ca^{2+}/Calmodulin (Boulay, 2002; Maroto et al., 2005; Miller, 2006; Montell, 2005; Singh.B et al., 2004; Tang et al., 2001; Vazquez et al., 2004; Zhang et al., 2001). The receptor-operated and store-operated pathways are the most intensively studied. In the receptor-operated pathway, when G-protein coupled receptor or receptor tyrosine kinase on the cell surface are activated by ligand binding, their corresponding downstream phospholipase C are activated to hydrolyze phosphatidylinositol 4,5-bisphophate (PIP2) into inositol 1,4,5-triphosphate (IP3) and diacylglycerol (DAG). The DAG can directly bind to and activate TRPC channels (Montell, 2005). In the store-operated pathway, when intracellular Ca^{2+} store (mostly refer to the endoplasmic reticulum) are released, for example under thapsigargin (inhibitor of Ca^{2+}-ATPase on the ER) treatment, the IP3 receptor or STIM1 on the ER can physically interact with TRPC channels on the plasma membrane and activate TRPC channels (Bolotina & Csutora, 2005; Ramsey et al., 2006; Varnai et al., 2009). It is worth mentioning that under different conditions, one single type of TRPC channels can have more than one activation pathways (Ding et al., 2010; Hofmann et al., 1999).

TRPC channels are found in a wide diversity of tissues and cells, including neurons, glial cells, smooth muscle cells, endothelial cells, kidney podocytes and tumor epithelial cells (Ahmmed & Malik, 2005; Aydar et al., 2009; El Boustany et al., 2008; Golovina, 2005; Guilbert et al., 2008; Heeringa et al., 2009; Jia et al., 2007; Reiser et al., 2005; Winn et al., 2005; S.L. Yang et al., 2009; Yu et al., 2003; Yu et al., 2004). They form functional channels as homotetramer or heterotetramer, as has been revealed that TRPC1, 4 and 5 can interact with each other and TRPC3, 6 and 7 can interact with each other to form functional channels (Hofmann et al., 2002; Strubing et al., 2001; Strubing et al., 2003). TRPC channels regulate neuronal survival, neurite development, synapse formation, axon guidance, endothelial permeability, cell migration, differentiation and proliferation (Ahmmed & Malik, 2005; Cai et al., 2006; Florio Pla et al., 2005; Jia et al., 2007; Li et al., 2005; Louis et al., 2008; Tai et al., 2008; Zhou et al., 2008;). Among the seven TRPC members, TRPC1 and TRPC6 have been reported to play important roles in glioma cell proliferation, migration and invasion, TRPC6 channels are also involved in tumor angiogenesis (Bomben et al., 2010; Bomben & Sontheimer, 2010; Chigurupati et al., 2010; Ding et al., 2010; Ge et al., 2009; Hamdollah Zadeh et al., 2008).

Channel	Cell type	Functions in glioma cells	Abnormal expression in glioma	Pharmacological or molecular antagonists	Ways of activation	Animal experiments or clinical trial	Distribution in normal tissues and cells
TRPC1	Cell line (D54MG)	Proliferation, cytokinesis, EGF-induced chemotaxis	Not known	SKF96365, RNAi		No	Heart, brain, testis, ovary,
TRPC6	Cell lines (U251, T98G, U87) and patient samples	Cell cycle progression,	High expression	SKF96365, DN-TRPC6, RNAi	PDGF	Yes, intracranially implanted glioma in nude mice	Neuronal cells, cardiac myocytes, smooth muscle cells, vascular endothelial cells, kidney podocytes
	Cell line (U373MG) and patient samples	Notch-induced invasion	High expression	SKF96365, RNAi	OAG	No	
TRPM2	Cell line (A172)	H_2O_2-induced cell death	Not known		Overexpression of wild type TRPM2	No	Brain
TRPM8	Cell line (DBTRG)	Menthol-induced cell migration	Not known		Menthol	No	Prostate, Trigeminal (TG), dorsal root gangalion (DRG)
TRPV1	Cell line (U373, U87) and patient samples	Capsaicin-induced cell death in TRPV1-high cells	Inversely correlated with glioma grade		Capsaicin	No	TG, DRG, urinary bladder
TRPV2	Cell line (U87) and patient samples	Negatively regulated proliferation	Inversely correlated with glioma grade	RNAi	Overexpression of wild type TRPV2	No	DRG, spinal cord (SC), brain, spleen, small and large intestine, vascular myocytes
Cav3.1	Cell lines (U87)	Promote proliferation	Not known	Mibefradil, NNC55-0396	Overexpression of wild type Cav3.1 α1 subunit	No	Vascular smooth muscle, fibroblasts, myocytes
	Cell lines (U87, U563, U251) and patient samples		Specific splicing form expressed in glioma cells			No	
BK	Cell lines (U251, U87)	Do not affect proliferation	A specific isoform highly expressed	Iberiotoxin, paxilline, penitrem A	NS1619	No	Neurons, smooth muscle cells

Channel	Cell type	Functions in glioma cells	Abnormal expression in glioma	Pharmacological or molecular antagonists	Ways of activation	Animal experiments or clinical trial	Distribution in normal tissues and cells
	Animal model	Increase the permeability of BTB		Iberiotoxin	NS1619	Yes, intracranial RG2 cell implantation in Wistar rat	
IK	Cell lines (U251, U87)	Do not affect proliferation, but promote cell migration	Not known	Clotrimazole and TRAM-34		No	Neurons, smooth muscle cells
	HUVEC, HMVEC	Promote angiogenesis		TRAM-34		Yes, in vivo matrigel plug assay in nude mice	
K_{ATP}	Cell lines (U251, U87)	Promote proliferation, cell cycle progression through G0/G1 phase	High expression	Tolbutamide	Diazoxide Minoxidil sulfate	Yes, subcutaneous coinjection of drugs with glioma cells in nude mice	Heart, skeletal muscle cells, pancreatic islet cells, vascular smooth muscle cells,
	Animal model	Increase permeability of BTB			Minoxidil sulfate	Yes, intracranial implanted GBM in nude mice	
TASK3		Negatively regulate cell survival	Not known	Bupivacaine, spermine	Isoflurane	No	Brain, kidney, liver, lung, colon, stomach, spleen, testis, skeletal muscle
hERG1	Cell lines (U138, A172) and patient samples	Modulate VEGF secretion	High expression	WAY		No	Heart, pancreas, colon
ASIC1	Cell line (D54MG)	Promote cell migration	Not known	Amiloride, psalmotoxin1 (PcTX-1)		No	CNS, PNS
ClC2	Cell line (D54MG)	Mediated Cl- current	High expression			No	
ClC3	Cell line (D54MG)	Mediate Cl- current required for M phase progression	High expression	Chlorotoxin		Yes, phase I clinical trial	Neurons
	Cell lines (STTG1, U251)	Cell invasion	High expression			No	

Table 1. Glioma-related ionic channels. The glioma-related ioninc channels are summarized in this table. Detailed information can be retrieved from the body text.

Channel	Subunit	Subunit assembly
TRP	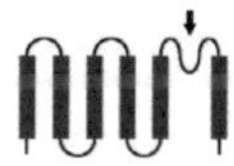	Tetramer
VGCC	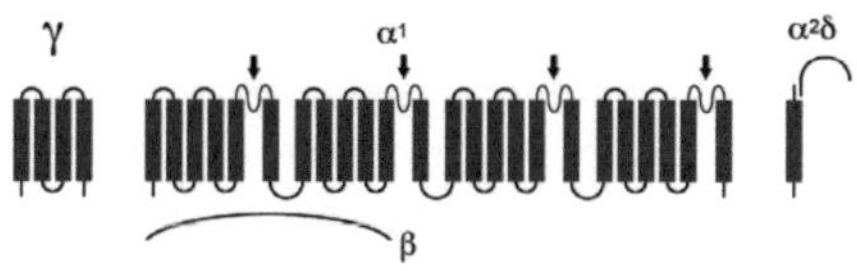	α1, β, α2δ, γ
BK	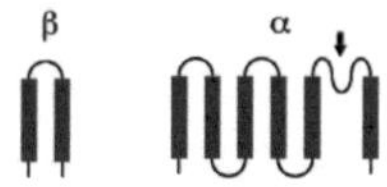	α x 4, β x 4
IK	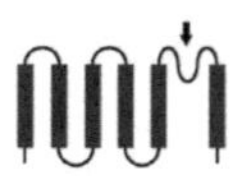	Tetramer
K_{ATP}	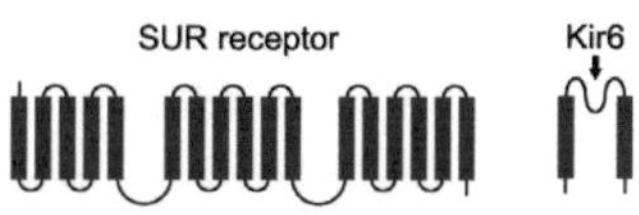	SUR receptor x 4, Kir6 x 4
TASK	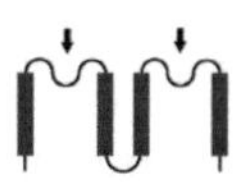	Dimer
hERG	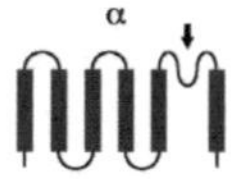	Tetramer
ASIC	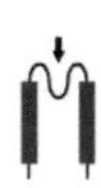	Tetramer
ClC	Complex structure, with 17 intramembrane domains	Dimer

Table 2. Schematic topology of subunit and subunit assembly of glioma-related ion channels. Transmembrane domains are represented as grey bars and pore-forming regions are indicated by the short arrows.

TRPC1 is the first TRPC member to be cloned (Wes et al., 1995). TRPC1 channels function in the regulation of neural stem cell proliferation, skeletal myoblast migration and differentiation, cell apoptosis and so on (Florio Pla et al., 2005; Louis et al., 2008; Bollimuntha et al., 2005). TRPC1 channels can be gated by receptor-operated pathway, store-operated pathway or even by mechanical stretch, depending on the cell types examined (Kim et al.,

2003; Maroto et al., 2005; Saleh et al., 2008). Glioma-related TRPC1 channels are involved in glioma cell proliferation and cell migration. In D54MG glioma cells, TRPC1 channels were gated by store-operated pathway. Pharmacological inhibition or shRNA-mediated suppression of TRPC1 channels inhibited glioma cell cytokinesis and resulted in multinucleated cells and eventually slowed glioma cell proliferation (Bomben & Sontheimer, 2010). Although Ca^{2+} signaling is important for cytokinesis in cell division, the channel through which the Ca^{2+} enters cells remains unknown. It is possible that TRPC1-mediated Ca^{2+} signaling is indispensable for cytokinesis in glioma cells, though the detailed molecular mechanism needs further exploration. Besides cytokinesis and proliferation, TRPC1 is also required for glioma cell migration. In response to the epidermal growth factor (EGF), TRPC1 protein was enriched in the leading edge of D54MG glioma cells and co-localized with lipid raft proteins. Inhibition of TRPC1 channels pharmacologically or by shRNA knockdown retarded EGF-induced cell migration, but did not affect the motility of un-stimulated cells. These results suggest that TRPC1 channels contribute to glioma chemotaxis in response to specific stimuli (Bomben et al., 2010).

Another TRPC channel member, TRPC6 channel is also essential for glioma progression. The TRPC6 channels are known to regulate axon growth cone turning (Li et al., 2005), survival of cerebellum granule neuron (Jia et al., 2007), dendrite development (Tai et al., 2008), synapse formation (Zhou et al., 2008), proliferation of pulmonary artery smooth muscle cells (Yu et al., 2004), cardiac myocytes (Kuwahara et al., 2006), vascular endothelial cells (Ge et al., 2009; Hamdollah Zadeh et al., 2008) and tumor cells (Cai et al., 2009; El Boustany et al., 2008; Thebault et al., 2006; Shi et al., 2009). Furthermore, TRPC6 functional mutations also contribute to the pathogenesis of a familiar renal disease named focal segmental glomerulosclerosis (Heeringa et al., 2009; Reiser et al., 2005; Winn et al., 2005). TRPC6 can be activated by receptor-operated pathway or by store-operated pathway as determined by different cell types. For example, in tumor cells, TRPC6 channels in most cases are store-operated and can be activated by thapsigargin or other ER Ca^{2+}-ATPase inhibitors (Ding et al., 2010; El Boustany et al., 2008), and in neuronal cells, TRPC6 channels are often receptor-operated and can be activated by neurotrophic factors or growth factors, such as brain-derived neurotrophic factor (BDNF) (Jia et al., 2007; Li et al., 2005).

The expression of TRPC6 was elevated in glioma tissues compared to normal brain tissues. By using neuronal marker, NeuN to distinguish normal neurons and normal glial cells in normal brain tissues, it was found that normal neurons expressed a high level of TRPC6, which was comparable to that in glioma cells, however in normal glial cells, the level of TRPC6 was barely detectable, suggesting that TRPC6 was specifically up-regulated in glioma cells, but not in neurons or in normal glial cells. Moreover, compared to low-grade glioma, TRPC6 expression level was even higher in GBM, suggesting that TRPC6 expression level was associated with glioma grade. TRPC3 is a closely related homolog to TRPC6, but unlike TRPC6, its expression level in glioma tissues was not significantly different from that of normal brain tissues. The selective up-regulation of TRPC6 channels in GBM implies the reliance of GBM tumor cell behavior on TRPC6 channels.

SKF96365 is a putative, but non-specific inhibitor for TRPC channels, treatment of glioma cells with SKF96365 could dramatically inhibit glioma cell proliferation. Specific inhibition of TRPC6 channels by a dominant-negative mutant channel (DN-TRPC6) (Hofmann et al.,

2002) or by RNA interference (RNAi) could also significantly inhibit glioma cell proliferation *in vitro* and in nude mice subcutaneous xenograft model. In nude mice intracranial xenograft model, DN-TRPC6 slowed the growth of tumors and significantly prolonged survival of tumor-bearing animals. Flowcytometry assay revealed that this inhibition of glioma cell proliferation was through arresting cell cycle in G2/M phase, not through induction of cell death, suggesting that TRPC6 channels are important for G2/M phase progression of glioma cells. Further analysis revealed that inhibition of TRPC6 channels down-regulated the expression of central cell cycle regulators, such as CDC25C, a phosphatase in activating CDC2/Cyclin B complex, which can drive cell cycle through G2/M phase (Boutros et al., 2007; Grana & Reddy, 1995). As has been known that Ca^{2+} signaling is essential for gene transcription (Greer & Greenberg, 2008), it is possible that TRPC6-mediated Ca^{2+} signaling contributes to the transcription of many cell cycle proteins in order to regulate glioma cell cycle progression.

As a Ca^{2+}-permeable channel in glioma cells, TRPC6 is functionally expressed. In U87-MG glioma cells, PDGF triggered a transient wave of intracellular Ca^{2+} elevation as reflected by Fura 2-AM Ca^{2+} image. This Ca^{2+} elevation was dramatically attenuated by SKF96365 perfusion, or by DN-TRPC6, or by TRPC6 RNAi, suggesting the contribution of TRPC6 channels to this induced Ca^{2+} wave. In Ca^{2+}-free medium, PDGF could only trigger a much smaller wave, but when Ca^{2+} was re-applied, the Ca^{2+} wave became much larger. When 2-APB (an IP3 receptor inhibitor blocking Ca^{2+} release from ER) (Maruyama et al., 1997) was present in the bath, PDGF-induced Ca^{2+} elevation was completely abolished. These results implied that PDGF might first trigger Ca^{2+} release from the ER and then through the store-operated pathway activate extracellular entry, which might through TRPC6 channels. It is known that when using cyclopiazonic acid (CPA, another ER Ca^{2+}-ATPase inhibitor as thapsigargin) (Demaurex et al., 1992) to deplete ER Ca^{2+} store under Ca^{2+}-free condition, Ca^{2+} re-application could induce the classical store-operated Ca^{2+} entry. Further experiments revealed that DN-TRPC6 could decrease the CPA-induced store-operated Ca^{2+} entry. This result clearly indicates that TRPC6 in glioma cells can be activated by PDGF and can mediate Ca^{2+} entry via the store-operated pathway. Since it has been well established that PDGF is a critical regulator for glioma tumorigenesis and development, these results indicated that TRPC6-mediated Ca^{2+} signaling might contribute to PDGF-induced glioma pathogenesis.

Besides cell proliferation and cell cycle, TRPC6 is also essential for hypoxia-induced glioma invasion and migration. Under hypoxia condition, Notch signaling pathway was activated and TRPC6 expression level increased in a Notch-dependent manner. Hypoxia treatment ($CoCl_2$ treatment) could activate TRPC6 channels and boost the ability of glioma proliferation and invasion. Inhibition of TRPC6 channels reversed the hypoxia-induced proliferation and invasion (Chigurupati et al., 2010). It is known that Notch signaling pathway is important for development and for maintaining cells in an undifferentiated state by regulating the transcription of many critical proteins (Artavanis-Tsakonas et al., 1999), these results suggest that Notch-induced TRPC6 expression may enhance undifferentiated state of glioma cells and therefore enhance the aggressiveness of glioma cells.

TRPC6 channels are also essential for angiogenesis, which is another important feature of malignant glioma (Wong & Brem, 2010). Human microvascular endothelial cell (HMVEC) is a good experimental model to study angiogenesis. In HMVECs, VEGF could trigger intracellular Ca^{2+} elevation and inhibition of TRPC6 channels by DN-TRPC6 alleviated VEGF-induced Ca^{2+} elevation. Meanwhile, DN-TRPC6 also inhibited the migration, sprouting and proliferation of HMVECs. On the contrary, overexpression of TRPC6 increased the migration and proliferation of HMVECs (Hamdollah Zadeh et al., 2008). In Human umbilical vein endothelial cells (HUVEC), similar phenomenon was observed. Inhibition of TRPC6 channels by SKF96365 or DN-TRPC6 arrested HUVEC cell cycle in G2/M phase and suppressed VEGF-induced cell proliferation and tube formation. Furthermore, inhibition of TRPCs abolished VEGF-, but not FGF-induced angiogenesis in the chick embryo chorioallantoic membrane (Ge et al., 2009). These results suggest that TRPC6 channels play an important role in VEGF-induced angiogenesis. Targeting TRPC6 in microvascular endothelial cells may inhibit the neo-angiogenesis of malignant glioma and eventually suppress tumor progression.

Based on the above basic findings, TRPC1 and TRPC6 channels could be potential drug targets in the therapy of malignant glioma. However, one major problem for TRPC channels as targets is that there is a severe lack of specific TRPC channel blockers. SKF96365 is a putative TRPC channel inhibitor, it can inhibit both TRPC1 and TRPC6 channels, but it can also inhibit many other types of channels and result in strong non-specific effect (Clapham, 2007; Fiorio Pla et al., 2005; Kim et al., 2003; Malkia et al., 2007; Mason et al., 1993; Merritt et al., 1990; Vazquez et al., 2004). Based on this situation, the currently available and efficient way of specifically inhibiting TRPC channels is to transfect cells with dominant-negative mutant form of specific channel proteins or with specific siRNA sequence to inhibit channel activity or knockdown gene expression. The DN-TRPC6 is a pore region-mutated channel, in which Leu678, Phe679 and Trp680 are mutated to Ala (Hofmann et al., 2002). DN-TRPC6 channel is impermeable, thus when overexpressed in glioma cell, DN-TRPC6 can chelate endogenous TRPC6 channels to form impermeable channel tetramers and achieve channel-specific blockade. Because TRPC6 can form functional tetramers with other TRPC channels, such as TRPC3, DN-TRPC6 also has certain side effects by inhibiting the activity of these TRPC6 binding channels. Besides DN-TRPC6, siRNA targeting TRPC6 is the most specific way of inhibiting TRPC6 channels without affecting other channel expression. Although channel dominant-negative and siRNA knockdown approaches are highly selective and have little side effects, the way of in vivo delivery of these nucleotide molecules will hinder their clinical use, because their inhibition effect largely relies on transfection efficiency. In order to get high transfection efficiency in cultured glioma cells, viral vectors have to be employed. In our publication, we used adenoviral vectors to deliver DN-TRPC6 and lentiviral vectors to deliver siRNA targeting TRPC6. Both these two types of vectors have high affinity to glioma cells and enable sufficient expression of DN-TRPC6 or siRNA to inhibit endogenous glioma TRPC6 channels (Ding et al., 2010). However, when systemically applied, the toxicities of virus will greatly restrict their usage, since adenovirus has high immunogenicity and lentivirus is genome integrative. Specific monoclonal antibody raised against the pore region of TRPC channels is another blockade approach. Such blockade antibody for TRPC5 channels has been reported. Monoclonal antibody against the third extracellular domain of TRPC5 was generated, by utilizing the specific recognition of antibody and antigen, this antibody can specifically bind to and inhibit TRPC5 channel activity (Xu et al., 2005). But such antibodies for TRPC1 or TRPC6 channels have not yet been reported. Therefore, in order to facilitate the clinical significance of TRPC channels in glioma therapy, developing specific blockers, especially small-molecule agents, to target TRPC1 and TRPC6 channels is an urgent need.

Besides the development of specific inhibitors, side effects of targeting TRPC channels also need a serious consideration. Since TRPC1 and TRPC6 channels have expression in many normal tissues and cells, especially in neuronal cells, cardiac myocytes, smooth muscle cells and vascular endothelial cells, side effects to these normal tissues and cells must be paid great attention to.

4.1.2 Implication of TRPM channels in glioma progression and therapy

The TRPM subfamily is composed of eight mammalian members, TRPM1 to TRPM8. Besides Ca^{2+} and Na^{+}, TRPM channels, such as TRPM6 and 7 channels are also permeable to Mg^{2+}. Different from other TRP channels, some TRPM members (TRPM2, 6 and 7) have enzyme activity in their C-terminal domain. TRPM2 has a ADP-ribose pyrophosphatase domain and TRPM6/7 have protein kinase domains. These TRPM channels are the so-called chanzymes (Montell, 2005). TRPM channels can be activated by menthol, cold temperature, osmolarity alteration and so on. TRPM channels function in temperature sensing, redox sensing, taste sensing, ischemia, neuronal cell survival and regulation of Mg^{2+} ion homeostasis (Aarts et al., 2003; Montell, 2005; Wei et al., 2007). TRPM2 and TRPM8 channels have been reported to be involved in glioma cell survival and cell migration.

TRPM2 channels can be activated by reactive oxygen species and mediate cell death in several types of cells (Kaneko et al., 2006; Miller, 2006). In A172 glioblastoma cells, TRPM2 channels could be targeted to the plasma membrane and mediate the Ca^{2+} influx induced by H_2O_2 treatment. This Ca^{2+} influx is important for H_2O_2-induced glioma cell death. However, overexpression of TRPM2 did not affect glioma cell proliferation, migration or invasion (Ishii et al., 2007). These results suggested that activation of TRPM2 channels can promote glioma cell death and that TRPM2 can be a candidate for glioblastoma therapy.

TRPM8 channels are also implicated in glioma migration. In DBTRG glioblastoma cells, menthol could activate Ca^{2+} entry and promote cell migration, and TRPM8 channels were found to mediate menthol-induced intracellular Ca^{2+} elevation and cell migration, suggesting that Ca^{2+} influx via TRPM8 is necessary for glioma cell migration in response to menthol stimuli (Wondergem et al., 2008).

4.1.3 Implication of TRPV channels in glioma progression and therapy

Mammalian cells have six TRPV subfamily members, TRPV1 to TRPV6. The TRPV channels can be activated by heat (>43°C) or warm temperature (30-39°C), membrane stretch, osmolarity alteration etc. Therefore, TRPV channels mainly function in sensing hot pain or warm temperature and osmolarity (Montell, 2005). In glioma cells, TRPV channels are also functionally expressed and TRPV1 and TRPV2 channels are involved in glioma cell death and proliferation.

In glioma cells, TRPV1 regulates capcaisin-induced cell death. TRPV1 expression level inversely correlated with glioma grade and in a majority of Grade IV glioblastoma, TRPV1 was markedly lost. Concordantly, capcaisin could only induce cell death in TRPV1 high expression cells, such as U373 cells, but not in TRPV1 low expression cells, such as U87 cells (Amantini et al., 2007). These results suggest that TRPV1 activation can promote glioma cell death and TRPV1 may be a good target for low-grade glioma, but not necessarily good for malignant glioma. The glioma-related TRPV2 channels are very much alike, its expression level was found to negatively correlate with glioma grade. Down-regulation of TRPV2 by RNA interference actually promoted U87MG glioma cell proliferation and rescued Fas-induced cell apoptosis. On the contrary, overexpression of TRPV2 in MZC glioma cells resulted in reduced cell viability and increased spontaneous and Fas-induced apoptosis (Nabissi et al., 2010).

The studies on glioma-related TRPM and TRPV channels suggest that activating these channels could inhibit glioma progression and further imply that agonists of these channels may serve as potential drugs for glioma therapy. TRPM8 channels are found to negatively regulate cell survival of prostate cancer and melanoma (Yamamura et al., 2008; Zhang & Barritt, 2004). Menthol, an activator of TRPM8 channels, can inhibit the growth of prostate cancer cells and melanoma cells and it seems to be a candidate drug also in glioma therapy. Since menthol is also an activator for many other pathways (Galeotti et al., 2002) and TRPM8 channels are functionally expressed in dorsal root ganglia (DRG) neurons (Montell, 2005), side effects of menthol in treating glioma have to be considered. Capsaicin is an ingredient of red chili peppers and an activator of TRPV1 channels. Capsaicin has been reported to possess anti-tumor activity, for example in prostate cancer and breast cancer, also in glioma (Sanchez et al., 2006; Mori et al., 2006; Thoennissen et al., 2010; Kim et al., 2010). Although the anti-tumor activity of capsaicin may not necessarily be through activation of TRPV1 channels (Ziglioli et al., 2009), capsaicin might be another potential anti-glioma drug and side effects to the DRG neurons should be considered, where TRPV1 channels are highly expressed.

4.2 Implication of voltage-gated Ca^{2+} channels (VGCC) in glioma progression and therapy

The VGCC are also a channel family including ten members. Each VGCC member is assembled through interaction of four subunits (Cavα_1, Cavβ, Cav$\alpha_2\delta$ and Cavγ) and each VGCC member is distinguished by their channel forming subunit, the Cavα_1 subunit. The Cavα_1 subunit consist of four transmembrane regions, each region contains six transmembrane domains. VGCC can be activated by membrane depolarization and based on physiological and pharmacological properties, VGCC members can be categorized as low-voltage activated VGCC including T-type VGCC (Cav3.1, Cav3.2 and Cav3.3) and high-voltage activated VGCC including, L-type (Cav1.1, Cav1.2, Cav1.3 and Cav1.4), N-type (Cav2.2), P/Q-type (Cav2.1) and R-type VGCC (Cav2.3) (Catterall, 2000). Functions of VGCC are involved in neuronal plasticity (e.g. long-term potentiation), exocytosis (e.g. Ca^{2+}-dependent release of neurotransmitters) and in many pathological processes such as pain (Bauer et al., 2002; Wang et al., 2004; Zamponi et al., 2009).

It has been known that T-type VGCC (Cav3.1) is involved in glioma cell proliferation. The Cav3.1 was found to express in both patient glioma tissues and in cultured glioma cell lines (U87, U563 and U251) and could promote glioma proliferation. Inhibition of Cav3.1 by its selective antagonist, mibefradil, could decrease its expression and suppressed glioma cell proliferation. Meanwhile, overexpression of Cav3.1 Cavα_1 subunit resulted in an increased cell proliferation (Panner et al., 2005), suggesting that Cav3.1 could actually promote glioma cell proliferation. Furthermore, our work showed that inhibition of Cav3.1 channels led to glioma cell cycle arrest in S phase (Ding et al., 2010), suggesting that this channel could be important for DNA synthesis or DNA damage repair. Inhibition of Cav3.1 may also sensitize glioma cells to irradiation. Interestingly, it has been found that besides previous known Cav3.1 $Cav\alpha_1$ splicing alternatives, glioma tissues seemed to express a novel splicing variant of $Cav\alpha_1$ subunit of Cav3.1 that was distinguished from normal brain tissues or fetal astrocytes (Latour et al., 2004). This finding implies that glioma-specific form of Cav3.1 might contribute to glioma pathogenesis and might be a unique target in glioma therapy.

Inhibition of T-type VGCC can be achieved by mibefradil, which is a synthetic small-molecule agent. Mibefradil is a widely used Ca^{2+} channel blocker and was once a drug for the treatment of hypertension (Ertel & Clozel, 1997; SoRelle, 1998). However, the potential use of mibefradil as therapeutic drug is greatly restricted by its lack of selectivity and its inhibition of other types of VGCCs, such as L-type VGCC (Mehrke et al., 1994; Bezprozvanny & Tsien, 1995). Since L-type VGCCs play important roles in many types of excitable cells (mainly myocytes and neurons) (Striessnig, 1999 & Greenberg, 1997), normal functions of skeletal/cardiac myocytes and the learning/memory abilities might be affected if T-type VGCC blockers can also interrupt the normal functions of L-type VGCC. Therefore, when targeting T-type VGCCs to treat glioma, these aspects must be seriously considered. In recent years, NNC55-0396 is synthesized as another inhibitor that is much more selective for T-type VGCC than mibefradil (Huang et al., 2004). In tumor research field, NNC55-0396 has been used to suppress human breast cancer cell proliferation in vitro (Taylor et al., 2008), but no studies on its use in glioma have yet been reported.

5. K^+, Na^+ channels and glioma

The K^+ channel family has 78 members and can be classified into four categories based on their activation mechanism and the number of transmembrane domains: inward-rectifying K^+ channels, two-pore K^+ channels, Ca^{2+}-activated K^+ channels and voltage-gated K^+ channels (Wulff et al., 2009). The K^+ channels play critical roles in cellular behavior and are involved in numerous biological processes, such as regulation of membrane potential and neuronal excitability and regulation of cell volume and cell proliferation (Bielanska et al., 2009; Grunnet et al., 2003; Jentsch, 2000; Trimarchi et al., 2002; Wang et al., 2007). The glioma-related K^+ channels include the BK and IK1 channels (Ca^{2+}-activated K^+ channels), ATP-sensitive K^+ channels (inward-rectifying K^+ channels), TASK3 (two-pore K^+ channels) and hERG1 (voltage-gated K^+ channels).

Na^+ channels are mostly voltage-gated, with a few ligand-activated Na^+ channels. Their primary function is to generate action potential in the nervous system and they are often involved in epilepsy and pain (Kohling, 2002; Lampert et al., 2010; Naundorf et al., 2006). In glioma cells, one type of ligand-activated Na^+ channels, the acid-sensing ion channels (ASIC, one type of the amiloride-sensitive Na^+ channel) is known to participate in glioma cell migration.

5.1 Implication of BK, IK1 channels in glioma cell proliferation and glioma therapy

The Ca^{2+}-activated K^+ channels include the big conductance channels (BK), intermediate conductance channels (IK) and small conductance channels (SK). BK channels are composed of four α subunits and four β subunits, IK and SK channels are composed of four pore-forming subunits and four calmodulin (Ledoux et al., 2006). BK channels and IK channels have been verified to express in glioma cell lines and primary glioma cells and can be properly activated to mediate K^+ current. Moreover, a specific BK channel isoform was found to be highly expressed in human glioma and was positively correlated with glioma grades (Liu et al., 2002). Inhibition of BK channels by its blocker iberiotoxin or paxilline suppressed U251 glioma cell migration. It was found that other BK channel blockers, paxilline and penitrem A, could also inhibit U251 and U87 cell proliferation (Abdullaev et al., 2010; Weaver et al., 2004; Weaver et al., 2006). However, in gene knockdown experiments, specific siRNA targeting BK channels failed to affect glioma cell proliferation, despite the siRNA could well down-regulate protein expression and inhibit channel current (Abdullaev et al., 2010). The inconsistency between pharmacological and molecular results suggests that BK channel pharmacological blockers might have some side effects or that BK channels do not to regulate glioma cell proliferation. As for IK1 channel, its blocker clotrimazole and TRAM-34 suppressed U251 and U87 cell proliferation, but the anti-proliferation effect failed to be repeated in siRNA knockdown experiments (Abdullaev et al., 2010). In another study, TRAM-34 or IK1 specific siRNA knockdown abolished CXCL12-induced glioma cell migration (Sciaccaluga et al., 2010). All these studies suggest that BK and IK1 channels do not participate in glioma cell proliferation, but IK1 channels indeed play a role in glioma cell migration. Moreover besides cell proliferation and migration, IK1 channels are found to regulate angiogenesis (Grgic et al., 2005). IK1 channels were expressed in HUVEC and HMVEC cells and could be stimulated by bFGF or VEGF to mediate K_{Ca} current. Blockade of IK1 channels by TRAM-34 suppressed bFGF- and VEGF-induced HUVEC or HMVEC cell proliferation. And in mice matrigel plug assay, administration of TRAM-34 could inhibit angiogenesis. This aspect concerning the in vivo use of TRAM-34 will be further discussed in the following section. Although BK channels do not seem to regulate cell proliferation, many studies have reported its role in regulating the permeability of blood-brain tumor barrier (BTB), which limits the chemotherapy agent delivery for glioma. This aspect will also be discussed in the following section.

Because BK and IK channels are essential for the regulation of smooth muscle contraction and neuronal excitability (McCarron et al., 2002; Vergara et al., 1998), side effects to smooth muscle cells and neurons must be considered.

5.2 Implication of ATP-sensitive K^+ channels (K_{ATP}) in glioma cell proliferation and glioma therapy

The K_{ATP} channels are consisted of two different types of subunits, the inward-rectifying K^+ channel member $K_{ir}6$ and sulfonylurea receptor (SUR) subunit (Akrouh et al., 2009). K_{ATP} channels are found to be important for glioma cell proliferation and cell cycle progression (Huang et al., 2009). Compard to normal glial cells, K_{ATP} channels were highly expressed in glioma cell lines and glioma tissue samples and inhibiting K_{ATP} channels by its blocker tolbutamide or by siRNA targeting $K_{ir}6.2$ subunit could decrease U251 and U87 glioma cell proliferation. Moreover, enhancing K_{ATP} channel activity by its opener diazoxide or by overexpressing $K_{ir}6.2$ or SUR1 subunit could increase glioma cell proliferation. The regulation of proliferation was through regulation of cell cycle progression because inhibition of K_{ATP} channels led to cell cycle arrest in G0/G1 phase. In animal experiments, subcutaneous co-injection of glioma cells with tolbutamide or with diazoxide could decrease or increase the growth of xenograft tumor, respectively. These results indicate K_{ATP} channels to be a potential target in glioma therapy.

K_{ATP} channels are mainly present in heart (Snyders, 1999), pancreatic cells (Bokvist et al., 1999) and smooth muscle cells (Quayle et al., 1997), side effects to these tissues and cells have to be considered.

5.3 Implication of two-pore domain K^+ channel TASK3 in glioma cell death and glioma therapy

The TASK3 (TWIK-related acid-sensitive K^+ channel, KCNK9) channel belongs to the two-pore domain K^+ channels (Enyedi & Czirjak, 2010). It is involved in regulating glioma cell death (Meuth et al., 2008). In high $[K^+]_{ex}$ medium, activation of TASK3 channel by its opener isoflurane resulted in a reduction of glioma cell survival and inhibition of TASK3 channel by its blocker bupivacaine or spermine could reverse isoflurane-induced cell death. These results suggest that under high K^+ environment, TASK3 channel activation actually promotes glioma cell death.

As a newly discovered gene, many normal functions of TASK3 remain to be discovered. But since TASK3 has been found to express in many organs, including brain, kidney, liver, lung, colon, stomach, spleen, testis and skeletal muscle (Kim et al., 2000), the side effect of targeting TASK3 channels has also to be considered.

5.4 Implication of hERG1 in glioma angiogenesis and glioma therapy

The hERG1 (human *ether a go-go* related) channels (KCNH2 or Kv11.1) belong to the voltage-gated K^+ channel family and are composed of four α subunits (Asher et al., 2010). hERG1 is overexpressed in many types of human cancers (Arcangeli, 2005). hERG1 is also overexpressed in human glioblastoma and is important for VEGF secretion in glioma cells (Masi et al., 2005). hERG1 current was recorded in primary glioma cells and by immunohistochemistry analysis, hERG1 was found to be highly expressed in glioblastoma multiforme. It is well known that secretion of angiogenic factors by glioma cells can promote angiogenesis and tumor malignancy. In U138 glioma cells which expressed functional hERG1 channels, channel blocker WAY could inhibit cellular VEGF secretion and this inhibition was not observed in A172 glioma cells, which did not express functional hERG1 channels. These results suggest that hERG1 channels may boost glioma malignancy by promoting angiogenic factor secretion and this channel is a possible target for anti-glioma therapy.

Side effects to heart, pancreas and colon should be considered, where hERG1 is abundantly expressed (Luo et al., 2008).

5.5 Implication of acid-sensing ion channels (ASIC) in glioma cell migration and glioma therapy

The ASIC channels are a group of amiloride-sensitive, voltage-independent Na^+ channels and can be activated by decreased pH. The ASIC channels are homotetrameric, which are assembled by the known subunits ASIC1a, ASIC1b, ASIC2a, ASIC2b, ASIC3 and ASIC4.

ASIC subunits have two transmembrane domains. Functions of ASIC channels involve perception of pain, ischaemic stroke, mechanosensation and so on (Krishtal et al., 2003; Wemmie et al., 2006).

ASIC channels are functionally expressed in glioma cells and contribute to glioma cell migration (Kapoor et al., 2009). In D54-MG glioma cells, ASIC1 was found to express higher than in primary human astrocytes. D54-MG glioma cells showed amiloride and psalmotoxin (ASIC inhibitors)-sensitive whole cell current under basal condition, indicating that glioma cells expressed functional ASICs. ASIC1 dominant-negative mutant transfection could decrease the whole cell current, and meanwhile, it also inhibited D54-MG cell migration as indicated by transwell assay. These results suggest that targeting ASIC1 channels might be another anti-glioma approach by disrupting glioma cell migration.

ASICs are widely expressed throughout the central nervous system and peripheral nervous system, targeting ASIC channels therefore should avoid side effects to the nervous system (Krishtal et al., 2003; Wemmie et al., 2006).

6. Cl^- channels and glioma

The Cl^- channel is a superfamily of ionic channels that are relatively poorly understood. They are either voltage-gated or ligand-gated. Three Cl^- channel families have been identified, the ClC, CFTR and ligand-gated GABA and glycine receptors. The ClC channels are dimerized from subunits, which might have 17 intra- or trans-membrane domains (Duran et al., 2010). Cl^- channels take function in the regulation of cell resting membrane potential, cell volume, cell migration, proliferation and differentiation. Two types of voltage-gated Cl^- channel family members 2 and 3 (ClC2 and 3) were found to functionally express in D54MG glioma cells (Olsen et al., 2003). ClC3 has been reported to be involved in glioma cell invasion and cell cycle progression. In D54MG glioma cells, ClC3 channels mediated the Cl^- current, which was required for pre-mitotic condensation (PMC) (Habela et al., 2008). PMC refers to obligatory cytoplasmic condensation process happened before mitotic phase and it is required for M phase progression. Besides cell cycle progression, ClC3 was also involved in STTG1 and U251 glioma cell invasion (Lui et al., 2010).

Chlorotoxin (CTX), a peptide from scorpion venom, is a small-conductance Cl^- channel blocker. CTX was found to specifically bind to the cell surface of glioma cell both in vitro and in vivo (Soroceanu et al., 1998), although the mechanism is still not clear. In vitro and in vivo delivery of CTX could well inhibit glioma invasion. This is because besides Cl^- channels, CTX has many other targets, for example matrix metalloproteinase 2 (MMP2), and it has been reported that specifically up-regulation of MMP2 in glioma cells accounted for the anti-invasive effect of CTX to glioma cells (Deshane et al., 2003). Iodine-131 labeled synthetic CTX (131I-TM-601) has been used for phase I clinical trial of treating recurrent malignant glioma (Mamelak et al., 2006). Intracavitary administration of 131I-TM-601 (0.25mg to 1 mg) was well tolerated with no observed toxicity. 131I-TM-601 could specifically bind to tumor tissues and was minimally taken by any other organ system. Furthermore, 131I-TM-601 treatment was proved to improve patient outcome to certain extent. Based upon these studies, CTX seems to be a potential drug for glioma targeting and therapy, although the working mechanism may not necessarily be through inhibiting Cl^- channels.

7. Ionic channels in brain tumor stem cells

In recent years, the concept of cancer stem cell (CSC) stands on the research focus (Gupta et al., 2009; Maitland & Collins, 2010; Takebe et al., 2010). CSCs are a population of cancer cells found in the tumor mass or hematological tumors. Unlike other cancer cells, CSCs possess the ability of reconstituting an entire tumor by giving rise to all cell types within the tumor, because CSCs have the characteristics of normal stem cells, which include the ability of self-renew, differentiation and proliferation. CSCs were firstly identified in leukemia (Bonnet & Dick, 1997), and were subsequently identified in many types of solid tumors, including brain (Singh. S et al., 2004), breast (Al-Hajj et al., 2003), ovarian (Zhang et al., 2008), colon (O'Brien et al., 2007), pancreatic (Li et al., 2007), prostate tumor (Maitland & Collins, 2008) and melanoma (Schatton et al., 2008) etc. CSCs have a completely different gene expression profile to other tumor cells, are extremely tumorigenic and are usually radiochemo-resistant. Although traditional therapy can kill most of the tumor cells, CSCs are considered to be mainly responsible for the relapse of tumor. The identification of brain tumor stem cells was first reported in 2004 (Singh. S et al., 2004). By dissecting primary surgical GBM or medulloblastoma samples, the authors have found that only the $CD133^+$ tumor cells within the tumor mass were capable of tumor initiation in SCID (severe combined immunodeficient) mouse brains. Injection of 100 $CD133^+$ cells was sufficient for xenograft tumor formation, whereas injection of 10^5 $CD133^-$ cells did not cause tumor formation. Importantly, the xenograft tumor histologically resembled the original tumor from patients. Further studies have revealed that the $CD133^+$ glioma cells promote glioma radioresistance and chemoresistance (Bao et al., 2006; Liu et al., 2006). Finding ways of targeting glioma stem cells are of great significance for therapy of malignant glioma.

As for targeting ionic channels, the implications of ionic channels in brain tumor stem cells have just begun to be understood. Many types of ionic channels seem to be highly expressed in brain tumor stem cells. In neuroblastoma cells, SH-SY5Y, CD133+ cells (cell population in which CD133+ cells% > 60%) were isolated as potential tumor stem cells, because CD133 is widely used as a cancer stem cell marker. In these $CD133^+$ cells, electrophysiological evidence indicated higher current density of large-conductance Ca^{2+}-activated K^+ channels (BK) and tetrodotoxin (TTX)-sensitive voltage-gated Na^+ channels than in $CD133^-$ cells. Furthermore, RT-PCR analysis showed that mRNA expression of BK and Nav1.7 was higher in $CD133^+$ cells than in $CD133^-$ cell (Park et al., 2010).

BCNU is a commonly used chemotherapeutic agent for glioblastoma therapy, but in primary glioma tumor mass, there is a subpopulation of BCNU-resistant glioma cells, which are stem-like cells, because the authors found that this subpopulations expressed CD133, CD117, CD90, CD71, and CD45 cell-surface markers, and had the capacity for multipotency (Kang & Kang, 2007). In the dissociated BCNU-resistant glioma stem cells, there was a high expression of several types of ionic channels, the chloride intracellular channels 1 (CLIC1) was one of these high expression channels. When using the Cl- channel blocker, 4,4'-diisothiocyanostilbene-2,2'-disulfonic acid (DIDS) in combination with BCNU, DIDS increased the apoptosis of BCNU-resistant glioma stem cells in vitro and augmented BCNU sensitivity ex vivo (Kang & Kang, 2008). These studies suggest that CLIC1 channel may contribute to the BCNU-resistance of glioma stem cells and blockade of this channel may enhance the BCNU-sensitivity of glioblastoma.

Although the relevance of ionic channels with glioma stem cells is still obscure, the present studies imply that the expression of some channels are abnormal in glioma stem cells and may contribute to the malignant feature of glioma stem cells. Blocking of these channels may facilitate chemo- or radio-therapy of glioblastoma.

8. Targeting ionic channels in animal models

As discussed above, many types of ionic channels regulate glioma cell behavior and control glioma progression. However, a large number of these studies are restricted to in vitro experiments, which mainly rely on the results obtained from cultured glioma cell lines. Although they shed lights on the concept that ionic channels play important roles in glioma progression, they only provide limited information as to whether these ionic channels can actually be targeted in vivo and whether these channel blockers exert side effects in systemic use. In this section, the in vivo targeting of ionic channels in animal tumor models will be discussed.

In the studies of TRPC6 and glioma cell proliferation and cell cycle progression, the anti-glioma effect of adenovirus-mediated DN-TRPC6 was tested in intracranial glioma xenograft model. U87MG glioma cells were infected by DN-TRPC6 before implantation. In this in vivo experiment, the animal bearing DN-TRPC6-infected glioma cells survived longer than the animals bearing GFP-infected glioma cells and suggested the potent anti-glioma effect of DN-TRPC6 (Ding et al., 2010). Nevertheless, from the clinical aspect, the most convincing way for delivering adenoviral DN-TRPC6 would be tail vein or in situ injection after the implanted tumor has reached certain size.

SKF96365 is a small-molecule blocker for TRPC channels. SKF96365 was developed in the early 1990s as a blocker for receptor-mediated Ca2+ entry, later it was found to block many types of TRP channels, including TRPC1, 3, 6 and 7. Additionally, it could block other types of TRP channels, such as TRPV2, TRPM8 and TRPP1 (Clapham, 2007; Fiorio Pla et al., 2005; Kim et al., 2003; Malkia et al., 2007; Mason et al., 1993; Merritt et al., 1990; Vazquez et al., 2004). Concerning glioma studies, SKF96365 has not been systemically used in animal models, but in the study of the implication of TRPC6 channels in gastric cancer progression, this drug has been applied intraperitoneally to suppress the subcutaneously implanted human gastric cancer cells in nude mice (6 weeks of age). SKF96365 was applied at the dose of 20 mg/kg daily for successive 5 days after 7 days of implantation and could apparently slow down the growth of xenograft. On the 51 day of implantation, the tumor volume in SKF96365-treated mice was approximately 20-30% smaller than in control mice. Meanwhile, physical conditions of the animals were not visibly deteriorating as compared to the animals receiving saline injection (Cai et al., 2009). The study suggested that SKF96365 at the above dose could be well tolerated by nude mice. However, the non-specificity of SKF96365 largely restricts the in vivo usage of SKF96365. New and specific TRPC6 channel blockers would be potential drugs for glioma therapy and the drug delivery approaches for treatment of glioma needs to be carefully designed. Because of the wide tissue distribution of TRPC6 channels, local rather than systemic delivery methods would be much desired.

IK channels regulate glioma progression. Clotrimazole is a putative inhibitor of IK channels (Jensen et al., 1998). Besides, it is also an inhibitor of cytochrome P-450 and translation initiation (Aktas et al., 1998; Ritter & Franklin, 1987). Application of clotrimazole suppressed proliferation of both human GBM cells and rat glioma cells (C6 and 9L). For in vivo experiments, either C6 or 9L cells were intracranially implanted into the brain of male Fischer-344 rats (between 250 and 300 g), and after 5 days, the animals were injected intraperitoneally daily with clotrimazole at the dose of 125mg/kg body weight for 8 consecutive days. This treatment caused a significant inhibition of intracranial tumor growth. Moreover, the survival of rats with 9L implantation were compared among clotrimazole, cisplatin (a commonly used chemotherapy agent for glioma) and combination of the two group and animals in the combination group survived longer than other groups (Khalid et al., 2005), suggesting that clotrimazole may enhance the glioma sensitivity to cisplatin, although conclusion has to be further verified and the mechanism remains to be revealed.

Although based on the current report, BK channels do not involve in glioma cell proliferation, it regulates the opening of blood-brain tumor barrier (BTB). NS1619 is the agonist of BK channels and iberiotoxin is a putative blocker of BK channels. The permeability of BTB was measured by rat glioma model, in which rat glioma cell line RG2 was intracranially implanted in female Wistar rat (180-200g). NS1619 (26.66 μg/kg/min) or iberitoxin (0.26 μg/kg/min) was co-infused with the radiotracer [^{14}C]α-aminoisobutyric acid ([^{14}C]-AIB) by intracarotid infusion. By using quantitative autoradiographic method to quantify the radioactivity in the tumor area, the BTB permeability for [^{14}C]-AIB could be accurately measured. By using this animal model, NS1619 was found to increase BTB permeability and iberiotoxin could decrease BTB permeability (Ningaraj et al., 2002). It was also found that infusion NS1619 with bradykinin could selectively enhance BTB permeability in brain tumors, not in normal brain (Hu et al., 2007). Moreover, iberiotoxin could reverse nitric oxide donors-induced increase in BTB permeability (Yin et al., 2008). NO can increase the vascular endothelial permeability and NO donors, such as L-arginine and hydroxyurea, could increase BTB permeability. These studies on the regulation of BTB permeability by BK channels suggest that pharmacologically regulating BK channel activity could potentially be used to improve glioma chemotherapy. The effectiveness and side effect of NS1619 and iberiotoxin remain to be verified in future animal experiments.

Besides BK channels, the K_{ATP} channel activator, minoxidil sulfate (MS) could also be used in vivo and increase the delivery of anti-glioma drugs such as temozolomide and herceptin by increasing the permeability of BTB. In this experiment model, MS (100 μg/kg/min for 15 min) was intravenously injected into nude rats with xenografted GBM. Temozolomide was labeled by [^{14}C], and herceptin was labeled by fluorescein and when they were coinjected, the drug delivery to the tumor was significantly increased, suggesting temozolomide or herceptin could be used in combination with MS to improve the effectiveness of standard chemotherapy (Ningaraj et al., 2009). Based on the present studies, different K^+ channel agonists can affect BTB permeability, including BK channel agonist and K_{ATP} agonists.

In a in vivo matrigel plug assay, which was used to examine angiogenesis in vivo, the IK channel blocker TRAM-34 was found to regulate angiogenesis (Grgic et al., 2005). In this experiment, standard matrigel supplemented with bFGF was implanted subcutaneously into the flank of C57/BL6 mice. Under control condition, the matrigel would get vascularized, but when the mice were treated daily with TRAM-34 (120mg/kg) intraperitoneally for two weeks, the vascularization would be decreased by approximately 85%, suggesting that TRAM-34 had anti-angiogenesis effect in vivo. Meanwhile, no visible side effects or macroscopic organ damage was observed. These results imply that TRAM-34 might exert anti-glioma effect in vivo by suppressing glioma angiogenesis and also imply the limited side effect of systemic use of TRAM-34. However, since TRAM-34 was delivered intraperitoneally in this study, whether TRAM-34 can pass the BTB remains to be further investigated.

As seen from the current available studies, several types of ionic channels are indeed potentially drug targets in treating glioma based on the in vivo data. The results obtained from the in situ (intracranial) glioma model seem to be much more convincing than the subcutaneous model, although different brain tumor in situ animal models may affect the final readout of these experiments (Barth & Kaur, 2009).

9. Chapter summary (At a glance)

Ionic channels play essential roles in glioma cell behavior, several types of Ca^{2+}, K^{+}, Na^{+} and Cl^{-} channels are potential therapeutic targets for malignant glioma.

TRP channels are newly found anti-glioma targets, some TRP channels are overtly expressed in human malignant glioma and they take function in glioma cell proliferation, migration or invasion.

Targeting several ionic channels might facilitate outcome of conventional chemo- or radio-therapy for malignant glioma.

Targeting ionic channels to treat malignant glioma remains in preclinical stage. Small-molecule compounds against ionic channels are experimentally tested in animal models. Glioma-related channel biology has to be more carefully studied before the possible clinical usage of channel drugs.

10. Summary and perspective

Many types of Ca^{2+}, K^{+}, Na^{+} and Cl^{-} channels have been implicated in glioma progression and serve as potential targets for malignant glioma therapy, but the studies linking ionic channels and glioma are a relatively new area in glioma therapy and very limited knowledge has been provided as to how ionic channels contribute to the glioma progression. Therefore, although the relation between ionic channels and glioma are getting clearer, there is still a long way to go to use ionic channels as potential drug targets in treating glioma. There are several major obstacles in this direction. First of all is the possible side effects of targeting ionic channels. Because ionic channels are rather universally expressed in different types of normal tissues, possible side effects have to be considered when targeting ionic channels to treat glioma. The cardiovascular system is the tissue that has to be considered in priority, because many types of ionic channels play important roles in regulating the normal functions of cardiovascular system. The possible side effects to nervous system also need great attention, because of the critical involvement of ionic channels in regulating normal neuronal function. Another obstacle is the permeability of BTB of these channel drugs. How they can be efficiently delivered to the glioma tumor tissue needs serious attention.

Because glioma is a multi-gene disease, combinative inhibition of multiple signal pathways is a promising strategy in glioma therapy. For example, simultaneous inhibition of EGFR and mTOR (Rao et al., 2005), RAF and mTOR (Hjelmeland et al., 2007) have been experimentally studied. However, the ionic channel-related signal pathways in glioma cells are poorly understood, and it is not known if there are certain pathways that are overtly activated to compensate the inhibition of specific channels. It would be ideal if we can target both the ionic channels and their compensatory pathways to maximize inhibition of glioma cells.

The ionic channels have several features as listed below, based on which the channel-targeting strategy could be theoretically justified. a). Ionic channels have membrane localization and are easily accessible to drugs, some types of channels have highly specific antagonists. b). Some types of channels have selective up-regulation in glioma cells. For example, TRPC6, KATP, hERG1 and ClC3 expression levels are very high in malignant glioma cells, but are low in normal glial cells or benign glioma cells. c). Channel blocker may boost the effect of standard glioma therapy. For example, TRPC6 blocker could be used as radiosensitizer for malignant glioma. Irradiation is a standard and effective therapy for malignant glioma and radiosensitizers could reduce the required irradiation dose and minimize damage to normal tissues. Inhibition of TRPC6 channels arrests glioma cell cycle in G2/M phase, which is an irradiation-sensitive phase, therefore, TRPC6 blocker may be a potential radiosensitizer for malignant glioma. d). Channel drugs can be used in combination with chemotherapy agents. Since several types of channel drugs can enhance the permeability of BTB, thus may facilitating the delivery of standard chemotherapy agents, such as temozolomide and BCNU.

11. Acknowledgement

This work was supported in part by the 973 program (2011CBA00400).

12. References

Aarts M, Iihara K, Wei WL, Xiong ZG, Arundine M, Cerwinski W, et al. (2003). *A key role for TRPM7 channels in anoxic neuronal death.* Cell;115(7):863-77. ISSN 0092-8674

Abdullaev IF, Rudkouskaya A, Mongin AA, Kuo YH. (2010). *Calcium-activated potassium channels BK and IK1 are functionally expressed in human gliomas but do not regulate cell proliferation.* PLoS One;5(8):e12304. ISSN 1932-6203

Ahmmed GU, Malik AB. (2005). *Functional role of TRPC channels in the regulation of endothelial permeability.* Pflugers Arch;451(1):131-42. ISSN 0031-6768

Akrouh A, Halcomb SE, Nichols CG, Sala-Rabanal M. (2009). *Molecular biology of K(ATP) channels and implications for health and disease.* IUBMB Life;61(10):971-8. ISSN 1521-6551 (Electronic), 1521-6543 (Linking)

Aktas H, Fluckiger R, Acosta JA, Savage JM, Palakurthi SS, Halperin JA. (1998). *Depletion of intracellular Ca2+ stores, phosphorylation of eIF2alpha, and sustained inhibition of translation initiation mediate the anticancer effects of clotrimazole.* Proc Natl Acad Sci U S A;95(14):8280-5. ISSN 0027-8424

Al-Hajj M, Wicha MS, Benito-Hernandez A, Morrison SJ, Clarke MF. (2003). *Prospective identification of tumorigenic breast cancer cells.* Proc Natl Acad Sci U S A;100(7):3983-8. ISSN 0027-8424

Amantini C, Mosca M, Nabissi M, Lucciarini R, Caprodossi S, Arcella A, et al. (2007). *Capsaicin-induced apoptosis of glioma cells is mediated by TRPV1 vanilloid receptor and requires p38 MAPK activation.* J Neurochem;102(3):977-90. ISSN 0022-3042

Arcangeli A. (2005). *Expression and role of hERG channels in cancer cells.* Novartis Found Symp;266:225-32; discussion 232-4. ISSN 1528-2511

Artavanis-Tsakonas S, Rand MD, Lake RJ. (1999). *Notch signaling: cell fate control and signal integration in development.* Science;284(5415):770-6. ISSN 0036-8075

Asher V, Sowter H, Shaw R, Bali A, Khan R. (2010). *Eag and HERG potassium channels as novel therapeutic targets in cancer.* World J Surg Oncol 2010;8:113. ISSN 1477-7819 (Electronic), 1477-7819 (Linking)

Aydar E, Yeo S, Djamgoz M, Palmer C. (2009). *Abnormal expression, localization and interaction of canonical transient receptor potential ion channels in human breast cancer cell lines and tissues: a potential target for breast cancer diagnosis and therapy.* Cancer Cell Int;9:23. ISSN 1475-2867

Bao S, Wu Q, McLendon RE, Hao Y, Shi Q, Hjelmeland AB, et al. (2006). *Glioma stem cells promote radioresistance by preferential activation of the DNA damage response.* Nature;444(7120):756-60. ISSN 1476-4687 (Electronic), 0028-0836 (Linking)

Barth, R. F. and B. Kaur (2009). *Rat brain tumor models in experimental neuro-oncology: the C6, 9L, T9, RG2, F98, BT4C, RT-2 and CNS-1 gliomas.* J Neurooncol 94(3): 299-312. ISSN 1573-7373 (Electronic), 0167-594X (Linking)

Bauer EP, Schafe GE, LeDoux JE. (2002). *NMDA receptors and L-type voltage-gated calcium channels contribute to long-term potentiation and different components of fear memory formation in the lateral amygdala.* J Neurosci;22(12):5239-49. ISSN 1529-2401 (Electronic), 0270-6474 (Linking)

Behin A, Hoang-Xuan K, Carpentier AF, Delattre JY. (2003). *Primary brain tumours in adults.* Lancet;361(9354):323-31. ISSN 0140-6736

Berridge MJ, Bootman MD, Roderick HL. (2003). *Calcium signalling: dynamics, homeostasis and remodelling.* Nat Rev Mol Cell Biol;4(7):517-29. ISSN 1471-0072

Bezprozvanny I, Tsien RW. (1995). *Voltage-dependent blockade of diverse types of voltage-gated Ca2+ channels expressed in Xenopus oocytes by the Ca2+ channel antagonist mibefradil (Ro 40-5967).* Mol Pharmacol;48(3):540-9. ISSN 0026-895X

Bielanska J, Hernandez-Losa J, Perez-Verdaguer M, Moline T, Somoza R, Ramon YCS, et al. (2009). *Voltage-dependent potassium channels Kv1.3 and Kv1.5 in human cancer.* Curr Cancer Drug Targets;9(8):904-14. ISSN 1873-5576 (Electronic), 1568-0096 (Linking)

Bode AM, Cho YY, Zheng D, Zhu F, Ericson ME, Ma WY, et al. (2009) *Transient receptor potential type vanilloid 1 suppresses skin carcinogenesis.* Cancer Res;69(3):905-13. ISSN 1538-7445 (Electronic), 0008-5472 (Linking)

Bokvist K, Olsen HL, Hoy M, Gotfredsen CF, Holmes WF, Buschard K, et al. (1999). *Characterisation of sulphonylurea and ATP-regulated K+ channels in rat pancreatic A-cells.* Pflugers Arch;438(4):428-36. ISSN 0031-6768

Bollimuntha S, Singh BB, Shavali S, Sharma SK, Ebadi M. (2005). *TRPC1-mediated inhibition of 1-methyl-4-phenylpyridinium ion neurotoxicity in human SH-SY5Y neuroblastoma cells.* J Biol Chem;280(3):2132-40. ISSN 0021-9258

Bolotina VM, Csutora P. (2005). *CIF and other mysteries of the store-operated Ca2+-entry pathway*. Trends Biochem Sci;30(7):378-87. ISSN 0968-0004

Bomben VC, Sontheimer H. (2010). *Disruption of transient receptor potential canonical channel 1 causes incomplete cytokinesis and slows the growth of human malignant gliomas*. Glia;58(10):1145-56. ISSN 1098-1136 (Electronic), 0894-1491 (Linking)

Bomben VC, Turner KL, Barclay TT, Sontheimer H. (2010). *Transient receptor potential canonical channels are essential for chemotactic migration of human malignant gliomas*. J Cell Physiol. ISSN 1097-4652 (Electronic), 0021-9541 (Linking)

Bonnet D, Dick JE. (1997). *Human acute myeloid leukemia is organized as a hierarchy that originates from a primitive hematopoietic cell*. Nat Med;3(7):730-7. ISSN 1078-8956

Boulay G. (2002). *Ca(2+)-calmodulin regulates receptor-operated Ca(2+) entry activity of TRPC6 in HEK-293 cells*. Cell Calcium;32(4):201-7. ISSN 0143-4160

Boutros R, Lobjois V, Ducommun B. (2007). *CDC25 phosphatases in cancer cells: key players? Good targets?* Nat Rev Cancer;7(7):495-507. ISSN 1474-175X

Brandes AA, Basso U, Pasetto LM, Ermani M. (2001). *New strategy developments in brain tumor therapy*. Curr Pharm Des;7(16):1553-80. ISSN 1381-6128

Burgoyne RD. (2007). *Neuronal calcium sensor proteins: generating diversity in neuronal Ca2+ signalling*. Nat Rev Neurosci;8(3):182-93. ISSN 1471-003X

Cai R, Ding X, Zhou K, Shi Y, Ge R, Ren G, et al. (2009). *Blockade of TRPC6 channels induced G2/M phase arrest and suppressed growth in human gastric cancer cells*. Int. J Cancer;125(10):2281-7. ISSN 1097-0215

Cai S, Fatherazi S, Presland RB, Belton CM, Roberts FA, Goodwin PC, et al. (2006). *Evidence that TRPC1 contributes to calcium-induced differentiation of human keratinocytes*. Pflugers Arch;452(1):43-52. ISSN 0031-6768

Catterall WA. (2000). *Structure and regulation of voltage-gated Ca2+ channels*. Annu Rev Cell Dev Biol;16:521-55. ISSN 1081-0706

Central Brain Tumor Registry of the United States, 2000-2004. *CBTRUS 2008 statistical report: primary brain tumors in the United States, 1998-2002*. (Accessed July 7, 2008, at http://www.cbtrus.org/reports/2007-2008/2007report.pdf.)

Chigurupati S, Venkataraman R, Barrera D, Naganathan A, Madan M, Paul L, et al. (2010). *Receptor channel TRPC6 is a key mediator of Notch-driven glioblastoma growth and invasiveness*. Cancer Res;70(1):418-27. ISSN 1538-7445

Clapham DE. (2007). *SnapShot: mammalian TRP channels*. Cell;129(1):220. ISSN 0092-8674

Cortright DN, Krause JE, Broom DC. (2007). *TRP channels and pain*. Biochim Biophys Acta;1772(8):978-88. ISSN 0006-3002

Cregg R, Momin A, Rugiero F, Wood JN, Zhao J. (2010). *Pain channelopathies*. J Physiol;588(Pt 11):1897-904. ISSN 1469-7793 (Electronic), 0022-3751 (Linking)

Demaurex N, Lew DP, Krause KH. (1992). *Cyclopiazonic acid depletes intracellular Ca2+ stores and activates an influx pathway for divalent cations in HL-60 cells*. J Biol Chem;267(4):2318-24. ISSN 0021-9258

Deshane J, Garner CC, Sontheimer H. (2003). *Chlorotoxin inhibits glioma cell invasion via matrix metalloproteinase-2*. J Biol Chem;278(6):4135-44. ISSN 0021-9258

Ding X, He Z, Zhou K, Cheng J, Yao H, Lu D, et al. (2010). *Essential role of TRPC6 channels in G2/M phase transition and development of human glioma.* J Natl Cancer Inst;102(14):1052-68. ISSN 1460-2105 (Electronic), 0027-8874 (Linking)

Duran C, Thompson CH, Xiao Q, Hartzell HC. (2010). *Chloride channels: often enigmatic, rarely predictable.* Annu Rev Physiol;72:95-121. ISSN 1545-1585 (Electronic), 0066-4278 (Linking)

El Boustany C, Bidaux G, Enfissi A, Delcourt P, Prevarskaya N, Capiod T. (2008). *Capacitative calcium entry and transient receptor potential canonical 6 expression control human hepatoma cell proliferation.* Hepatology;47(6):2068-77. ISSN 1527-3350

Enyedi P, Czirjak G. (2010) *Molecular background of leak K+ currents: two-pore domain potassium channels.* Physiol Rev 2010;90(2):559-605. ISSN 1522-1210 (Electronic), 0031-9333 (Linking)

Ertel SI, Clozel JP. (1997). *Mibefradil (Ro 40-5967): the first selective T-type Ca2+ channel blocker.* Expert Opin Investig Drugs;6(5):569-82. ISSN 1744-7658 (Electronic), 1354-3784 (Linking)

Fiorio Pla A, Maric D, Brazer SC, Giacobini P, Liu X, Chang YH, et al. (2005). *Canonical transient receptor potential 1 plays a role in basic fibroblast growth factor (bFGF)/FGF receptor-1-induced Ca2+ entry and embryonic rat neural stem cell proliferation.* J Neurosci;25(10):2687-701. ISSN 1529-2401

Flourakis M, Lehen'kyi V, Beck B, Raphael M, Vandenberghe M, Abeele FV, et al. (2010) *Orai1 contributes to the establishment of an apoptosis-resistant phenotype in prostate cancer cells.* Cell Death Dis;1(9):e75. ISSN 2041-4889 (Electronic)

Galeotti N, Di Cesare Mannelli L, Mazzanti G, Bartolini A, Ghelardini C. (2002). *Menthol: a natural analgesic compound.* Neurosci Lett;322(3):145-8. ISSN 0304-3940

Ge R, Tai Y, Sun Y, Zhou K, Yang S, Cheng T, et al. (2009). *Critical role of TRPC6 channels in VEGF-mediated angiogenesis.* Cancer Lett;283(1):43-51. ISSN 1872-7980

Golovina VA. (2005). *Visualization of localized store-operated calcium entry in mouse astrocytes. Close proximity to the endoplasmic reticulum.* J Physiol;564(Pt 3):737-49. ISSN 0022-3751

Grana X, Reddy EP. (1995). *Cell cycle control in mammalian cells: role of cyclins, cyclin dependent kinases (CDKs), growth suppressor genes and cyclin-dependent kinase inhibitors (CKIs).* Oncogene;11(2):211-9. ISSN 0950-9232

Greenberg DA. (1997). *Calcium channels in neurological disease.* Ann Neurol;42(3):275-82. ISSN 0364-5134

Greer PL, Greenberg ME. (2008). *From synapse to nucleus: calcium-dependent gene transcription in the control of synapse development and function.* Neuron;59(6):846-60. ISSN 1097-4199 (Electronic), 0896-6273 (Linking)

Grgic I, Eichler I, Heinau P, Si H, Brakemeier S, Hoyer J, et al. (2005). *Selective blockade of the intermediate-conductance Ca2+-activated K+ channel suppresses proliferation of microvascular and macrovascular endothelial cells and angiogenesis in vivo.* Arterioscler Thromb Vasc Biol;25(4):704-9. ISSN 1524-4636 (Electronic), 1079-5642 (Linking)

Grunnet M, Jespersen T, MacAulay N, Jorgensen NK, Schmitt N, Pongs O, et al. (2003). *KCNQ1 channels sense small changes in cell volume.* J Physiol;549(Pt 2):419-27. ISSN 0022-3751

Guilbert A, Dhennin-Duthille I, Hiani YE, Haren N, Khorsi H, Sevestre H, et al. (2008). *Expression of TRPC6 channels in human epithelial breast cancer cells.* BMC Cancer;8:125. ISSN 1471-2407

Gupta PB, Chaffer CL, Weinberg RA. (2009). *Cancer stem cells: mirage or reality?* Nat Med;15(9):1010-2. ISSN 1546-170X (Electronic), 1078-8956 (Linking)

Habela CW, Olsen ML, Sontheimer H. (2008). *ClC3 is a critical regulator of the cell cycle in normal and malignant glial cells.* J Neurosci;28(37):9205-17. ISSN 1529-2401 (Electronic), 0270-6474 (Linking)

Hamdollah Zadeh MA, Glass CA, Magnussen A, Hancox JC, Bates DO. (2008). *VEGF-mediated elevated intracellular calcium and angiogenesis in human microvascular endothelial cells in vitro are inhibited by dominant negative TRPC6.* Microcirculation;15(7):605-14. ISSN 1549-8719

Heeringa SF, Moller CC, Du J, Yue L, Hinkes B, Chernin G, et al. (2009). *A novel TRPC6 mutation that causes childhood FSGS.* PLoS One;4(11):e7771. ISSN 1932-6203

Hjelmeland AB, Lattimore KP, Fee BE, Shi Q, Wickman S, Keir ST, et al. (2007) *The combination of novel low molecular weight inhibitors of RAF (LBT613) and target of rapamycin (RAD001) decreases glioma proliferation and invasion.* Mol Cancer Ther;6(9):2449-57. ISSN 1535-7163 (Print), 1535-7163 (Linking)

Hofmann T, Obukhov AG, Schaefer M, Harteneck C, Gudermann T, Schultz G. (1999). *Direct activation of human TRPC6 and TRPC3 channels by diacylglycerol.* Nature;397(6716):259-63. ISSN 0028-0836

Hofmann T, Schaefer M, Schultz G, Gudermann T. (2002). *Subunit composition of mammalian transient receptor potential channels in living cells.* Proc Natl Acad Sci U S A;99(11):7461-6. ISSN 0027-8424

Holzer P. (2011) *Transient receptor potential (TRP) channels as drug targets for diseases of the digestive system.* Pharmacol Ther. (in press) ISSN 1879-016X (Electronic), 0163-7258 (Linking)

House CD, Vaske CJ, Schwartz AM, Obias V, Frank B, Luu T, et al. (2010) *Voltage-gated Na+ channel SCN5A is a key regulator of a gene transcriptional network that controls colon cancer invasion.* Cancer Res;70(17):6957-67. ISSN 1538-7445 (Electronic), 0008-5472 (Linking)

Hu J, Yuan X, Ko MK, Yin D, Sacapano MR, Wang X, et al. (2007). *Calcium-activated potassium channels mediated blood-brain tumor barrier opening in a rat metastatic brain tumor model.* Mol Cancer;6:22. ISSN 1476-4598

Huang L, Keyser BM, Tagmose TM, Hansen JB, Taylor JT, Zhuang H, et al. (2004). *NNC 55-0396 [(1S,2S)-2-(2-(N-[(3-benzimidazol-2-yl)propyl]-N-methylamino)ethyl)-6-fluo ro-1,2,3,4-tetrahydro-1-isopropyl-2-naphtyl cyclopropanecarboxylate dihydrochloride]: a new selective inhibitor of T-type calcium channels.* J Pharmacol Exp Ther;309(1):193-9. ISSN 0022-3565

Huang L, Li B, Li W, Guo H, Zou F. (2009). *ATP-sensitive potassium channels control glioma cells proliferation by regulating ERK activity.* Carcinogenesis;30(5):737-44. ISSN 1460-2180 (Electronic), 0143-3334 (Linking)

Huse JT, Holland EC. (2010). *Targeting brain cancer: advances in the molecular pathology of malignant glioma and medulloblastoma.* Nat Rev Cancer;10(5):319-31. ISSN 1474-1768 (Electronic), 1474-175X (Linking)

Ishii M, Oyama A, Hagiwara T, Miyazaki A, Mori Y, Kiuchi Y, et al. (2007). *Facilitation of H2O2-induced A172 human glioblastoma cell death by insertion of oxidative stress-sensitive TRPM2 channels.* Anticancer Res;27(6B):3987-92. ISSN 0250-7005

Ishiuchi S, Tsuzuki K, Yoshida Y, Yamada N, Hagimura N, Okado H, et al. (2002). *Blockage of Ca(2+)-permeable AMPA receptors suppresses migration and induces apoptosis in human glioblastoma cells.* Nat Med;8(9):971-8. ISSN 1078-8956

Jang HS, Lal S, Greenwood JA. (2010). *Calpain 2 is required for glioblastoma cell invasion: regulation of matrix metalloproteinase 2.* Neurochem Res;35(11):1796-804. ISSN 1573-6903 (Electronic), 0364-3190 (Linking)

Jang SH, Choi SY, Ryu PD, Lee SY. (2010) *Anti-proliferative effect of Kv1.3 blockers in A549 human lung adenocarcinoma in vitro and in vivo.* Eur J Pharmacol;651(1-3):26-32. ISSN 1879-0712 (Electronic), 0014-2999 (Linking)

Jensen BS, Strobaek D, Christophersen P, Jorgensen TD, Hansen C, Silahtaroglu A, et al. (1998). *Characterization of the cloned human intermediate-conductance Ca2+-activated K+ channel.* Am J Physiol;275(3 Pt 1):C848-56. ISSN 0002-9513

Jentsch TJ. (2000). *Neuronal KCNQ potassium channels: physiology and role in disease.* Nat Rev Neurosci;1(1):21-30. ISSN 1471-003X

Jia Y, Zhou J, Tai Y, Wang Y. (2007). *TRPC channels promote cerebellar granule neuron survival.* Nat Neurosci;10(5):559-67. ISSN 1097-6256

Kaneko S, Kawakami S, Hara Y, Wakamori M, Itoh E, Minami T, et al. (2006). *A critical role of TRPM2 in neuronal cell death by hydrogen peroxide.* J Pharmacol Sci;101(1):66-76. ISSN 1347-8613

Kang MK, Kang SK. (2007). *Tumorigenesis of chemotherapeutic drug-resistant cancer stem-like cells in brain glioma.* Stem Cells Dev;16(5):837-47. ISSN 1547-3287

Kang MK, Kang SK. (2008). *Pharmacologic blockade of chloride channel synergistically enhances apoptosis of chemotherapeutic drug-resistant cancer stem cells.* Biochem Biophys Res Commun;373(4):539-44. ISSN 1090-2104 (Electronic), 0006-291X (Linking)

Kapoor N, Bartoszewski R, Qadri YJ, Bebok Z, Bubien JK, Fuller CM, et al. (2009). *Knockdown of ASIC1 and epithelial sodium channel subunits inhibits glioblastoma whole cell current and cell migration.* J Biol Chem;284(36):24526-41. ISSN 0021-9258

Khalid MH, Tokunaga Y, Caputy AJ, Walters E. (2005). *Inhibition of tumor growth and prolonged survival of rats with intracranial gliomas following administration of clotrimazole.* J Neurosurg;103(1):79-86. ISSN 0022-3085

Kim JY, Kim EH, Kim SU, Kwon TK, Choi KS. (2010). *Capsaicin sensitizes malignant glioma cells to TRAIL-mediated apoptosis via DR5 upregulation and survivin downregulation.* Carcinogenesis;31(3):367-75. ISSN 1460-2180 (Electronic), 0143-3334 (Linking)

Kim SJ, Kim YS, Yuan JP, Petralia RS, Worley PF, Linden DJ. (2003). *Activation of the TRPC1 cation channel by metabotropic glutamate receptor mGluR1.* Nature;426(6964):285-91. ISSN 1476-4687

Kim Y, Bang H, Kim D. (2000). *TASK-3, a new member of the tandem pore K(+) channel family.* J Biol Chem;275(13):9340-7. ISSN 0021-9258

Kohling R. (2002). *Voltage-gated sodium channels in epilepsy*. Epilepsia;43(11):1278-95. ISSN 0013-9580

Krishtal O. (2003). *The ASICs: signaling molecules? Modulators?* Trends Neurosci;26(9):477-83. ISSN 0166-2236

Kunzelmann K. (2005). *Ion channels and cancer*. J Membr Biol;205(3):159-73. ISSN 0022-2631

Kuwahara K, Wang Y, McAnally J, Richardson JA, Bassel-Duby R, Hill JA, et al. (2006). *TRPC6 fulfills a calcineurin signaling circuit during pathologic cardiac remodeling*. J Clin Invest;116(12):3114-26. ISSN 0021-9738

Lampert A, O'Reilly AO, Reeh P, Leffler A. (2010). *Sodium channelopathies and pain*. Pflugers Arch;460(2):249-63. ISSN 1432-2013 (Electronic), 0031-6768 (Linking)

Latour I, Louw DF, Beedle AM, Hamid J, Sutherland GR, Zamponi GW. (2004). *Expression of T-type calcium channel splice variants in human glioma*. Glia;48(2):112-9. ISSN 0894-1491

Ledoux J, Werner ME, Brayden JE, Nelson MT. (2006). *Calcium-activated potassium channels and the regulation of vascular tone*. Physiology (Bethesda) 2006;21:69-78. ISSN 1548-9213 (Print), 1548-9221 (Linking)

Lee US, Cui J. (2010). *BK channel activation: structural and functional insights*. Trends Neurosci;33(9):415-23. ISSN 1878-108X (Electronic), 0166-2236 (Linking)

Li C, Heidt DG, Dalerba P, Burant CF, Zhang L, Adsay V, et al. (2007). *Identification of pancreatic cancer stem cells*. Cancer Res;67(3):1030-7. ISSN 0008-5472

Li Y, Jia YC, Cui K, Li N, Zheng ZY, Wang YZ, et al. (2005). *Essential role of TRPC channels in the guidance of nerve growth cones by brain-derived neurotrophic factor*. Nature;434(7035):894-8. ISSN 1476-4687

Liu G, Yuan X, Zeng Z, Tunici P, Ng H, Abdulkadir IR, et al. (2006). *Analysis of gene expression and chemoresistance of CD133+ cancer stem cells in glioblastoma*. Mol Cancer;5:67. ISSN 1476-4598

Liu X, Chang Y, Reinhart PH, Sontheimer H. (2002). *Cloning and characterization of glioma BK, a novel BK channel isoform highly expressed in human glioma cells*. J Neurosci;22(5):1840-9. ISSN 1529-2401 (Electronic), 0270-6474 (Linking)

Louis M, Zanou N, Van Schoor M, Gailly P. (2008). *TRPC1 regulates skeletal myoblast migration and differentiation*. J Cell Sci;121(Pt 23):3951-9. ISSN 0021-9533

Lui VC, Lung SS, Pu JK, Hung KN, Leung GK. (2010). *Invasion of human glioma cells is regulated by multiple chloride channels including ClC-3*. Anticancer Res;30(11):4515-24. ISSN 1791-7530 (Electronic), 0250-7005 (Linking)

Luo X, Xiao J, Lin H, Lu Y, Yang B, Wang Z. (2008). *Genomic structure, transcriptional control, and tissue distribution of HERG1 and KCNQ1 genes*. Am J Physiol Heart Circ Physiol;294(3):H1371-80. ISSN 0363-6135

Maitland NJ, Collins AT. (2008). *Prostate cancer stem cells: a new target for therapy*. J Clin Oncol;26(17):2862-70. ISSN 1527-7755 (Electronic), 0732-183X (Linking)

Maitland NJ, Collins AT. (2010). *Cancer stem cells - A therapeutic target?* Curr Opin Mol Ther;12(6):662-73. ISSN 2040-3445 (Electronic), 1464-8431 (Linking)

Malkia A, Madrid R, Meseguer V, de la Pena E, Valero M, Belmonte C, et al. (2007). *Bidirectional shifts of TRPM8 channel gating by temperature and chemical agents modulate the cold sensitivity of mammalian thermoreceptors.* J Physiol;581(Pt 1):155-74. ISSN 0022-3751

Mamelak AN, Rosenfeld S, Bucholz R, Raubitschek A, Nabors LB, Fiveash JB, et al. (2006). *Phase I single-dose study of intracavitary-administered iodine-131-TM-601 in adults with recurrent high-grade glioma.* J Clin Oncol;24(22):3644-50. ISSN 1527-7755 (Electronic), 0732-183X (Linking)

Maroto R, Raso A, Wood TG, Kurosky A, Martinac B, Hamill OP. (2005). *TRPC1 forms the stretch-activated cation channel in vertebrate cells.* Nat Cell Biol;7(2):179-85. ISSN 1465-7392

Maruyama T, Kanaji T, Nakade S, Kanno T, Mikoshiba K. (1997). *2APB, 2-aminoethoxydiphenyl borate, a membrane-penetrable modulator of Ins(1,4,5)P3-induced Ca2+ release.* J Biochem;122(3):498-505. ISSN 0021-924X

Masi A, Becchetti A, Restano-Cassulini R, Polvani S, Hofmann G, Buccoliero AM, et al. (2005). *hERG1 channels are overexpressed in glioblastoma multiforme and modulate VEGF secretion in glioblastoma cell lines.* Br J Cancer;93(7):781-92. ISSN 0007-0920

Mason MJ, Mayer B, Hymel LJ. (1993). *Inhibition of Ca2+ transport pathways in thymic lymphocytes by econazole, miconazole, and SKF 96365.* Am J Physiol;264(3 Pt 1):C654-62. ISSN 0002-9513

McCarron JG, Bradley KN, Muir TC. (2002). *Ca2+ signalling and Ca2+-activated K+ channels in smooth muscle.* Novartis Found Symp;246:52-64; discussion 64-70, 221-7. ISSN 1528-2511

Mehrke G, Zong XG, Flockerzi V, Hofmann F. (1994). *The Ca(++)-channel blocker Ro 40-5967 blocks differently T-type and L-type Ca++ channels.* J Pharmacol Exp Ther;271(3):1483-8. ISSN 0022-3565

Merritt JE, Armstrong WP, Benham CD, Hallam TJ, Jacob R, Jaxa-Chamiec A, et al. (1990). *SK&F 96365, a novel inhibitor of receptor-mediated calcium entry.* Biochem J;271(2):515-22. ISSN 0264-6021

Meuth SG, Herrmann AM, Ip CW, Kanyshkova T, Bittner S, Weishaupt A, et al. (2008). *The two-pore domain potassium channel TASK3 functionally impacts glioma cell death.* J Neurooncol;87(3):263-70. ISSN 0167-594X

Miller BA. (2006). *The role of TRP channels in oxidative stress-induced cell death.* J Membr Biol;209(1):31-41. ISSN 0022-2631

Montell C. (2005). *The TRP superfamily of cation channels.* Sci STKE;2005(272):re3. ISSN 1525-8882

Mori A, Lehmann S, O'Kelly J, Kumagai T, Desmond JC, Pervan M, et al. (2006). *Capsaicin, a component of red peppers, inhibits the growth of androgen-independent, p53 mutant prostate cancer cells.* Cancer Res;66(6):3222-9. ISSN 0008-5472

Nabissi M, Morelli MB, Amantini C, Farfariello V, Ricci-Vitiani L, Caprodossi S, et al. (2010). *TRPV2 channel negatively controls glioma cell proliferation and resistance to Fas-induced apoptosis in ERK-dependent manner.* Carcinogenesis;31(5):794-803. ISSN 1460-2180 (Electronic), 0143-3334 (Linking)

Naundorf B, Wolf F, Volgushev M. (2006). *Unique features of action potential initiation in cortical neurons.* Nature;440(7087):1060-3. ISSN 1476-4687 (Electronic), 0028-0836 (Linking)

Ningaraj NS, Rao M, Hashizume K, Asotra K, Black KL. (2002). *Regulation of blood-brain tumor barrier permeability by calcium-activated potassium channels.* J Pharmacol Exp Ther;301(3):838-51. ISSN 0022-3565

Ningaraj NS, Sankpal UT, Khaitan D, Meister EA, Vats T. (2009). *Activation of KATP channels increases anticancer drug delivery to brain tumors and survival.* Eur J Pharmacol;602(2-3):188-93. ISSN 1879-0712 (Electronic), 0014-2999 (Linking)

O'Brien CA, Pollett A, Gallinger S, Dick JE. (2007). *A human colon cancer cell capable of initiating tumour growth in immunodeficient mice.* Nature;445(7123):106-10. ISSN 1476-4687 (Electronic), 0028-0836 (Linking)

Olsen ML, Schade S, Lyons SA, Amaral MD, Sontheimer H. (2003). *Expression of voltage-gated chloride channels in human glioma cells.* J Neurosci;23(13):5572-82. ISSN 1529-2401 (Electronic), 0270-6474 (Linking)

Onohara N, Nishida M, Inoue R, Kobayashi H, Sumimoto H, Sato Y, et al. (2006). *TRPC3 and TRPC6 are essential for angiotensin II-induced cardiac hypertrophy.* EMBO J;25(22):5305-16. ISSN 0261-4189

Panner A, Cribbs LL, Zainelli GM, Origitano TC, Singh S, Wurster RD. (2005). *Variation of T-type calcium channel protein expression affects cell division of cultured tumor cells.* Cell Calcium;37(2):105-19. ISSN 0143-4160

Park JH, Park SJ, Chung MK, Jung KH, Choi MR, Kim Y, et al. (2010). *High expression of large-conductance Ca2+-activated K+ channel in the CD133+ subpopulation of SH-SY5Y neuroblastoma cells.* Biochem Biophys Res Commun;396(3):637-42. ISSN 1090-2104 (Electronic), 0006-291X (Linking)

Quayle JM, Nelson MT, Standen NB. (1997). *ATP-sensitive and inwardly rectifying potassium channels in smooth muscle.* Physiol Rev;77(4):1165-232. ISSN 0031-9333

Ramsey IS, Delling M, Clapham DE. (2006). *An introduction to TRP channels.* Annu Rev Physiol;68:619-47. ISSN 0066-4278

Rao RD, Mladek AC, Lamont JD, Goble JM, Erlichman C, James CD, et al. (2005) *Disruption of parallel and converging signaling pathways contributes to the synergistic antitumor effects of simultaneous mTOR and EGFR inhibition in GBM cells.* Neoplasia;7(10):921-9. ISSN 1522-8002 (Print), 1476-5586 (Linking)

Reiser J, Polu KR, Moller CC, Kenlan P, Altintas MM, Wei C, et al. (2005). *TRPC6 is a glomerular slit diaphragm-associated channel required for normal renal function.* Nat Genet;37(7):739-44. ISSN 1061-4036

Ritter JK, Franklin MR. (1987). *Clotrimazole induction of cytochrome P-450: dose-differentiated isozyme induction.* Mol Pharmacol;31(2):135-9. ISSN 0026-895X

Roderick HL, Cook SJ. (2008). *Ca2+ signalling checkpoints in cancer: remodelling Ca2+ for cancer cell proliferation and survival.* Nat Rev Cancer;8(5):361-75. ISSN 1474-1768

Saleh SN, Albert AP, Peppiatt-Wildman CM, Large WA. (2008). *Diverse properties of store-operated TRPC channels activated by protein kinase C in vascular myocytes.* J Physiol;586(10):2463-76. ISSN 1469-7793

Sanchez AM, Sanchez MG, Malagarie-Cazenave S, Olea N, Diaz-Laviada I. (2006). *Induction of apoptosis in prostate tumor PC-3 cells and inhibition of xenograft prostate tumor growth by the vanilloid capsaicin.* Apoptosis;11(1):89-99. ISSN 1360-8185

Schatton T, Murphy GF, Frank NY, Yamaura K, Waaga-Gasser AM, Gasser M, et al. (2008). *Identification of cells initiating human melanomas.* Nature;451(7176):345-9. ISSN 1476-4687 (Electronic), 0028-0836 (Linking)

Sciaccaluga M, Fioretti B, Catacuzzeno L, Pagani F, Bertollini C, Rosito M, et al. (2010). *CXCL12-induced glioblastoma cell migration requires intermediate conductance Ca2+-activated K+ channel activity.* Am J Physiol Cell Physiol;299(1):C175-84. ISSN 1522-1563 (Electronic), 0363-6143 (Linking)

Shi Y, Ding X, He ZH, Zhou KC, Wang Q, Wang YZ. (2009). *Critical role of TRPC6 channels in G2 phase transition and the development of human oesophageal cancer.* Gut;58(11):1443-50. ISSN 1468-3288

Singh BB, Lockwich TP, Bandyopadhyay BC, Liu X, Bollimuntha S, Brazer SC, et al. (2004). *VAMP2-dependent exocytosis regulates plasma membrane insertion of TRPC3 channels and contributes to agonist-stimulated Ca2+ influx.* Mol Cell;15(4):635-46. ISSN 1097-2765

Singh SK, Hawkins C, Clarke ID, Squire JA, Bayani J, Hide T, et al. (2004). *Identification of human brain tumour initiating cells.* Nature;432(7015):396-401. ISSN 1476-4687 (Electronic), 0028-0836 (Linking)

Snyders DJ. (1999). *Structure and function of cardiac potassium channels.* Cardiovasc Res;42(2):377-90. ISSN 0008-6363

SoRelle R. (1998). *Withdrawal of Posicor from market.* Circulation;98(9):831-2. ISSN 0009-7322

Soroceanu L, Gillespie Y, Khazaeli MB, Sontheimer H. (1998). *Use of chlorotoxin for targeting of primary brain tumors.* Cancer Res;58(21):4871-9. ISSN 0008-5472

Striessnig J. (1999). *Pharmacology, structure and function of cardiac L-type Ca(2+) channels.* Cell Physiol Biochem;9(4-5):242-69. ISSN 1015-8987

Strubing C, Krapivinsky G, Krapivinsky L, Clapham DE. (2001). *TRPC1 and TRPC5 form a novel cation channel in mammalian brain.* Neuron;29(3):645-55. ISSN 0896-6273

Strubing C, Krapivinsky G, Krapivinsky L, Clapham DE. (2003). *Formation of novel TRPC channels by complex subunit interactions in embryonic brain.* J Biol Chem;278(40):39014-9. ISSN 0021-9258

Stupp R, Mason WP, van den Bent MJ, Weller M, Fisher B, Taphoorn MJ, et al. (2005). *Radiotherapy plus concomitant and adjuvant temozolomide for glioblastoma.* N Engl J Med;352(10):987-96. ISSN 1533-4406 (Electronic), 0028-4793 (Linking)

Tai Y, Feng S, Ge R, Du W, Zhang X, He Z, et al. (2008). *TRPC6 channels promote dendritic growth via the CaMKIV-CREB pathway.* J Cell Sci;121(Pt 14):2301-7. ISSN 0021-9533

Takebe N, Harris PJ, Warren RQ, Ivy SP. (2010). *Targeting cancer stem cells by inhibiting Wnt, Notch, and Hedgehog pathways.* Nat Rev Clin Oncol;8(2):97-106. ISSN 1759-4782 (Electronic), 1759-4774 (Linking)

Tang J, Lin Y, Zhang Z, Tikunova S, Birnbaumer L, Zhu MX. (2001). *Identification of common binding sites for calmodulin and inositol 1,4,5-trisphosphate receptors on the carboxyl termini of trp channels.* J Biol Chem;276(24):21303-10. ISSN 0021-9258

Taylor JT, Huang L, Pottle JE, Liu K, Yang Y, Zeng X, et al. (2008). *Selective blockade of T-type Ca2+ channels suppresses human breast cancer cell proliferation.* Cancer Lett;267(1):116-24. ISSN 0304-3835

Thebault S, Flourakis M, Vanoverberghe K, Vandermoere F, Roudbaraki M, Lehen'kyi V, et al. (2006). *Differential role of transient receptor potential channels in Ca2+ entry and proliferation of prostate cancer epithelial cells.* Cancer Res;66(4):2038-47. ISSN 0008-5472

Thoennissen NH, O'Kelly J, Lu D, Iwanski GB, La DT, Abbassi S, et al. (2010). *Capsaicin causes cell-cycle arrest and apoptosis in ER-positive and -negative breast cancer cells by modulating the EGFR/HER-2 pathway.* Oncogene;29(2):285-96. ISSN 1476-5594 (Electronic), 0950-9232 (Linking)

Trimarchi JR, Liu L, Smith PJ, Keefe DL. (2002). *Apoptosis recruits two-pore domain potassium channels used for homeostatic volume regulation.* Am J Physiol Cell Physiol;282(3):C588-94. ISSN 0363-6143

Varnai P, Hunyady L, Balla T. (2009). *STIM and Orai: the long-awaited constituents of store-operated calcium entry.* Trends Pharmacol Sci;30(3):118-28. ISSN 0165-6147

Vazquez G, Wedel BJ, Aziz O, Trebak M, Putney JW, Jr. (2004). *The mammalian TRPC cation channels.* Biochim Biophys Acta;1742(1-3):21-36. ISSN 0006-3002

Vergara C, Latorre R, Marrion NV, Adelman JP. (1998). *Calcium-activated potassium channels.* Curr Opin Neurobiol;8(3):321-9. ISSN 0959-4388

Wang MC, Dolphin A, Kitmitto A. (2004). *L-type voltage-gated calcium channels: understanding function through structure.* FEBS Lett;564(3):245-50. ISSN 0014-5793

Wang ZH, Shen B, Yao HL, Jia YC, Ren J, Feng YJ, et al. (2007). *Blockage of intermediate-conductance-Ca(2+) -activated K(+) channels inhibits progression of human endometrial cancer.* Oncogene;26(35):5107-14. ISSN 0950-9232

Weaver AK, Bomben VC, Sontheimer H. (2006). *Expression and function of calcium-activated potassium channels in human glioma cells.* Glia;54(3):223-33. ISSN 0894-1491

Weaver AK, Liu X, Sontheimer H. (2004). *Role for calcium-activated potassium channels (BK) in growth control of human malignant glioma cells.* J Neurosci Res;78(2):224-34. ISSN 0360-4012

Wei WL, Sun HS, Olah ME, Sun X, Czerwinska E, Czerwinski W, et al. (2007). *TRPM7 channels in hippocampal neurons detect levels of extracellular divalent cations.* Proc Natl Acad Sci U S A;104(41):16323-8. ISSN 0027-8424

Wemmie JA, Price MP, Welsh MJ. (2006). *Acid-sensing ion channels: advances, questions and therapeutic opportunities.* Trends Neurosci;29(10):578-86. ISSN 0166-2236

Wen PY, Kesari S. (2008). *Malignant gliomas in adults.* N Engl J Med;359(5):492-507. ISSN 1533-4406 (Electronic), 0028-4793 (Linking)

Wes PD, Chevesich J, Jeromin A, Rosenberg C, Stetten G, Montell C. (1995). *TRPC1, a human homolog of a Drosophila store-operated channel.* Proc Natl Acad Sci U S A;92(21):9652-6. ISSN 0027-8424

Winn MP, Conlon PJ, Lynn KL, Farrington MK, Creazzo T, Hawkins AF, et al. (2005). *A mutation in the TRPC6 cation channel causes familial focal segmental glomerulosclerosis.* Science;308(5729):1801-4. ISSN 1095-9203

Wondergem R, Ecay TW, Mahieu F, Owsianik G, Nilius B. (2008). *HGF/SF and menthol increase human glioblastoma cell calcium and migration.* Biochem Biophys Res Commun;372(1):210-5. ISSN 1090-2104 (Electronic), 0006-291X (Linking)

Wong ET, Brem S. (2010). *Taming glioblastoma by targeting angiogenesis: 3 years later.* J Clin Oncol;29(2):124-6. ISSN 1527-7755 (Electronic), 0732-183X (Linking)

Wulff H, Castle NA, Pardo LA. (2009). *Voltage-gated potassium channels as therapeutic targets.* Nat Rev Drug Discov;8(12):982-1001. ISSN 1474-1784 (Electronic), 1474-1776 (Linking)

Xu SZ, Zeng F, Lei M, Li J, Gao B, Xiong C, et al. (2005). *Generation of functional ion-channel tools by E3 targeting*. Nat Biotechnol;23(10):1289-93. ISSN 1087-0156

Yamamura H, Ugawa S, Ueda T, Morita A, Shimada S. (2008). *TRPM8 activation suppresses cellular viability in human melanoma*. Am J Physiol Cell Physiol;295(2):C296-301. ISSN 0363-6143

Yang S, Zhang JJ, Huang XY. (2009) *Orai1 and STIM1 are critical for breast tumor cell migration and metastasis*. Cancer Cell;15(2):124-34. ISSN 1878-3686 (Electronic), 1535-6108 (Linking)

Yang SL, Cao Q, Zhou KC, Feng YJ, Wang YZ. (2009). *Transient receptor potential channel C3 contributes to the progression of human ovarian cancer*. Oncogene;28(10):1320-8. ISSN 1476-5594

Yin D, Wang X, Konda BM, Ong JM, Hu J, Sacapano MR, et al. (2008). *Increase in brain tumor permeability in glioma-bearing rats with nitric oxide donors*. Clin Cancer Res;14(12):4002-9. ISSN 1078-0432

Yu Y, Fantozzi I, Remillard CV, Landsberg JW, Kunichika N, Platoshyn O, et al. (2004). *Enhanced expression of transient receptor potential channels in idiopathic pulmonary arterial hypertension*. Proc Natl Acad Sci U S A;101(38):13861-6. ISSN 0027-8424

Yu Y, Sweeney M, Zhang S, Platoshyn O, Landsberg J, Rothman A, et al. (2003). *PDGF stimulates pulmonary vascular smooth muscle cell proliferation by upregulating TRPC6 expression*. Am J Physiol Cell Physiol;284(2):C316-30. ISSN 0363-6143

Zamponi GW, Lewis RJ, Todorovic SM, Arneric SP, Snutch TP. (2009). *Role of voltage-gated calcium channels in ascending pain pathways*. Brain Res Rev;60(1):84-9. ISSN 0165-0173

Zhang L, Barritt GJ. (2004). *Evidence that TRPM8 is an androgen-dependent Ca2+ channel required for the survival of prostate cancer cells*. Cancer Res;64(22):8365-73. ISSN 0008-5472

Zhang S, Balch C, Chan MW, Lai HC, Matei D, Schilder JM, et al. (2008). *Identification and characterization of ovarian cancer-initiating cells from primary human tumors*. Cancer Res;68(11):4311-20. ISSN 1538-7445 (Electronic), 0008-5472 (Linking)

Zhang X, Bertaso F, Yoo JW, Baumgartel K, Clancy SM, Lee V, et al. Deletion of the potassium channel Kv12.2 causes hippocampal hyperexcitability and epilepsy. Nat Neurosci 2010;13(9):1056-8. ISSN 1546-1726 (Electronic), 1097-6256 (Linking)

Zhang Z, Tang J, Tikunova S, Johnson JD, Chen Z, Qin N, et al. (2001). *Activation of Trp3 by inositol 1,4,5-trisphosphate receptors through displacement of inhibitory calmodulin from a common binding domain*. Proc Natl Acad Sci U S A;98(6):3168-73. ISSN 0027-8424

Zhou J, Du W, Zhou K, Tai Y, Yao H, Jia Y, et al. (2008). *Critical role of TRPC6 channels in the formation of excitatory synapses*. Nat Neurosci;11(7):741-3. ISSN 1097-6256

Ziglioli F, Frattini A, Maestroni U, Dinale F, Ciufifeda M, Cortellini P. (2009). *Vanilloid-mediated apoptosis in prostate cancer cells through a TRPV-1 dependent and a TRPV-1-independent mechanism*. Acta Biomed;80(1):13-20. ISSN 0392-4203